With thanks [...]
to the Visit[...],
and best wishes
Doy [...]
dear, Oct '93

Frontiers of Medicine

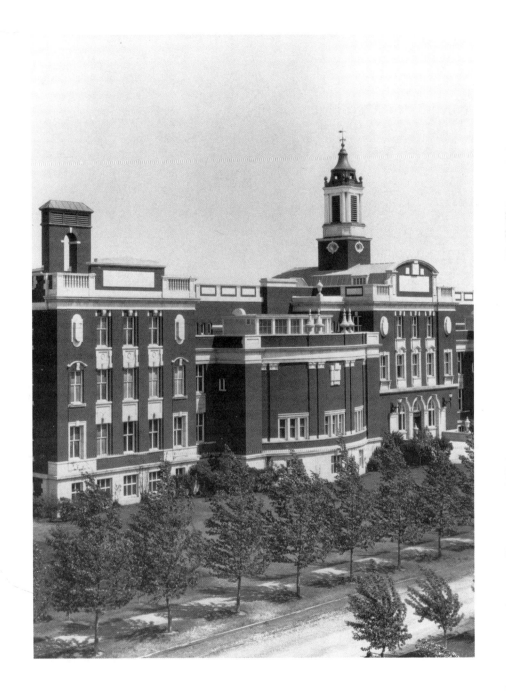

FRONTIERS OF MEDICINE

A HISTORY OF MEDICAL
EDUCATION AND RESEARCH
AT THE UNIVERSITY OF ALBERTA

ELISE A. CORBET

 University of Alberta Press

First published by
The University of Alberta Press
141 Athabasca Hall
Edmonton
Alberta T6G 2E8
1990

Canadian Cataloguing in Publication Data

Corbet, Elise A.
  Frontiers of medicine

  Includes bibliographical references.
  ISBN 0-88864-231-8

  1. University of Alberta. Faculty of Medicine—
History.   2. Medical education—Alberta—History.
I. Title.
R749.U552C67 1990   610'.7'11712334   C90-091673-7

Typesetting by Pièce de Résistance Ltée., Edmonton, Alberta, Canada
Printed in Canada by D.W. Friesen & Sons Ltd.
Designed by Steve Tate

Contents

Tables

Foreword

THE PREPARATION of a written history of the Faculty of Medicine at the
University of Alberta immediately became a high priority when staff, students, and alumni began to plan for the seventy-fifth anniversary of our
medical school. 'Living history' is certainly an apt description for history
that you can see around you and which involves people known personally
to many still alive. Such is the history of the Faculty of Medicine at the
University of Alberta. In the context of the dynamic development of western
Canada and of biomedical science, medical education and health care in
the twentieth century, the medical school has moved in one lifetime from
a gleam in the eye of Henry Marshall Tory and his small band of colleagues
and students in a frontier city, to a beautiful and complex Health Sciences
Centre with an international reputation in many fields of patient care, education and research. Is it any wonder that those personally familiar with these
developments wished to see them thoroughly documented?

On behalf of the Faculty, I wish to express my appreciation to Dr.
Robert Fraser, Dr. Peter Allen, Dr. Tim Cameron, Dr. Louis Francescutti,
Dr. Donald Wilson and Dr. Carl Betke (Historic Sites Service, Alberta
Culture and Multiculturalism), for conducting this history project in honor
of our seventy-fifth anniversary (1913-1988). We are particularly grate-
ful to Mrs. Elise Corbet who plunged into the project with enthusiasm and

has skillfully captured the spirit of our predecessors and the eras through which the Faculty has evolved.

We expect that this History will recall many happy memories for our alumni and will excite present and future generations of students, as well as the community we serve, about our medical school. The Faculty of Medicine at the University of Alberta is proud of its past, enthusiastic about the present, and prepared for the challenges of the twenty-first century. We hope that you will enjoy this historical account of our growth and development during the emergence of western Canada and of Canadian medical education, research and health care.

Douglas R. Wilson, M.D., FRCPC
Dean

Preface

TO RECORD the full story of the hundreds of faculty and staff, the thousands of students and the hundreds of thousands of patients, each of whom played a part in the development of this major academic medical centre, is a formidable task. Many of the anecdotes of the early efforts to establish a first class medical school, remote from the world's major medical centres, will, of necessity, live on only in the memories of those associated with the institution in its formative years. Each generation will have its own memories of the challenges and rewards, of the frustrations and successes, and of the talents and idiosyncrasies of their colleagues in the development of this vast enterprise.

It is also important, however, to examine that record and draw from it the provincial themes that will provide a comprehensive understanding of the Faculty of Medicine's evolution at the University of Alberta. Current and future members of the faculty, as well as people more generally interested in the development of modern health care, will profit from attention to its historical roots. Here, then, will be found the highlights and the long term trends in a fascinating story of the efforts of dedicated and compassionate professionals of many disciplines working together toward a common goal — the pursuit of excellence in patient care, research and the "provision of doctors for tomorrow."

D.F. (Tim) Cameron M.D., F.R.C.P.C., F.A.C.A.
Dean, Faculty of Medicine, University of Alberta, 1974-1983

Acknowledgements

There are many people who supported me with their encouragement, enthusiasm and expertise during the research and writing of this manuscript. To them all, I extend my thanks and appreciation.

In the first place, I would like to thank the Archives Committee of the Faculty of Medicine for giving me the opportunity to write this history of the University of Alberta's medical school, and participate in it's 75th anniversary. Dr. Robert S. Fraser, chairman of the committee, and his colleagues, Drs. Peter Allen, Tim Cameron, Louis Francescutti and Donald Wilson, were unfailingly helpful and patient as they guided me through such matters as the intricacies of scientific advances and medical terminology. The members of this committee reviewed the manuscript as it developed, and I am grateful to them for their advice and suggestions. Dr. Carl Betke, Chief of Research, Historic Sites Service, the Department of Culture and Multiculturism of the Province of Alberta, was also part of this committee, and was of inestimable assistance in a variety of different ways during the entire course of the production of this book.

Dean Wilson and his staff suffered gladly my many questions and requests, and all those I met during my research activities at the medical school expressed great interest and gave willingly of their time and knowledge. I am grateful to those whom I interviewed; they shared their memories and insights with me and helped me to develop a feeling for the medical school over the years and the changes which took place. I remember with great pleasure an interview with the late Dr. J.S. (Smitty) Gardner, whose powers of mimicry brought so many people to life.

Bryan Corbett and his staff at the University of Alberta Archives, particularly Trude McLaren, were of immense help in guiding me through the large collections of material and photographs which were relevant to this project. I would also like to thank the staff of the Provincial Archives of Alberta, and the Glenbow-Alberta Institute.

I am grateful to Drs. Janice Dickin McGinnis and Thomas Brown, who encouraged me to undertake this project and suggested some guidelines for research. And lastly, my thanks to Lindsay Moir for the development of the Index, an important adjunct to any book of this nature.

Finally, we acknowledge and appreciate the financial assistance of the Alberta Medical Foundation and the Alberta Historical Resources Foundation towards the publication of this history.

Introduction

Who is responsible for the establishment of a faculty of medicine at this university, and why did the school become necessary? Frankly we are not sure. Those who have been questioned have each a different answer. All who were most intimately concerned are now alive and it is for future students (when the pioneers are safely dead) to determine to whom credit is due.

THUS BEGAN a history of the Medical Students' Club, written in 1929 by J.M. Large, D.G. Revell and E.F. Cain,[1] and now held in the archives of the University of Alberta. This manuscript, however, goes on to provide a good part of the answer:

It is also significant that the original plans of the university made ample provision for a medical school, its laboratories, hospital and clinics. This could have been done only by one who had early foreseen the necessity for a faculty of medicine. It is impossible in any inquiry into the early days of this university to forget the predominant, and dominant, part played by its first president.

Now that "the pioneers are safely dead," the truth of the last sentence remains. During the twenty years that Henry Marshall Tory presided over the University of Alberta, he did indeed control all aspects of the institution and his word was law. The University of Alberta opened its doors in 1908, just three years after the birth of the province and during the ground swell of a developing boom period. A new university in a new province during the settlement period needed a person of Tory's calibre, with the knowledge, the energy, and, above all, the determination to get it off the ground and to keep it going. It was not an easy task, and Tory had to fight for support in the community. Frank Oliver, the editor of the *Edmonton Journal*, is reputed to have said, "That man Tory must be crazy. We don't need any college here at all; if we did, it would be to turn out horse-doctors."[2]

Tory was a scientist by training and came to Edmonton from McGill University in Montreal, where he taught physics. He was also intimately involved in developing higher institutions of learning and, according to Robert C. Wallace, his successor as president of the University of Alberta, was "a builder — of institutions, of the spread of scientific knowledge, of international goodwill. He delighted in seeing things grow. He was less interested if for any reason growth could not be continued."[3] Although well established at McGill, Tory could not resist the challenge of building a university from scratch in a young and newly settled part of the country, with the opportunity to put into practice his ideas concerning the development of a publicly funded university.

From the beginning, Tory envisioned a university that offered not only the traditional humanities, classics and philosophy but also the professions: law, engineering, medicine, agriculture, architecture and accounting. In his view, a developing province needed to produce its own professionals, from among its own citizens, and not draw on those from more established parts of the country who would bring their own values. The professionals, the future leaders of the province, should be drawn from local people who knew the country and were familiar with its needs. Tory lost no time in developing professional faculties. In 1912, he established the Faculty of Law and the following year the Faculty of Applied Science (Engineering) and Medicine. Despite the onset of World War I, he continued the expansion programme and added the Faculty of Agriculture in 1915. By 1922 the university campus included five major buildings, as well as an adjacent teaching hospital, and had ambitious plans for the future.

Such rapid development took place in the small town of Strathcona, on the edge of the frontier, where methods of communication, transportation and industrial development were in their infancy. One of the first professors, William Hardy Alexander, called it a "remote backwater of Empire." When the Canadian Pacific Railway built a spur line north from

Calgary in 1891, it terminated the line on the south side of the North Saskatchewan River, where the community of Strathcona developed around the terminus. For many years, the rail link to the main transcontinental CPR line at Calgary was the major method of transportation for settlers to the district. Passengers for Edmonton and other communities on the north side of the river had to travel across the river by ferry, or via the Low Level Bridge after its completion in 1902. Not until 1913, after Edmonton and Strathcona had merged and the construction of the High Level Bridge was complete, did the CPR rail line begin to carry passengers northward across the river. The town of Strathcona, initially known as South Edmonton, was incorporated in 1899, and the community flourished in its role at the railhead for more than a dozen years. It maintained a completely separate existence from Edmonton, having its own city council, public school board, newspaper and hospital (Strathcona Hospital). Its own MLA, A.C. Rutherford, happened to be the premier of the province as well as the minister of education. Over the years the "twin cities," separated by a formidable physical barrier, a river with banks 200 feet high, developed a keen rivalry.

Strathcona was a small community, however, essentially clustered around the CPR depot on 103rd Street, and when Rutherford purchased the portion of land known as River Lot No. 5 as a site for the university, the location received mixed reviews. It was at least a mile west of the outskirts of the town, west of a plot of land cultivated by a pioneer farmer named Armand Garneau (later a residential district bearing his name). A thick growth of native willow and poplar, straggling bushes and tall grasses covered the university site. The land was marshy, crossed by Indian trails, and bordered by large areas of unsettled land to the west and south. Until construction began on the first university building in 1910, no roads connected the site to Strathcona, and it would be many years before any were paved. Across the river in Edmonton, the opulent new legislature building was under construction, towering above the old fur trading post of Fort Edmonton.

The medical profession was in a primitive stage of organization and professionalism as well. Most of the early physicians in what would become Alberta came with the institutions that played a large part in the exploitation and settlement of the West: the Hudson's Bay Company, the North-West Mounted Police and the Canadian Pacific Railway. Others were employed by the dominion government to care for the native population. Following the turn of the century, when the trickle of settlers began to turn into a flood, medical practitioners also began to migrate westward and to set up in private practice in the new urban communities. They found few hospitals and laboratories. Most practitioners treated patients in their homes, often travelling many miles over unimproved roads on horseback, by democrat, or by sleigh in the wintertime. It was not until the 1920s that a network of railways made travel around the province easier, and even the advent of the motor car offered few advantages, as roads were all but impassable during the winter and spring.

The College of Physicians and Surgeons of the North West Territories had been established in 1886, and after the formation of Alberta and Saskatchewan in 1905, each province formed its own college.[4] J.D. Lafferty of Calgary, who had been registrar of the North West Territories College, was appointed registrar of the College of Physicians and Surgeons of Alberta (CPSA). One of the chief concerns of the college at this time was to enforce the registration and licensing qualifications of those practising medicine in Alberta. At its first meeting in October 1906, the college established an education committee and decided upon the subjects for examination. Local practitioners in selected areas of the province conducted examinations in the subjects listed below with the required pass marks.[5]

Anatomy 50%
Chemistry 25%
Physiology and histology 40%
Materia medica and therapeutics 60%
Medical jurisprudence and toxicology 40%
Pathology and bacteriology 50%
Surgery 60%
Obstetrics 60%
Diseases of women and children 60%
Theory and practice of medicine 60%
Sanitary science and hygiene 50%

As can be seen, a lower standard was acceptable in the medical sciences; nevertheless, a considerable number failed the examinations, but without the support of government regulations there was little to stop them from continuing to practise. Some of those who practised did not even attempt the examinations, including many who had received no formalized medical training and who practised some form of ''irregular'' medicine. Most of these practitioners lived in rural areas.

The college spent a great deal of time in efforts to protect the public from "charlatans and other fakers," but it had a difficult time enforcing its own regulations with neither the provincial government nor the public on its side. Subsequently, the legislature passed the Medical Professional Act, which required practising physicians to obtain a licence from the CPSA, but it remained difficult to bring unlicensed practitioners to court. Alberta was an agricultural province with a widely scattered population. Only 25% of the people lived in cities; yet urban communities claimed 55% of the doctors. Those who lived in rural and isolated areas were happy to use the services of anyone with a modicum of medical knowledge. A large proportion of the rural population was made up of immigrants, who brought with them their customs for dealing with illness, childbirth and disease; customs that were generally not based on currently accepted scientific medical practices. Registered doctors themselves were not above employing unlicensed practitioners to serve as locums when they wanted to take a holiday, and many a fourth- or fifth-year medical student took the opportunity to acquire "hands-on" experience by spending the summer vacation in this way.

"Chiropractors, faith-curists, christian scientists and such fakers" were a constant source of irritation to the medical profession in the early days, and continued to be so for many years. Many of the practitioners of these different "branches" of medicine, such as osteopaths and naturopaths, were graduates of schools in the United States and came with diplomas, but in many cases they were still unable to pass the required examinations for licensure in Alberta. There is some reason to believe, however, that examining doctors made it extremely difficult for them to succeed so as to keep them out of the province. Over the years, several complaints of unfairness were charged against the examining board.[6]

Between October 1915 and September 1916, three years after the establishment of the medical school, eleven people were found guilty of practising medicine while unregistered. They were fined $50 and costs, or one month in jail.[7] Ten years later, in the mid-1920s, "irregular" practitioners still practised in the province, and a few were charged. Nick Markowsky, accused of bloodletting at St. Paul de Metis, claimed to have a licence for such treatment. He treated a consumptive, who had been sent home from hospital as incurable, by "cutting the veins in his legs." When the patient died, Markowsky was charged with unlawfully practising surgery. "If he hadn't died," said Markowsky in his own defence, "I know I could have cured him." He was found guilty and fined $25 and costs.[8]

A.J.L. Olson of Camrose used the initials N.D. (Naturopathic Doctor) after his name to signify a diploma from a school of naturopathy in Cedar Rapids, Iowa. He treated nervous diseases, using "a little each of chiropractic, osteopathic, mechano-therapy and naturopathy," and charged according to the patient's ability to pay. Olson, who advertised himself as a "Drugless Physician," was charged with practising without a licence, pleaded guilty and was fined $50 and costs. He then moved to another town and continued to practise until he was charged again. Purveyors of proprietary and patent medicines often claimed to be "specialists" who could cure "stubborn diseases" without recourse to an operation. A homeopath near Cardston said he could treat rheumatism and asthma by massage and his own medicine and did a good business among the natives of the area. A trained nurse who lived near Acme used her home as a hospital and treated patients there. It was, however, difficult to get sufficient information concerning her activities as "the roads were in poor condition."

It was often difficult, because of physical conditions, to obtain sufficient information to lay charges, and in addition few people would give evidence of such activities. Furthermore, if charges were laid against an "irregular" and the culprit found guilty, there was little to stop him or her moving on to another community and setting up shop there. While irregular practitioners probably effected few cures, they also did little harm to their patients, except by relieving them of some hard-earned money. People were accustomed to using traditional (old wives') remedies for whatever ailed them, and most were unaccustomed to using the services of a trained doctor. Before the days of scientific medicine, trained physicians themselves had few methods of curing illnesses beyond surgery and a few harsh drugs. The only answer seemed to be the education of the public, to encourage them to look closely at the qualifications of their doctor and to understand the value of university training. Here, the University of Alberta and its new medical school assisted directly. From 1912 on, the responsibility for the qualifying examinations was turned over to the university, and after the inauguration of the medical school, members of the faculty conducted most of the examinations. In addition, the presence of a provincial medical school gave a certain impetus to the spread of knowledge concerning the qualifications of accredited medical practitioners and the value of seeking professional medical assistance.

It was within this societal and medical framework that Alberta's medical school was born. President Tory experienced sustained opposition from some local members of the medical profession to his plans to start a medical school. Many felt that the province was not ready for such an ambitious undertaking, that it could produce no more than a second-rate institution, given the lack of staff and the facilities available. For many years the children of local physicians who wished to enter medicine went East to their fathers' *alma maters* for training. However, Tory's co-operation in the fight against "irregular" practitioners prompted a grudging support for the medical school from the CPSA and the medical community. Its presence supported the general contention of the profession that entry into its ranks must be through a university education and that common standards of qualification were a necessary requirement.

The CPSA kept a close eye on the activities of the province's medical school in its early years, on the entrance requirements and on the curriculum. In a statement to the Senate of the university, the college affirmed its opinion

>...that the Alberta standards of education of medical students should be so framed as to equal the highest similar and corresponding standards in any Canadian university and that if necessary the Alberta curriculum should be revised accordingly and that extension of the medical curriculum should be made from time to time in order to meet and maintain an approved and established standard.[9]

Certain members of the provincial legislature opposed the introduction of a medical school as well, mainly on account of its cost. In such a new province there were few people or corporations sufficiently wealthy to provide grants or bequests to educational institutions; so the school would have to be supported totally by public funds. Medical schools are extremely expensive if they are to achieve a reputable standing. Saskatchewan, a province in a similar situation as Alberta, did not start even a limited two-year programme until 1926, and it was another twenty years before it was extended to a full degree-granting programme. British Columbia, a much older province, and one that had institutions of higher education as early as the1880s, did not establish a medical school until 1949. The medical fraternity in that province felt that any earlier time had been too soon. Nevertheless, Tory's determination to include professional schools in the University of Alberta was not to be gainsaid. A faculty of medicine was part of his dream of a full-fledged university, and he nurtured it. He chose the faculty members and, despite his somewhat limited medical knowledge, became closely involved with curriculum planning and the overseeing of the day-to-day activities.

President Tory laid the groundwork well. While the school offered only the first three years of a degree-granting programme initially, within ten years the full medical course was in place, and the medical faculty received a Grade A rating from the Education Committee of the American Medical Association. The school attracted a core of well-qualified and dedicated professionals who remained loyal to the medical school through many difficult years of declining budgets and indifference on the part of the provincial government. It survived two world wars and a major economic depression and emerged with the strength to enhance its commitment to medical education. While the focus of the medical school in its first thirty years was to train general practitioners, following World War II, the initiation of a postgraduate programme enabled graduates to take further training and qualify for a fellowship in a specialty with the Royal College of Physicians and Surgeons of Canada.

The difficulties of the 1950s and 1960s fell into a much different category as the school struggled to adapt to sweeping medical and societal changes. The implementation of universal medical health care required a significant increase in the number of doctors and placed greater emphasis on medical research. An increasingly sophisticated and urban population demanded improvements in medical care, and to satisfy these demands medical educators sought innovative educational methods and improvements to the professional standards. During these two decades, the school faced the problems of increased enrolment, with inadequate facilities, and the development of research programmes in all departments. The faculty added full-time academic physicians, changed the curriculum to reduce the emphasis on didactic lecturing, introduced students to hands-on patient care earlier in the programme, and admitted students to all aspects of the administration of the programme.

The University of Alberta's medical school grew rapidly during the 1970s and the 1980s. Together with medical educators across the North American continent, Alberta's administrators adopted the concept of a health sciences centre that would incorporate all health-related faculties and schools together with a teaching hospital. The advent of the Alberta Heritage Foundation for Medical Research made significant changes in the role of the medical school. It not only created opportunities for a tremendous expansion in research activities but also attracted medical scientists from around the world. It broadened the international reputation of the school as well as the medical education available to its students. Both these developments fulfilled Tory's ambitions for the infant school—that it would become an important clinical centre and a well-known venue for medical research.

PART I

CHAPTER 1

The Early Years

1913-1921

IN 1912, a group of twenty-five science students at the fledgling University of Alberta signed a petition requesting the Senate to institute a faculty of medicine. Henry Marshall Tory, president of the university, presented the petition to the Senate at its meeting in April of that year and gave it his complete support. Medical practitioners arriving in the rapidly developing West, he said, preferred to settle in the larger urban centres, and those settlers who lived in small communities and rural areas had little access to a physician. If the farming families in the outlying districts were to receive adequate medical care, then it was necessary to train doctors in Alberta. Those who had been raised here understood the needs of the people of the province, and after their training would return and settle in the local communities in which they had lived. Tory's persuasive arguments, coupled with the students' petition, led the Senate to agree to the establishment of a medical school as soon as faculty members and a curriculum could be put in place.

For President Tory, the introduction of a medical school within the framework of the University of Alberta was a long-cherished dream, and he had been laying the groundwork for several years. Tory's concept of a provincial university included the early introduction of professional faculties, so that young Albertans could be trained in the professions without incurring the expense of travelling to eastern universities. Before he accepted the position of president of the new university, Tory discussed the subject in detail with representatives of the provincial government and received their approval for the concept.

A university act was among the bills passed at the first sitting of Alberta's legislature in 1906. Premier A.C. Rutherford, who was also the Minister of Education, proposed the legislation, as he was anxious that the new province should begin planning a system of higher education. With the act in place, Rutherford, a lawyer and graduate of McGill University, turned to members of that institution for advice and assistance in this venture.

One of these was Henry Marshall Tory, one of Canada's most brilliant educationalists. Tory received his M.A. in 1895, a D.Sc. in 1903, and was a gold medallist in mathematics and physics. In 1906, he was a professor of physics at McGill; but he also specialized in problems associated with university expansion and was working in Vancouver on proposals for setting up the McGill University College of British Columbia. He broke his train journey between Montreal and Vancouver on several occasions to meet with educationalists and provincial politicians in Alberta. They discussed the future development of a provincial university, and Tory expressed his definite views about educational institutions in the newly developing western provinces.

Despite his ordination as a methodist minister, Tory was a committed centralist and strongly opposed denominational colleges. If a university in the new province was to achieve a standing and reputation in the rest of Canada it must, in his view, have complete and direct control over all educational standards and examinations in the province, be the sole degree-granting institution, and set its own matriculation entrance requirements. Competition from other educational institutions, he opined, would restrict development for all and hold back the opportunity for educational growth in the province. "Centralization should be the watchword of higher work, it costs the country less in the end and is a thousand times more efficient." [1]

Tory felt strongly that an educational institution supported by the public purse should offer "practical" subjects that would be of direct benefit to those who helped fund it. Many older universities in the country began as schools of philosophy, classics and languages, and it was only after many years that they added professional faculties. The "classical" university would not fulfil the needs of a newly settled country. The largely immigrant population demanded tangible results from its university, that is, doctors, lawyers and engineers to serve the public, as well as the opportunity for their sons and daughters to train for these professions locally. Yet, Tory also adhered to tradition, and it is significant that when the university began it offered only the humanities and students were required to wear gowns. "We must use tradition as a guide, and take from it the best that it contains as a lead for us in our work," he told the Senate at its first meeting in 1908.[2]

Rutherford and Tory met on several occasions to discuss plans for a provincial university, and Tory visited both Edmonton and Calgary, where he met many influential citizens, including several medical practitioners. As a result, the second session of the legislature, in 1907, amended the University Act to grant authority, by order-in-council, for the appointment of the "first or an acting president," to set his salary and term of office, and to "alter or vary such term of office."[3] Rutherford then offered the position to Tory—and he accepted. On 1 January 1908, the university, which had no staff, no students and no buildings, at least had a president.

Henry Marshall Tory was a dynamic individual with great energy, determination, indomitable optimism, strong ideas, and a certain ruthlessness of character, which tended to ride roughshod over those who did not agree with him or wished to move more slowly. In recommending Tory to Rutherford, A.P. Low, director of the Geological Survey of Canada, said:

> Tory is by far the best suited...his personality will appeal to the western people...he is not the "frock-coat type" of professor, but rather the type of a western rustler. He is a man to meet and impress all classes of the community...and is strong enough to do without the frills often necessary for weaker individuals...[4]

According to a later president, Robert Newton,

> Tory identified himself completely with any enterprise he undertook, and by his energy and drive usually dominated it...no one in the university questioned his decisions, even if they sometimes had private reservations. This applied to the Board of Governors and even the provincial government."[5]

Site of the New University

Even before Tory's appointment as president, he and Rutherford had discussed the choice of a site for the university. Calgary, which had lost out in its bid to become the capital of the new province, was actively promoting that city as the locale for the provincial university. Premier Rutherford, however, had other ideas. His political constituency was Strathcona, on the south side of the North Saskatchewan River, across from the capital city. As Edmonton had been named the capital and Calgary was to be the home of the provincial Normal (teachers' training) School, he felt that Strathcona should have the provincial university. Furthermore, Strathcona was the terminal of the Canadian Pacific Railway line from Calgary, and was therefore more centrally situated for students coming from the south as well as the north.

Rutherford selected the site, which bordered on the south bank of the North Saskatchewan River, and personally conducted the negotiations for purchase. The property, consisting of 258 acres, was part of an estate administered by three women living in southern Ontario. They offered it for sale at a price of $150,000.[6] The university site was in its natural state, covered with "cottonwood, birch, willow, poplar, saskatoon, choke-cherry, wild rose, honeysuckle, clematis, cranberry and hazel-nut."[7] The choice was not universally approved. It would be difficult for students from Edmonton to reach it, and it was, in fact, some distance from the centre of Strathcona, the west part of the site being outside the town limits. Indeed, the river lot to the east of it was owned and farmed by a pioneer named Armand Garneau. Because of the site's relative inaccessibility, the first buildings to be constructed were residence halls.

In 1907, the provincial government also established a provincial laboratory in Edmonton, an event that had a direct bearing on the eventual development of a medical faculty at the University of Alberta. The North West Territories government had maintained a laboratory in its capital, Regina, and the Saskatchewan government took over its operation after it became a province in 1905. With rapid growth in population in both Alberta and Saskatchewan, the Regina laboratory could not serve the needs of both provinces adequately; thus, the Alberta government established its own laboratory in Edmonton, under the auspices of the Department of Agriculture. Daniel G. Revell, who was its first director, came well recommended. Dr. R.G. Brett, a Banff medical practitioner who was a member of the first Senate of the university and would later become the Lieutenant-Governor of the province, wrote to a friend at the University of Chicago, where Revell was teaching in the anatomy department. "I would advise Dr. Revell," he wrote, "to send an application both to Premier Rutherford and to the Council of Physicians and Surgeons of which I am president. I would be pleased to lend him what assistance I can."[8] Not surprisingly, Revell obtained the position and arrived in Edmonton in August 1907 "to organize the Provincial Laboratory, which from its inception was regarded as the nucleus of a medical faculty."[9] Revell set up the laboratory in the basement of the Terrace Building, the first provincial government building.

Early in 1908, Tory arrived in Edmonton to take up his duties as president of the University of Alberta. In that first year as president, he organised Convocation and the first Senate, hired four professors and began discussions with architects concerning the university buildings. He also travelled the length and breadth of the province promoting the new provincial university—a university for all and not just for those who lived within close proximity to Strathcona. He urged prospective university students to consider the University of Alberta, and some forty-five registered in the first year. Tory encountered a certain resistance, however, from principals of some of the high schools he visited, who felt the enterprise was premature and preferred to encourage their students to enter their own *alma maters*, principally McGill, Toronto and Queen's.[10] Nevertheless, with forty-five students and four professors, the Senate agreed with Tory that classes could commence in the Faculty of Arts and Science in the fall of that first year. These were held on the top floor of what was then known as the Duggan Street School, later to be renamed the Queen Alexandra School.

To expedite matters, the Senate appointed an executive committee, with a mandate to investigate and plan the future development of the university. Both Tory and Rutherford were members of this executive committee, which recommended, as early as June 1909, the establishment of faculties in law and medicine at an early date. The full Senate concurred.[11] Meanwhile, during the same year, at a meeting of a newly formed Alberta Medical Association held in Calgary, the subject of a medical school in Alberta was raised, briefly discussed, and dropped, because those members present concluded that the time was "not ripe for such a venture."[12] They felt that the province did not have the resources, in manpower or facilities, to warrant the establishment of a medical school.

In 1910, Premier Rutherford was forced to resign when scandals erupted concerning financial mismanagement of railway construction in northern Alberta. Tory lost a staunch ally. The Liberal government had a large majority and Rutherford's resignation did not lead to its defeat, but the Lieutenant-Governor appointed a new premier to form a government. Arthur Sifton, previously Alberta's Chief Justice, was uncommunicative and reserved, and Tory had to use all his energies to win him over. The change in leadership came at a particularly bad time for Tory. Although construction had started on the first university building, the legislature had not yet voted the money to pay for it. Furthermore, a new university act was before the legislature, and it faced strong opposition. R.B. Bennett, a future Prime Minister of Canada, had been elected to the legislature as a Conservative, representing Calgary. One of the most eloquent debaters in the province, and an opponent of Tory from the outset, Bennett proposed a bill to institute a university in Calgary. Tory would later state that this was "one of the gravest and most anxious times of my life," when the university came extremely close to being split into several sections throughout the province. It was saved because he was "absolutely unyielding in the matter."[13]

The bill to establish a university in Calgary was backed by a petition signed by one hundred Calgarians. The chief promoter was Thomas Blow, a medical doctor and real estate developer, and later a member of the Alberta legislature. Members of the legislature debated the bill and, after various amendments, established Calgary College, but denied it degree-granting status.[14] Classes began in 1912 in the Public Library, but without the power to grant degrees, and the loss of staff and students due to the first world war, Calgary College folded within three years. As far as Calgarians were concerned, it was Tory who had used his influence to subvert this project. Although he denied this, he had certainly made clear his stand against the decentralization of higher education. Tory continued to promote the concept of the University of Alberta for all Albertans, and frequently quoted statistics to prove that southern Alberta was well represented in the student body. Yet, consistently fewer students from Calgary than from Edmonton would enter the medical faculty, though both cities were of a comparable size.

The new University Act, approved at the same sitting of the legislature in 1910, set up a board of governors to be responsible for the business management and administration of the university. This included the handling of money, investments, the supervision of the buildings and grounds, and staff appointments; however, the act also stipulated that "no person shall be appointed...unless he has first been nominated for the position...by the President of the University."[15] Although the powers of the Senate were correspondingly reduced, it retained sole responsibility for the academic work of the university, including discipline, curricula, student regulation, and the conferring of degrees. The new act also empowered the Senate to conduct examinations for candidates applying for registration in the various professions in Alberta.[16] By mutual agreement with the professional bodies in the province, the university set and conducted examinations, and thus maintained the standards of entrance to all professions in Alberta. As far as the medical profession was concerned, President Tory, together with Drs. W.D. Ferris and W.S. Galbraith, both members of the Senate, discussed this issue with the College of Physicians and Surgeons of Alberta. At its inaugural meeting in 1906, the college had set up an education committee to appoint examiners and set pass marks, and had since then examined incoming practitioners for licensure.[17] From 1912 onward, the university appointed the examiners and set the questions, thus effectively controlling the academic standards of the medical profession in the province.[18]

In this way, the university was able to assist the profession in preventing the admission of what were known as "irregular practitioners." The university assisted the CPSA in educating the public, by identifying those who were scientifically trained to university standards, and differentiating them from those who subscribed to the many unscientific theories of medical practice prevalent at the time. Tory used his considerable powers of persuasion to have the Medical Professional Act amended to make it more difficult for "irregulars" to practise in Alberta; thus, he was able to obtain the support, albeit sometimes unwillingly given, of the College of Physicians and Surgeons for his plans for a medical school. In an effort to achieve a common standard of qualification for admission to the profession throughout the country, the Medical Council of Canada was established by federal legislation in 1912. It also attempted to achieve a commonality in entrance requirements, curriculum and facilities for Canadian medical schools.[19] When it sought the sole right to conduct examinations in all provinces, the CPSA refused,

> on account of the extreme difficulty we of Alberta have had in so arranging a suitable standard for the Medical Profession in conflict with Quacks and Charletons [sic], we deem it unwise at the present as yet to surrender to the Medical Council of Canada the sole right to conduct examinations allowing entry.[20]

The college felt that the administration of qualifying examinations by the University of Alberta was of greater help in improving the standard of medical practitioners in the province.

Plans for a University Hospital

As plans for a faculty of medicine at the university began to take shape, Tory associated himself with hospital facilities in both Edmonton and

Strathcona. Initially, he endeavoured to promote the idea of a hospital on the north side of the High Level Bridge, in the general area of the new legislature buildings, that would serve the citizens of both Edmonton and Strathcona and also be close enough to the university to serve as a teaching hospital for a medical school. This venture fell through, as both the medical practitioners and the citizens of Edmonton wanted their own hospital, one that would be administered by city council, not the university.[21]

The increasing power of the University of Alberta and its president met with some resistance, as shown in the preceding instance. He met with opposition from members of both the public and the legislature, who questioned the "unrestrained" growth of the university and its use of public funds; they accused Tory of pushing through his plans regardless of financial or public support; and suggested that the need for a medical faculty was born "in the ambitious and overheated brain of the President."[22] In the press, he was sometimes described as a dreamer—a visionary who wanted to "grab everything in sight."[23] His plans for a teaching hospital led to controversial debates on the topic of medical students practising on, and at the expense of, the poor and the indigent.

But Tory was not deterred and set his sights on Strathcona Hospital. Strathcona council recognized the need for a larger hospital than existed at the time, and had received taxpayers' authority to build a new hospital in 1907. For economic reasons, construction did not take place, but Tory revived interest in the project with an offer of land on the university site. In January 1912, after lengthy discussions, Strathcona council and the university's Board of Governors eventually reached agreement and signed a lease. The university provided land on the condition that the council build a hospital, at a minimum cost of $100,000, and that it would become a teaching hospital when a faculty of medicine was established. The terms of the lease stated explicitly that the site was to be used for a hospital building only; that the plans and specifications had first to be approved by the university; and that once the teaching of medicine began at the university, management and control would be turned over to the university, which would then take over the debenture debt.[24] Concurrently with these negotiations, in 1911 and 1912, discussions concerning the amalgamation of Strathcona and Edmonton, were also taking place. The lease was signed shortly before the date of amalgamation, and it was the council of the combined cities that then became committed to the construction of the hospital, the total costs of which, including construction, equipment and furniture, amounted to more than $350,000.[25]

Another step towards the establishment of a medical school took place in 1911 with the removal of the Provincial Laboratory from its original home in the basement of the Terrace Building on the north side of the river to the recently completed Athabasca Hall, the first of the university buildings to be constructed. Revell was still the Director and Provincial Bacteriologist and "had no small part in its transfer to the University, which [he] believed was in the mutual interest of these two organizations."[26] He supervised the move across the river and set up the laboratory in the north wing of the new building. Such a move was not a simple matter. Everything was loaded onto wagons and taken across the river by ferry, then transported up the steep hill to Strathcona, and finally along a trail to Athabasca Hall. The journey was made even worse by the condition of the muddy roads: the "prairie gumbo" clung tenaciously to the wagon wheels. With this move, the Provincial Laboratory came under the joint jurisdiction of the university and the provincial government, and would provide the basis for future departments of pathology and bacteriology when the medical school was established, and also provide teachers for the medical sciences.[27]

Tory forged ahead with his plans for the continued growth of the university, and the establishment of professional faculties. A law faculty and an extension department were added in 1912, and a faculty of applied science (engineering) early in 1913. The next step was a faculty of medicine, and everything was now in place. A hospital, the Provincial Laboratory and the College of Physicians and Surgeons of Alberta were all on side. A statement in the legislature by Peter Gunn, the MLA for Lac Ste. Anne, endorsing a medical school that would train doctors for the rural areas of the province, together with the petition from a group of students, provided public support. There is reason to believe that Tory himself instigated the petition, suggesting to some students that such an action would promote the establishment of a medical school at the university.[28] The Senate had little option but to sanction Tory's recommendation that the time was now ripe to start a faculty of medicine. The first year of the programme, essentially a premedical year, was offered in 1913-14; the first and second year, the premedical year plus the first medical science year, in 1914-15; and all three years in 1915-16.

The Faculty of Medicine of the University of Alberta began at a time when standards and improvements in medical education were under close scrutiny throughout North America. In 1910, the Carnegie Institute commissioned Abraham Flexner, a professional educator, to make a study of medical schools in the United States and Canada. He visited most of the medical schools in the United States and all those in Canada, described and rated them, and in many cases offered severe criticisms. Improvements in medical education had been taking place in a number of schools long before the publication of this report;[29] nevertheless, its recommendations served as a basis for continued and more widespread improvements in all schools. Flexner recommended that all medical schools affiliate with a university, as it was there that basic sciences were readily available for hands-on scientific training in the initial years of a medical student's education. Other recommendations included high admission standards; the university to be the degree-granting institution rather than the medical school; two years of study in medical sciences followed by two years of clinical training; and the encouragment of scholarly research. Medical education on the North American continent followed, for many years, Flexner's basic "two and two" curriculum.[30]

Tory agreed completely with these views. In an address to the Congress on Medical Education held in Chicago in February 1926, he stated that,

> the real struggle for modern medicine began when biology, physics and chemistry invaded the domain of medical instruction and demanded a place with anatomy and physiology.[31]

These fundamental sciences, he continued, should be taught as university subjects by those who were masters of their subject and not by medical practitioners to whom they were merely incidental. In the new era of "scientific medicine," medical students should be taught that the study of medical sciences was "fundamental to the understanding and treatment of disease." Tory also felt that a university affiliation would help maintain the standing of the medical profession within the province, by applying rigorous university standards in all subjects of the curriculum. A scientist himself, Tory was not a subscriber to the "medicine as an art" theory; he felt that a good bedside manner was fine, provided that it was accompanied by sound scientific knowledge.[32]

Alberta's medical school was the first in Canada to originate within the framework of an established university,[33] and as it opened its doors in the wake of the Flexner Report, it was in a position to base its initial curriculum upon the recommendations of that document. The quality of medical schools in both Canada and the United States varied considerably, and following the publication of the Flexner Report in 1910, schools received an A, B or C rating from the American Medical Association's

Council on Medical Education. University administrators, anxious to improve the standards in their schools, exerted great pressure on their medical faculties to achieve a high standing, preferably a Class A rating, which would be recognized by the public as well as by aspiring medical students.[34]

While it has been generally assumed that only the first three years of a five-year programme were originally planned at the University of Alberta, it is not clear from the literature that this was so. With the completion of Strathcona Hospital in the summer of 1913, it is likely that Tory envisioned a full five-year medical programme at the University of Alberta right from the start. In his report to the legislature in June 1913, Tory announced the establishment of a medical faculty and stated that arrangements would be made with eastern universities for the last two years of the course, "should these not be offered in the University of Alberta on the completion of the first three."[35] Tory wrote to Dr. George Adami, professor of pathology at McGill, in December 1914 that it was:

> ... not yet decided whether to extend the course beyond the first three years of a five year course.... We intend asking McGill to accept our first three years work and if we can get amicable agreement, probably will not try to go further - particularly if hard times continue.[36]

When the Senate agreed to establish a medical faculty in 1912, "boom" conditions still existed in Alberta. During that year, in fact, immigration into the province reached a high that, on a proportional basis, has never been surpassed. The future looked exceedingly bright for the young province. Just a year later, however, in 1913, the "boom" collapsed, wheat prices fell, and immigration figures began to decline. Alberta's future prosperity was no longer assured.[37] World War I broke out in 1914, a traumatic occurrence that became a watershed in Alberta's history. Men, and some women, both students and faculty, went to war, and national and provincial economies geared up to fight a war, not to build educational institutions. Student enrolment, which had been increasing steadily since 1908, stagnated during the war years. Those faculty members who remained were called upon to do double duty, and in 1916 the medical school lost its clinical facilities when the dominion government took over the Strathcona Hospital to provide hospital care for wounded soldiers. It was impossible to complete the full medical course under such conditions.

Initially, there were only two medically trained doctors on the Medical

Faculty Council. Daniel G. Revell, professor of anatomy, and Heber H. Moshier, professor of physiology, were both graduates of the University of Toronto medical school. Over the first three years, they developed and refined the curriculum, which was based on "The Model Medical Curriculum" that had been prepared by a committee of "100 leading educators of the United States and Canada" and published under the direction of the Council on Medical Education of the American Medical Association.[38] The first year was a premedical programme and included courses in chemistry, physics, biology, zoology and French or German. In 1913, many of the high schools of the province lacked the facilities to teach science subjects that required laboratory equipment. Entrance to university, therefore, followed junior matriculation, Grade XI, and the premedical year covered senior matriculation courses.

The second year was the first professional year, during which the university offered instruction in such medical sciences as anatomy, physiology, organic chemistry, biochemistry, pharmacy and materia medica (pharmacology). Third-year studies included senior courses in anatomy, physiology and pharmacology, as well as bacteriology, pathology and an introduction to clinical medicine and surgery.[39] The curriculum was typical of that offered in other medical schools in Canada and, after 1915 was accepted by both McGill and the University of Toronto. Graduates of the three years given in Alberta were accepted at these two eastern universities without further examination.

The First Faculty Members

Dr. Daniel G. Revell was the first member of the medical faculty to be hired specifically for the medical school—the other professors were already employed by the university in their own disciplines. He was also the only medical doctor on the faculty council that first year. Revell graduated initially in arts and taught school for several years before returning to the University of Toronto to take a medical degree. Older than his fellow medical students, he had demonstrated a quiet, studious and dignified manner that earned him the affectionate nickname of "Daddy," which would remain with him throughout his career. After graduating, he went to the University of Chicago where he took a fellowship in anatomy, helped establish an anatomy department, and was later appointed a professor. There, together with two of his colleagues, he wrote a textbook entitled *A Laboratory Manual of Anatomy.*[40]

Soon after his appointment as professor of anatomy at the University of Alberta's medical school, Revell resigned his position as Director of the Provincial Laboratory as he wished to enter private practice. He had developed a hearing problem, however, and this proved a major obstacle to a satisfactory medical practice. For the same reason, he was considered unfit for overseas service in the army, but he did join the Royal Canadian Army Medical Corps and served at the Strathcona Hospital as pathologist for the Edmonton area. At the same time, he carried on his teaching duties at the medical school. Revell would teach anatomy to hundreds of medical students before his retirement in 1937 at the age of sixty-eight—a retirement that he did not seek and did not want.[41] Revell was a gentle person, who taught his subject in meticulous detail—sometimes to the distraction of his students. His method of examining the students was to place a selection of bones, often dinosaur bones, under a sheet and require the student to identify them by touch alone.[42] He was a man with eclectic interests, including painting, nature study and etymology, and these sometimes took precedence over anatomy in his lectures; the students could readily steer him off topic by some judicious questioning.[43] Throughout his career, he co-operated with both the Saskatchewan and Alberta police departments in the scientific examination of documents and the identification of handwriting.[44]

The second medical practitioner to join the faculty was Heber H. Moshier, who had been practising in Calgary. A young, vibrant individual, he was appointed professor of physiology but he also taught pathology and clinical medicine and organized the Student Medical Service where he cared for sick students himself. In 1916, when universities across the country formed field ambulance units for service at the front, Moshier volunteered to organize a unit manned by students from the four western universities, and to take it to the Somme in France. Just a few months before the war ended, Moshier, by then a lieutenant-colonel, was killed instantly when he was hit by a piece of shrapnel while driving an ambulance. He was just twenty-seven years old and his early death was a great loss to the young medical school. The Volunteer Overseas Medical Officers' Association of Edmonton subsequently donated a medal in his name to the medical school, to be awarded to the final year student with the highest average standing in all subjects of the medical curriculum.[45] Known as the Moshier Memorial Award, it is still the highest award of the medical school.

Allan C. Rankin, a McGill graduate in medicine and public health, succeeded Revell as Director of the Provincial Laboratory in 1914 and was appointed professor of bacteriology in the same year. Rankin came directly to Edmonton from Siam [Thailand], where he was the chief bacteriologist. He was in Edmonton only a short time, however, a matter of just a few months, before war was declared. As he had previously served in Canada's militia, he immediately offered his services and went overseas with the first Canadian contingent. It was October 1919 before he returned, and the following year he was appointed dean.[46]

During his absence, Heber C. Jamieson served as acting Director of the Provincial Laboratory, and also received an appointment to the Faculty of Medicine. Another University of Toronto graduate, Jamieson practised medicine in Edmonton. During the first few years, he taught bacteriology and a clinical laboratory course, and later gave a course in medical history. He had a great love for the history of medicine and offered an annual prize to the medical school for the best essay on that subject. Jamieson was a kind, unconventional man, with a gentlemanly manner—who perhaps imbibed a little too freely—but was of the old school of medical practitioners, and rarely demanded payment from his patients, particularly if he knew they were unable to pay.[47] He is perhaps best remembered for his book *Early Medicine in Alberta, The First Seventy-Five Years*, published by the Alberta Division of the Canadian Medical Association in 1947.

J. Bertram Collip, who would later bring great fame to Alberta's medical school through his participation in the purification of insulin, arrived in 1915. Another graduate of the University of Toronto, Collip graduated in arts and science with honours in physiology and biochemistry. He then studied as a fellow and research scholar, received his Ph.D. in biochemistry, and had already attracted attention in the new field of biochemistry before his arrival in Alberta. Collip lectured in biochemistry and physiology, and during the final years of the war, he, Revell and Jamieson virtually held the school together.

By 1914, four medical science departments were established within the Faculty of Medicine: anatomy under Revell, physiology and pharmacology under Moshier, and bacteriology under Rankin. Medical students also received instruction in chemistry, biology and physics, which were part of the Faculty of Arts and Science, and their professors in these subjects were also members of the Medical Faculty Council. Students in the Faculty of Arts and Science also took courses in anatomy and physiology, applied science students studied bacteriology, and, obviously, pharmacy students took courses in the department of pharmacology. The medical school was, therefore, closely interwoven into the academic structure of the university. Expansion plans for the immediate future called for an increase in the number of instructors, but did not include the addition of any new clinical departments.[48]

The curriculum included only two clinical courses, one in medicine, the other in surgery, and both were in the third year. Initially conducted at the Strathcona Hospital, they moved across the river to the Royal Alexandra Hospital after 1916 when the former became a military hospital. Initially, the laboratory courses were offered on the third floor of Pembina Hall, the third residence building, newly completed in 1914. Later, they transferred to the Power Plant, and the anatomy laboratories were small rooms along one side of the top floor. Revell liked this arrangement. Each room was large enough for four students and the central dissecting table, for the "silent, best atlas of anatomy," and Revell felt that the students worked better and more independently than if they were all in one large room with its attendant distractions.[49] Equipment in the anatomy laboratories in 1915 included compound and dissecting microscopes for each student, microtomes, charts, models, and prepared specimens for study. Each room was well lit and supplied with hot and cold water.[50] An initial problem in the department of anatomy was the provision of sufficient cadavers for use in the anatomy laboratories. This was solved by an amendment to the University Act in 1913, which stipulated that the bodies of those who died in publicly supported institutions and whose bodies were not claimed should be made available to the university "for anatomical purposes and for scientific instruction and research."

The First Students

Twenty-seven students registered for the first year in 1913, and all were male. One of them, at least, Walter Morrish, found some of the first year courses "weren't too useful and were a great waste of time...but...if you wanted to be a doctor you must follow the prescribed course and ask no questions." Morrish, like many of the others in his class, was older than the average first-year university student, was well-travelled and anxious to get on with the "real" medical courses.[51] As would be expected, there were some problems that first year, mostly occasioned by the lateness or nonarrival of equipment that had been ordered from Great Britain. "There have been disappointments," wrote the president of the first class, "and we believe that none have felt them more keenly than Dr. Tory, but these have been due to unforeseen delay in the arrival of equipment." He also reported that the class planned to furnish a room in the new South Side (Strathcona) Hospital, which had been significantly assisted by a generous donation from Tory.[52]

The geographical background of this first medical class belied Tory's assumption that the medical students would be mainly from small communities in the province. Of the twenty-seven, seven were from Edmonton, two from Calgary, but only seven from smaller centres in Alberta. Nine of them came from other parts of Canada: from British Columbia, New Brunswick, Ontario and Saskatchewan; and two from England.[53]

University regulations stipulated that students who did not have family or relatives with whom they could live in Edmonton had to live in residence.[54] For those who lived on the north side of the river, travel to and from the university was quite an expedition. Although the High Level Bridge was completed in 1913, the lower deck was not yet opened. Students could cross the railway level of the bridge on the girders, dodging any oncoming trains, or they could walk across the frozen river during the winter. The more conventional route was to take a streetcar across the Low Level Bridge, up 99th Street and along Whyte Avenue to 109th Street, and then walk about a mile through bush to the residence halls where the classes took place.[55]

Fees were $50 for the first year, and $75 for each of the second and third years. They did not increase until 1920, when the first year increased to $75, and subsequent years rose to $100. Room and board in the residence halls cost $40 a month.[56] There was no financial assistance, and most students had to work during the summer in order to pay their fees. The only scholarships available were five awards of $50 each offered by the College of Physicians and Surgeons of Alberta.[57]

Of the first twenty-seven students, only sixteen registered for the second year in 1914, and two of these were newcomers—one from Michigan and the other from McGill University in Montreal. By this time, war had been declared and no doubt some had enlisted, two were repeating their year, and others "were unable to return." Eleven students, three of them women, registered in the first year, so there were still just twenty-seven students in the medical school; however, there were new and additional faces among the faculty. Gordon C. Gray, who was a gold medallist from the University of Toronto, assisted Moshier in physiology; Leighton C. Conn, from McGill, instructed in anatomy; and Morton Hall, from Toronto, taught pathology. After long delays, new apparatus and equipment for the physiological and histological laboratories finally arrived from England, and Heber Jamieson, after teaching a half-year course in bacteriology, went to New York to study new instructional methods for use in well-equipped laboratories. While the students "generally conceded that first-class medical schools are not usually established in a year, or five years," they began to feel more satisfied with the instruction they were receiving.[58] Dr. Revell, according to Morrish, while not a "natural teacher,"

> was the mainstay of the year... [and]... his pioneer work laid the foundation for the excellent medical school which has become favourably known all over the world.... All in all the medical courses added up to a fairly sound introduction... [and]... compared favourably with the courses given then in McGill and Toronto.[59]

Those who went on to eastern universities for their clinical years generally fitted in well academically, and two of them received gold medals in their final years at McGill.[60]

Some of the students in these early years would return to Alberta and make their mark in the Faculty of Medicine. One of these was John W. Scott, who would become the third dean of the school. After he completed his third year, in 1917, he had the opportunity to remain for another year as a demonstrator in physiology and, at the same time work towards an additional science degree as well as his M.D. He chose, instead, to enlist in the Tank Corps, and later completed his course at McGill.[61]

Another was Harold Vango. A Cockney, he had emigrated from England and worked on the grounds of the University of Alberta when Revell first met him. Impressed with his capabilities, Revell employed him as a technician in his laboratory, and later encouraged him to enrol in medical school. After his three years at Alberta, Vango went on to McGill, where he graduated in 1922. After internship in Montreal and postgraduate studies in Edinburgh and Vienna, Vango returned to Alberta where he joined the faculty as a member of the pathology department. Later, he returned to Britain and Europe to conduct research in medical jurisprudence, a field in which few people had great expertise at that time, and taught courses in this subject upon his return. A promising future was in store for him when, in 1932, he cut himself while performing an autopsy and died a few days later of streptococcal septicaemia.[62]

World War I

At the outbreak of World War I, the university was just about to commence its seventh year of existence and the medical school its second. The problems that were to ensue over the next four years were difficult enough for older universities and schools; yet the University of Alberta not only survived but also contributed in tangible ways to the successful conclusion of that war. Altogether, some 484 people went into active service, mainly students, but also faculty members and other employees, and eighty-two were killed in action. Two of these were members of the first medical class in 1913—P.N. McNally and John Hammond died in action in France in 1918.[63] As the student body had numbered only 440 when war was declared, this was a remarkable contribution. The Canadian Officers Training Corps (COTC) was established in the university immediately after the declaration of war and would remain a part of university life until its dissolution in 1968. In the first year, 144 students enlisted for training in the COTC, and khaki uniforms became a common sight on campus as the war dragged on. Medical students who took military medical corps work through the COTC received a bonus of 10% on their final mark,[64] and during the war years military training supplanted physical education.[65]

A Western Universities' Battalion (the 196th Battalion, Canadian Expeditionary Force) established in 1916, consisted of four companies, one from each of the four western provincial universities. Alberta's company was "housed and fed and trained on university grounds."[66] Later that year, Moshier, by then a captain in the army, organized the 11th Field Ambulance Unit of the Canadian Army Medical Corps, and the university calendar of 1917 listed some twenty-nine students in this unit, of whom sixteen were medical students. Those second- and third-year students who served in the Field Ambulance Corps received university credit for work done while serving at the front. Medical officers of the Royal Canadian Army Medical Corps gave them the instruction needed to complete their course to the end of their respective years. A certificate issued by the medical officer was sufficient authority for the university to grant the student a pass for that year.[67]

Total registration in the medical school during the years of the first world war remained fairly stable: forty-four in 1914, forty-two in 1915, thirty-six in 1916, and forty-eight in 1917. In 1918, with the end of the war in sight and as soldiers began to return from the front, registration increased sharply to eighty-six. In 1919, when the war was over and the wartime army had been demobilised, seventy-six students registered in the first year alone, and those who had interrupted their studies to join the services swelled the numbers in the second and third years.[68] The massive increase in registration in 1918 and 1919 occurred throughout all faculties of the university and included many students who had joined the services when, under normal circumstances, they would have entered university. There were enormous problems in assimilating such large numbers into a university that had seen little growth in buildings or equipment. Furthermore, returned soldiers were entirely different from the typical prewar university student; they were not only older in years but their experiences of life and death on the battlefield made them considerably more mature in their attitudes and expectations. Conventional excuses and platitudes were not acceptable to them.[69] Changes had to, and did, take place.

As classes were small in number during the war, they could be well accommodated in the space available at the time. Construction of the Arts Building had been delayed because of the war, and although it was eventually completed in 1916 the university was still ill-equipped to handle the large registration of the immediate postwar years. Space for both tuition and accommodation was at a premium. Even though all three residence buildings were used solely for residents by 1921, the university was no longer able to accommodate all those who applied. More than one hundred were refused accommodation.[70]

In the medical school, the first order of priority was the appointment of a dean. Revell, because of his long and close association with the development of the school since its inception, fully expected to be appointed dean. In August 1918, he wrote to W.A.R. Kerr, Dean of the Faculty of Arts and Science, who was Acting President while Tory served in England during the latter years of the war.

> Attention should also be drawn to the very real risk we are running in the failure to make effective provision for those important duties which properly belong under a deanship of medical students. In simple fairness to our students and to McGill and Toronto Universities, which accept our students, we should not continue to jeopardize our rating, and incidentally theirs, in the classification of medical colleges in America. A low rating once suffered would be a stigma on us for all time, and great labor, expense and pains would be necessary to replace our rating with a higher revised standing.[71]

But Tory was not to be rushed into a decision. From England, he wrote to Kerr, ''that there is no man at present on our staff that I would think for one moment of appointing.'' He had, he said, discussed the matter with Rankin, who was also still in England. Both of them were seeking a likely candidate in that country, preferably someone on the clinical side of medicine or an educational specialist who would devote his whole time to administration.[72] But highly competent people in these fields, as in all others, were in great demand as all universities struggled to meet the needs of a rapid increase in registration following the war. When Rankin was appointed dean in 1920, Revell felt that the decision had been influenced by both Rankin and Tory having been trained at McGill, whereas he was a Toronto graduate.[73] In a time period, and in an area, where university graduates were fairly limited in number, loyalty and allegiance to one's *alma mater* were important matters. While the small group that had held the medical school together during the war years was made up predominantly of graduates from the University of Toronto, postwar appointments went largely to McGill graduates. By 1921, Alberta's medical school had a distinct McGill flavour, with all its Osler and Edinburgh traditions of a strong emphasis on bedside teaching.

Construction of the Medical Building
Meanwhile, in 1918, a representative of the Council on Medical Education and Hospitals of the American Medical Association had visited the medical school and offered a few suggestions for improvement. Given the exigencies of wartime and the shortage of faculty members, these could not be implemented. The following year, N.P. Colwell, secretary of the council, made a follow-up inspection, and during his visit addressed the medical students. He pointed out that the American Medical Association found it necessary to grade schools "in order to eliminate the fakes that have arisen, due to the demand for doctors since the war."[74] Colwell's report, dated 5 November 1919, was not sent to the university until the end of May 1920, when Tory was back in full charge. The report outlined several deficiencies: overcrowding; a limited supply of laboratory equipment; insufficient full-time and well-qualified staff; little opportunity for research; an inadequate library; minimum educational standards; a university year of only twenty-eight weeks; and the absence of a medical museum. The report offered various suggestions for improvement and ended with the words: "The chief hope in preparing and sending this report is that it may be of assistance in the efforts you are undoubtedly making to develop a high class medical school in Alberta."[75]

In his lengthy reply to this report, Tory commented that he "was somewhat startled at its content." And, indeed, in the six months that it had taken the American Medical Association to forward its report, many of the noted deficiencies had already been corrected, and plans for other improvements were under way. A new medical building, which would include adequate and well-equipped laboratories, as well as a library and a museum, was already under construction. Additional staff, both full-time and part-time, had been hired, and although some positions remained to be filled, Tory was actively seeking additional personnel. As far as the entrance requirements were concerned, Tory stated that Alberta's matriculation standard was identical to that of Toronto and McGill, both of which were Class A medical schools and accepted Alberta students without further examination. He did concede, however, that after 1923 senior matriculation would be required for entrance into all Canada's medical schools, including Alberta's. He also agreed that Alberta's term was shorter than those in the United States, "but on account of the distances which our students travel we intensify our work during the year."[76]

In December 1919, soon after his return to Edmonton, and just one month after the AMA inspection took place, Tory reported to the government that,

> there is an urgent need for a Medical Building to house our medical faculty, which should include space for the Public Health Laboratories and also for the Department of Chemistry. The latter department is so very much over-crowded as to make the proper conduct of the laboratory work exceedingly difficult.[77]

The following year, in his annual report to the legislature, Tory commented that,

> The Anatomy, Chemistry and Physics Laboratories were so crowded that it was with great difficulty that we got through the year without a serious breakdown. The Board of Governors therefore authorised the immediate construction of a new building to contain these departments.[78]

Armed with preliminary plans for a new building, the executive committee of the Board of Governors met with certain members of the government, including the premier, the provincial treasurer, and the ministers of education and municipalities. They discussed the problems occasioned by the large registration, as well as the plans for a medical building, and received almost immediate approval from the government to start work on a building to house the medical faculty. Detailed plans and specifications had not been prepared and there were, therefore, no firm estimates of the costs of construction or equipment. The reason for such haste was to expedite construction so that at least part of the building would be available for use by the fall of 1920.[79] The building inspector's report stated that the value placed on the building at the time the permit was taken out was $750,000, but a subsequent auditor's report, in January 1922, showed that construction costs exceeded one million dollars and equipment costs amounted to well over $65,000.

R.G. Brett, the president of the College of Physicians and Surgeons of Alberta and a member of the University Senate, laid the cornerstone in 1920, and construction began forthwith; but it was the fall of 1921 before the building was ready for occupancy. The Medical Building, a handsome neoclassical building, was given an architectural style that conformed with other buildings on the campus. It faced south on 89th Avenue, forming the south side of a quadrangle of university buildings. It was such a fine looking building that Tory later expressed the wish that he had chosen a site on the north side of the quadrangle so that it could be viewed from across the river.[80] Two large lecture theatres, situated on each side of the front entrance, had curved outside walls, giving an interesting and unusual aspect to the front façade of the building. These lecture theatres seated two hundred students, were two storeys in height, and could be entered from both the first and second floors. The building was designed in such a way that it could be readily expanded when numbers warranted. The structure would only be complete when three wings were added at the back—an east, west and central wing. The Medical Building was, however, the last building of any substantial size to be constructed on the university campus for some thirty years, and it was not until 1946 that a start was made on the construction of the first wing.

All the departments of the medical faculty moved in, as well as the chemistry department and the Provincial Laboratory. Cadavers were brought in through a specially constructed and secluded entryway, and transported by a nonstop elevator to the anatomy department on the third floor of the building. The main anatomy laboratory was one large room with space enough for eight dissecting tables. Revell was not pleased with this plan. His years of teaching in single-unit dissecting rooms in the Power House had shown him the advantages of such a system, and he would, in the years ahead, make repeated attempts to get approval for the division of this one large room into smaller units.[81] Biochemistry occupied the west half of the same floor and included "a spacious animal room which is well-lighted, heated and ventilated."[82] For the first time, the medical school had its own library, display cabinets in the corridors for museum exhibits, and even a common room for students.

With a new building in place, a dean appointed, and respected members of the medical and educational fraternities employed on the faculty, the Faculty of Medicine finally achieved its coveted Class A rating in November 1922. In his letter to Tory, Colwell said that ''the high ideals under which you have thus far developed your medical school give ample assurance that in its further development, these ideals will still prevail.'' Tory, the medical students and faculty members were jubilant. The University of Alberta's medical school was, according to Tory,

> ...the only medical school between Winnipeg and Peking, the only university in Canada with a hospital entirely under its control and direction...[and]...in ten years would develop into an important clinical centre ....[83]

* * * * *

CHAPTER 2

The Years of Struggle

The twenties and the thirties

THE YEARS immediately following the war were exciting ones for the young school, even though fraught with tension, problems and concern about its future. There were high points: the Class A rating, the opening of the Medical Building, an endowment of half a million dollars from the Rockefeller Foundation, the extension of the programme to a full-degree course, and the pride and excitement of having one of its own faculty members involved with the dramatic discovery of insulin.

Several major events took place during this postwar period to solidify and strengthen the role of the Faculty of Medicine within the framework of the University of Alberta. Construction of a building specifically for the school itself spelled stability and progress, as did the appointment of new faculty members, some on a full-time basis. When the Department of National Defence gave up its lease on the Strathcona Hospital in 1922, Tory's vision of a university teaching hospital was finally realized. Changes in the curriculum at Toronto's and McGill's medical schools necessitated changes in Alberta's curriculum as well, and gradually the clinical years were added to the programme. The first class to earn an M.D. (Alberta) graduated in 1925.

All these developments will be explored in this chapter, but first they have to be set within the framework of the political and economic situation in Alberta. In 1921, Albertans went to the polls and elected a new government, a "farmers' government." As is their wont, when Albertans decide to change governments, they do so decisively. In this instance, they replaced the Liberals with the United Farmers of Alberta, a pseudopolitical party that won thirty-eight seats in a sixty-one-seat legislature. Alberta's penchant for third-party politics, and its frequent disenchantment with the old-line parties, was already under way.

The new premier, Herbert Greenfield, and many of his colleagues were not enthusiastic supporters of Tory and his expansionist ideas for the university. Generally speaking, the farming community at this time felt that the university was for children of the well-to-do, who should support it with their fees.[1] Tory was away at the time of the election in 1921 and Kerr wired him the unexpected results. Later, he wrote, "I know it is hard having, so to speak, to start all over again to make converts of a new lot of men, but perhaps conversion this time will be easier than in the former instance."[2] This would not prove to be the case. Each year, the government instructed the Board of Governors to trim expenditures to the bone, and still cut the proposed budgets even more. This occurred in the 1920s as well as in the 1930s as economic conditions deteriorated. The university vote of $474,890 in 1922 was reduced to $433,281 in 1923, and to $414,000 in 1924, which forced the closure of the architectural school and the release of several staff members.[3]

As for the medical school, the new government was skeptical at best about its value to Alberta and uneasy about the province's ability to pay for it. It was expensive, second only to the Faculty of Agriculture. The benefits of the latter to the people of Alberta, most of whom were involved with agriculture in one form or another, were more obvious and relevant to the new legislators. Over the years, they made numerous and detailed enquiries about the costs of running a medical school: the Medical Building and its cost overrun, staff members and their salaries, and the costs of the necessary clinical facilities. Against this they weighed the income derived from student fees and the return to the people of Alberta in the services of the medical school graduates.

By this time, Alberta's economy was dependent upon a single export crop—wheat. Wheat prices and yields remained high during the war years, and as a result farmers invested in more land and put more and more of their acreage into wheat production. They also invested in mechanization, and as a result many carried a heavy debt load to mortgage lenders and farm equipment companies. The price of wheat fell after the war and remained unstable until the mid-twenties when prices and yields started to rise again. It was a short lived period of prosperity, however, for both prices and yields fell in 1929. In 1930, although production was much higher the price fell so drastically that the return to the farmer was even less than in 1929.

Wheat had risen to a high of $2.00 a bushel in the late1920s. In 1932, it brought 34¢. With the collapse of the mainstay of the province's economy, secondary and service industries, dependent upon the wheat economy, suffered accordingly. Unemployment rose, while many farm families faced starvation and the loss of their land. "Relief" became a way of life for large numbers of people. Whereas the industrialized world began to pull out of the depression by the mid-1930s, drought, wind and dust storms, and grasshopper plagues added to the problems of the prairie provinces.

Neither Liberal nor Conservative governments in Ottawa seemed able to alleviate the drastic conditions on the prairies, and the UFA government in Alberta provided no answers either. This left the field open for a third-party again, and in the 1935 provincial election poverty-stricken Albertans elected another new government. The Social Credit party elected a total of fifty-six members in a sixty-three-seat legislature, and the UFA was wiped out, returning not a single candidate. The new party offered a simplistic monetary theory—nevertheless almost no one understood it—but he people were prepared to try anything if it would bring them out of the severe economic conditions that had prevailed for so long.[4]

The new premier, William Aberhart, was a schoolteacher who had been principal of Crescent Heights High School in Calgary for many years. He had, therefore, an obvious interest in education. President Wallace invited all the MLAs to "spend an evening at the university," and provided cars to bring them to Athabasca Hall for supper with the male students in residence. A tour of the university followed, beginning with the Medical Building.[5] But it was to no avail. The economic exigencies of the province precluded any increase in the university's budget. The Annual Report of the university for the following year stated that,

> The University of Alberta continues to grow ... [but] ... accommodation and general equipment are not growing with it. No new construction has taken place since the erection of the Medical Building.... It is seventeen years since the Provincial Treasury has afforded any easement of the increasingly crowded conditions. Government has always been cordial and sympathetic to our needs...but has not seen its way clear to accede to our requests.[6]

The only advantage provided to the university during these lean years was the opportunity to conduct its own affairs—and survive as best it could—without any political interference from the government.[7] As the 1930s drew to a close another war was on the horizon, which would bring problems of a different but equally distressing nature.

* * * * *

Throughout these two decades, the medical school was not entirely dependent upon student fees and government grants. It also received the interest on an endowment of $500,000 from the Rockefeller Foundation. There is a story, obviously originating with Tory himself, that credits the Rockefeller grant with saving the medical school from extinction in the early 1920s. On a particular morning in 1923, so the story goes, Premier Herbert Greenfield went to see Tory in his office at the university, specifically to tell him that he could not continue with his plans to establish a medical school. Quite simply, the province could not afford it. By chance a cheque for half a million dollars from the Rockefeller Foundation had arrived in that morning's mail, the interest on which was to be used specifically for the further development of the medical school. Tory waved the cheque triumphantly in the air, at which point Greenfield got up without saying a word and left the office, never to mention the matter again.[8]

It makes a good story, and the essence of it bears some resemblance to what happened. In fact, Tory was not even in Edmonton when the cheque arrived; he was in Regina, on his way to eastern Canada, and received news of its arrival by telegram from Kerr. In addition, the medical school had been receiving a yearly grant from the Rockefeller Foundation for three years. In 1920, the foundation awarded a grant of five million dollars to assist with the development of medical education in Canada. McGill, Toronto and Dalhousie each received a million. Other medical schools in the country became eligible for assistance once they had shown sufficient progress, and in the meantime received token financial aid.

Flexner's report on medical education had advocated the use of full-time professors for the clinical years of the medical programme—faculty members whose first duty would be to their teaching and their students. However proficient part-time teachers might be, their first responsibility would always remain with their practice and their patients. The Rockefeller Foundation, which now employed Flexner, promoted the recommendations of the Flexner Report, particularly with regard to the appointment of full-time clinical staff. Tory agreed strongly with this principle, although the full-time concept was by no means universally accepted, particularly by small and less affluent schools.[9] The University of Alberta, therefore, applied to the Rockefeller Foundation for financial assistance specifically to hire more full-time professors and to develop the clinical years of the programme. To assist the university in this purpose, the Foundation awarded a yearly grant of $25,000 (which amounted to $28,000 with exchange), the interest on half a million dollars.[10] With the completion of the Medical Building, clinical facilities established at its own university hospital, the appointment of full-time clinical faculty members, and the Class A rating, the Foundation turned over the full sum of $500,000 in 1923, to be administered by the university itself. It was an endowment, but only the interest could be used.

The first notification of the full approval of the grant from the Foundation arrived by telegram from E.M. Embree, secretary of the Rockefeller Foundation, in December 1923.

> Appropriation of $500,000 made for endowment of Medical School. We are ready to make payment at once. Will you advise whether you prefer to have us purchase Canadian currency in New York or deposit same to your account leaving purchase of exchange or investment entirely for action by the University.[11]

Kerr turned the question over to Tory, who wired back that it should be sent in American dollars so that the university could take advantage of the exchange rate. The full grant, in Canadian currency, amounted to $512,299.69.[12]

Expansion to a Full Degree-granting Programme

It would seem evident that plans to extend the three-year course into a full programme took place over a number of years but were always dependent upon receiving a Rockefeller Foundation grant. Tory's wish to select a dean who was a clinician signifies that as early as 1919 he was contemplating the addition of the clinical years. It must have been envisaged when the government decided, in such haste, to construct the Medical Building in 1920. There is also reason to believe that the virulent influenza epidemic, which swept through the western world in 1918-19, heightened the demand for increased professional medical care in the West, and gave added support to the need for a full medical course in the minds of some members of the legislature.[13] In addition, both McGill's and the University of Toronto's medical faculties made changes in their curricula in 1919-20 that directly affected Alberta students. Both universities extended their medical courses from five years to six, a premedical year followed by a five-year medical programme. This meant that Alberta students would be required to spend three years at an eastern university to complete their degree, unless similar changes took place in the Alberta curriculum. The Senate, therefore, approved the addition of a fourth year to the programme in 1920.[14]

This change to a six-year course created a hardship for those returned soldiers whose education was interrupted when they enlisted in the services. They had originally entered a five-year medical programme, had interrupted this to go and fight for their country, and now it seemed their graduation would be put back yet another year because of the recent extension of the programme. This hardly seemed a fair way to treat those who had chosen to serve their country, and Kerr wrote, expressing these views, to both Toronto and McGill. Both replied that they would honour those ex-servicemen who had initially enrolled in a five-year programme and would enable them to complete their course in that time, an arrangement that affected their own returning soldiers as well as those returning to Alberta.[15]

The first few years after the war were hectic, and the curriculum went through many changes and additions. There were two streams of students going through the programme—those whose course had been interrupted by military service were on the old five-year programme, whereas new entrants, whether they planned on staying at Alberta to complete their degree or on going to the East, were on the new six-year programme. In 1921, the third-year class consisted of forty-two veteran students in the five-year programme and only fourteen regular students who were in the six-year programme. In 1922, the larger group went on to eastern universities and the smaller group stayed and embarked upon the new fourth-year course. Some of these went to the East after the fourth year; others remained to complete their course in the new fifth and sixth years.[16]

Over the next several years, a number of students still left Alberta midway through their course to complete their degree at eastern universities. McGill and Toronto were the "elite" schools in Canada, and a degree from one of them carried more weight when applying for postgraduate training or to American licensing boards.[17] They could also offer better and more broadly based clinical facilities than were available at the University of Alberta Hospital. Given the limited facilities in Edmonton, Tory himself agreed that the school could "only guarantee to carry forward a limited number of [students] to the degree."[18]

Embarking upon the full programme required full-time professors in both medicine and surgery. Drs. Egerton L. Pope and Frank Hamilton Mewburn received these appointments. While the terms of their appointments denied them a regular medical practice, they were able to carry on a consulting practice, taking only those cases referred to them by the profession. Each received a salary of $5,000 a year, and Pope, at any rate, earned an equivalent amount from consulting fees.[19] Mewburn, who headed the department of surgery, had attended McGill University, where Sir William Osler's teaching made a lasting impression upon him. Following graduation, he headed west. His associations with the military began almost at once when he was appointed to the Base Military Hospital in Winnipeg during the North-West Rebellion of 1885. Following this episode, Mewburn headed even further west and settled in Lethbridge as assistant surgeon to the North-West Mounted Police and medical officer for the North West Coal and Navigation Company. Surgery was always his main interest, and he followed the advances in this branch of medicine—largely through medical literature—with great determination but some difficulty, given the isolation of the area. After twenty-seven years in Lethbridge, he moved to Calgary and limited his practice to surgery.

Following the declaration of war in 1914, Mewburn, then fifty-six years old, wired the Minister of National Defence offering his services. The minister thanked Mewburn for his offer, but regretted that he was too old. Mewburn wired back, "Reference your wire - go to hell! I am going anyway." And go he did. He spent the war years as chief of the Surgical Division of the Canadian military hospital in Taplow, England, where he achieved the rank of colonel and was awarded the Order of the British Empire. Shortly after his return to Calgary, he accepted the position at the new medical school in Edmonton. Always referred to as "The Colonel," Mewburn was a colourful character, whose language could best be termed "earthy," a forceful and enthusiastic person with a violent temper, and a slow and careful surgeon who was completely "patient-centred."[20] When he died in 1929, representatives of the government and the military, as well as the medical fraternity attended his funeral. A couple of years later, the Medical Students' Club presented a gold medal, known as the Mewburn Memorial Medal, to be awarded to the student with the highest standing in surgery.[21]

Dr. Egerton L. Pope, a totally different type of person, was appointed full-time head of the department of medicine and medical director of student medical services. Also a McGill graduate, Pope took postgraduate training in London, and then practised in Winnipeg and taught at the Manitoba medical college. He was a unique character, always flawlessly dressed in a cutaway coat, pin-striped trousers and spats, an upturned stiff collar, and highly polished shoes. He carried a cane or an umbrella and wore a top hat. His hair was well brushed and glossy (the students strongly suspected it was dyed), and he wore a pince-nez, attached by a long ribbon to his jacket. His own chauffeur drove him to class in a large limousine, and when he arrived at the Medical Building, usually late, he was often accompanied by a small poodle dog. His manner was dignified and courtly, and he spoke with perfect diction. Artistic by nature, he painted and did needlepoint. He was also a Greek scholar and frequently quoted from mythology. He based his lectures on William Osler's *The Principles and Practice of Medicine*, first published in 1892, but personalized them with his own aphorisms.[22]

One of the students in the first graduating class, Leone McGregor Hellstedt, wrote of him,

> ...Dr. Pope came as professor of medicine and really inspired us all. I thought he was the most fascinating and cultivated man I had ever seen and I more or less worshipped him as well as his subject. I read Osler's medicine from cover to cover in order to be able to answer his questions. No other professor in my six years of medicine made such an impression on me. His lectures were masterpieces, his clinic was well run ....[23]

Pope remained with the school until his retirement in 1944.

Two such contrasting individuals had much to offer the students, and they were supported by a number of part-time professors, medical practitioners from the community who lectured or demonstrated in specific fields.[24] One of these, Dr. Leighton C. Conn, fitted somewhere between part-time and full-time status, in that he was permitted a hospital practice as well as a consulting practice.[25] Conn was the gold medallist in his year at McGill and, always interested in teaching, he felt the newly developing West would afford him greater opportunities. He arrived in Edmonton in 1913, set up in practice and started as a demonstrator in the department of anatomy in the Faculty of Medicine in 1914. With the addition of the clinical years, Conn was appointed head of the department of obstetrics and gynaecology and remained with that department until his early death in 1941. He was an excellent teacher, strict and thorough, whom the students both admired and feared. Everyone tried to sit in the back row, as far away as possible from his probing questions. He attended every delivery when students were present and afterwards discussed the case with them in detail, asking questions such as "How would you have dealt with this if you were in a small cabin in the bush, miles from any medical supplies?"[26]

There had been full-time professors in the basic medical sciences almost since the school began. Both Revell and Rankin were full-time appointments to the university, in that they served both the Provincial Laboratory and the Faculty of Medicine. Dr. John J. Ower, who would become a dominant member of the faculty and its second dean, joined the staff in September 1919. Another graduate of McGill, Ower accepted a full-time position as professor of pathology and provincial serologist. Ower was not altogether well liked by his colleagues, and some students found him autocratic and intimidating, although a good and fair teacher. He was sarcastic, had a gruff exterior and was difficult to get to know. He demanded much of his students; but he was also extremely helpful to them and entertained them in his home, and many kept in touch with him for years after they graduated. He was also one of the few members of the faculty who accepted women as *bona fide* members of the medical profession, respecting their professional knowledge and abilities in the same way as he did those of their male counterparts. In 1929, he was offered a position in the pathology department of Toronto's Western Hospital with a position on the staff of the University of Toronto, at a salary of $7,500, considerably more than he received at the University of Alberta. It was a distinct honour to be offered such a position and signifies his high reputation in Canadian medicine; yet Ower did not want to leave Alberta and instead used the offer to negotiate an increase in his salary. This was successful to some degree, and although he did not receive the $7,500 he would have received at Toronto, he elected to remain in Alberta.[27]

Another full-time professor in the medical sciences who became a pillar of the medical school was Dr. Ralph Shaner. He joined the faculty in 1921 as an assistant to Revell. Shaner, a brilliant anatomist, was one of the few Americans on staff. He came from the Harvard Medical School, where he had received his Ph.D., and instructed in the department of histology. He, too, had opportunities to move on to more prestigious schools but elected to remain at Alberta. The year following his appointment, he received the offer of an assistant professorship at Stanford University. After considerable thought, he decided to turn it down,

> I have just come from a big institution to a small one, where my responsibility is greater and where I can develop an individuality. When I arrived

I found the technical apparatus quite complete but the class teaching materials in an undeveloped condition. I have worked hard all winter collecting histological and neurological material, embryos, and museum exhibits. In so doing I gave up time for research. Since classes have ceased, I have turned to the last in earnest and am regaining momentum. My future status will be largely determined by the work I turn out the next ten years. To leave here now would mean last year all over again and another year lost from original work... one ought to stay more than one year at a place and make one's mark before passing on to the next.[28]

He would receive other offers over the years, but he turned them all down, despite his relationship with Revell, which was strained at best. Shaner's interests were mainly in research, and he found Revell's experience and interest in that area to be "very slender." "Alberta is a fine place for one who has a good start elsewhere," said Shaner, "but not the place to give one a good start."[29] He achieved an international reputation with his research in cardiac embryology, was often asked to review Ph.D. and masters theses from McGill as an "outside authority," and was an excellent teacher. After his first year, he asked his students for written criticisms of his courses. A number complied and all were laudatory, some suggesting only minor adjustments.[30] Until his retirement in 1961, Shaner taught every medical student who went through the University of Alberta. After the first few years, he did not give examinations in neuro-anatomy, as the only person he had failed in that subject went on to become chief of neurosurgery in a prestigious Boston clinic. This so unnerved him that he resolved never to set an examination again.[31]

Other full-time appointments to the scientific departments included Evan Greene and Ardrey W. Downs. The former was a McGill graduate who came west in 1905, setting up practice in the young community of Strathcona. He began teaching in the anatomy department in 1919 on a part-time basis; but after a serious illness caused him to give up his practice, he continued as a full-time teacher.[32] Downs received his M.D. from the University of Pennsylvania in 1904 and later received an appointment to the teaching staff at McGill. There he received a D.Sc. for research into the physiological aspects of gas warfare. Just a year later, Tory persuaded him to come to Alberta and head up the department of physiology and biochemistry.[33] In his first year, he developed his lecture notes and, from all accounts, never changed them during the remainder of his teaching career at the University of Alberta.[34]

Many of these professors were comparatively young men at the time of their appointments and most lived in the Garneau district. They formed a closely knit group, and their social as well as their academic lives revolved around the university. Medical faculty wives became involved with such activities as raising money for the hospital.[35] Classes were small, and this gave professors the opportunity to know their students as individuals and to assess their aptitudes for the profession. Many faculty members entertained the senior classes at their homes, for dinner and conversation, and were in turn entertained by the students. A close relationship often developed, although always on the formal basis of teacher and student. Ower's diaries made several references to outings and social gatherings with students.

As well as appointments to the faculty, the school required adequate clinical facilities before the programme could be extended. The Department of National Defence took over Strathcona Hospital in 1916, for the care of returned soldiers, and after the war extended the lease on a year-by-year basis. Finally, in November 1922, under the terms of a joint agreement among the University of Alberta, the City of Edmonton and the Dominion Government, the city transferred all its interests in the hospital to the university, upon payment of $150,000 in debentures. At the same time, the university agreed to construct an annex to the hospital, for the care and treatment of ex-servicemen, which was known as the Soldiers Civil Re-establishment (SCR) wing. It was located directly north and west of the main hospital, and the two buildings combined became the University of Alberta Hospital, with a total of 175 beds. The university paid $25,000 a year to the hospital board for the use of its facilities, and the Dominion Government paid a monthly stipend based on a rate of $3 a day for each SCR patient.

From its inception, the medical school's objective was to prepare students for general practice. They needed, therefore, the opportunity for contact with the everyday illnesses and accidents that the general practitioner would meet most frequently in a family practice. An "out-door clinic," that offered free service for those who attended with everyday "walk-in" medical problems, provided a good experience for the students. The clinic was at the University Hospital but attracted few people; it was located too far from the more populated parts of the city. So, in 1924, the faculty opened an outdoor clinic in the downtown area, in the McLeod House at 99th Street and 103rd Avenue,[36] where the students received some of their clinical training. In addition, a few staff members of the General, Royal Alexandra and Misericordia hospitals received appointments to the faculty of the medical school and held clinics for medical students.[37]

Most clinical teaching, however, took place at the University of Alberta Hospital, and its board consisted of Deans Rankin and Kerr; Archibald West, the university bursar; Dr. R.T. Washburn, superintendent of the hospital; with President Tory in the chair. It was a "closed" general teaching hospital,[38] with a staff appointed by the hospital board on the recommendation of the Medical Advisory Board. The members of this latter board were Drs. Mewburn, Ower and Jamieson, and those doctors appointed to the hospital were all members of the Faculty of Medicine. The head of the department of medicine at the school was also the head of the department of medicine at the hospital.

A representative of the American College of Surgeons visited the University of Alberta Hospital in 1924 and gave it a favourable report. "This hospital is by far the best west of Toronto...the type of work done in this institution is of a superior quality...a young and ambitious staff has great plans for its future."[39] A couple of years later, in 1926, the education committee of the American Medical Association rated the hospital as suitable for internships, which meant that graduate students who interned there would receive credit for their work throughout the United States and Canada. Only five other hospitals in Canada had an equivalent rating at that time.[40]

A steady decline in income over the next several years, however, led to severe budgetary problems. Typically, university teaching hospitals admitted a large number of indigent or nonpaying patients to provide sufficient clinical material for teaching purposes,[41] but paying patients who consented also served as "teaching material" at the University of Alberta Hospital. Although the Alberta government subsidized the beds used by indigent patients, the amount was insufficient to enable the hospital to maintain a balanced budget. Each year, the losses increased and became a constant drain on the already tight university budget. The loss in 1923 was $11,649; in 1924, $10,633; in 1925, $37,632, and for the first six months of 1926, $12,033, making a total accrued debt of over $50,000.[42]

Acting President Kerr and the Chancellor of the university, Chief Justice Stuart, met with Premier Brownlee to discuss the alarmingly large deficit at the hospital, of which the government was previously unaware. The premier proposed that the government take over the hospital as a provincial enterprise and meet its deficit out of the public purse, but in this event the government should have representation on the board so that it could monitor finances on a regular basis.[43] The members of the hospital board saw no major objections to this proposal, in fact it was greeted with some relief, as it would relieve the university of much of its fiscal responsibility. They wished to safeguard the interests of the medical school, however, in so far as teaching facilities and medical appointments to the hospital were concerned.[44] After several months of negotiation, the provincial government assumed financial responsibility for the hospital in 1929. The composition of the new board consisted of three members appointed by the government and three by the university. President Robert C. Wallace chaired the new board, which included Dean Rankin and Harry H. Cooper as the university's appointments, and M.R. Bow, Deputy Minister of Health; W.B. Milne, Supervisor of Hospital Affairs; and John Gillespie, founder of his own grain company, as the government appointees.[45] The hospital remained "closed" and appointments were made on the recommendation of the Medical Advisory Board as before. The latter board, now considerably expanded, consisted of Drs. E.L. Pope, A.R. Munroe, L.C. Conn, H.H. Hepburn, Harold Orr, R. Proctor, Emerson Smith and W.A. Wilson, and was responsible for hospital practice.[46]

With clinical facilities available and professional staff appointed, the full-degree programme could proceed. The first class graduated in 1925. There were eleven new M.D.s, "ten sturdy men and one enchanting woman," according to Pope. It was a momentous occasion, and no one was prouder than President Tory. The occasion was celebrated with a banquet at the Macdonald Hotel. Members of the faculty were present, of course, and many prominent members of the profession. It was an all-male affair, though, so the "enchanting woman" could not attend, even though she had won the Moshier Memorial Award as top student of her class. Dr. Pope gave the toast to the graduates and asked that they "remain in this great dominion and help in its reconstruction."[47]

At this time, success in the final year of the University of Alberta medical school entitled the graduate to register with the CPSA and practise medicine in the province without further examination. To practise outside the province, however, it was necessary to take the Medical Council of Canada (MCC) examinations. During this period, the MCC made several attempts to interest medical schools across the country in holding what were called "conjoint" examinations, which would combine the university final examinations with the licensing examinations of the MCC. This was part of a continuing effort by the MCC to achieve a uniform standard of medical education across the country. A conjoint examination was a perennial subject for discussion at Faculty Council meetings, and the

University of Alberta consistently opposed the concept. It felt that they would interfere with the autonomy of the university, in that the examinations for a medical degree would eventually pass out of the control of both the medical school and the university.[48]

Under the terms of the Canadian Medical Act, the standard of the MCC licensing examinations had to be no lower than the highest provincial qualifying examinations, or, in other words, the highest standard in Canada.[49] Of the eleven successful graduates in Alberta's first year, eight took the MCC examinations, and seven were successful. The eighth failed in one subject only. The 1926 class, however, did not fare so well. Fourteen graduates wrote the examinations; but only six passed all subjects, the rest failed in one or more. This was a 47% pass rate and compared unfavourably with other medical schools in Canada: Manitoba—85%; Queen's—77%; Western Ontario—75%; Toronto—74%; and McGill—56.2%.[50] As the years went by, however, Alberta graduates improved and eventually compared well with those of other schools. In 1930, Alberta students had the highest average for marks in the written examinations, although they usually did better in their orals, and in 1932,

TABLE 1: THE MEDICAL COUNCIL OF CANADA EXAMINATIONS[51] JUNE 1935

	Average in All Subjects Combined Written & Oral	Number of Students	Passed	Referred	Rejected
Alberta	71.24%	33	31	2	0
Dalhousie	70.88%	11	10	1	0
McGill	69.97%	43	41	1	1
Western Ontario	69.70%	34	34	0	0
Manitoba	68.91%	40	36	4	0
Toronto	67.78%	110	104	6	0
Queen's	67.56%	44	38	6	0

twenty-two out of twenty-four were successful.[52] The results in 1935, when Alberta had the highest average in combined written and oral examinations, are shown in Table 1. In this year, Alberta students did consistently well in their oral examinations and were above and well above average in all subjects, particularly in pathology and bacteriology; but in their written examinations, they were average or below average, particularly in obstetrics and gynaecology and surgery.

Advent of "Reporting Clubs"

Alberta's graduates compared favourably with other medical schools in the country despite its extreme isolation from both the Canadian medical establishment and the well-known American medical schools in the midwest. Few guest lecturers included Edmonton on their itineraries, and it was too far away geographically and too close to the frontier syndrome to attract large scale medical meetings. Under such conditions it was difficult for faculty members to keep up with new ideas and concepts, research activities, and developments in medical practices and education. The library subscribed to several medical journals, but the process of circulating these was slow and cumbersome. Ower, particularly, was acutely aware of the isolation of the University of Alberta medical college, and to combat this situation, he suggested the formation of a "Medical Journal Reporting Club"—"to keep abreast of medical progress by systematic reading of current literature."[53] The membership included representatives from the surgical, medical and medical science departments, and each member "gave an abstract of some recent scientific article in his own field that he thought might interest the others. Questions and discussion followed."

Ower hosted the first meeting at his home on 28 September 1920, and the charter members were J.B. Collip, L.C. Conn, Evan Greene, H.H. Hepburn, Heber Jamieson, D.B. Leitch, A.R. Munroe and Dean Rankin. They decided to keep the membership small and initially met in each other's home, where the host's wife prepared dinner. After a while, they found that a good dinner—and probably a drink or two—were not conducive to controversial discussions, so they decided to move the meeting place to the Macdonald Hotel "and partake of more austere alimentation." From time to time, they changed their locale, as the costs and quality of meals rose and fell; but Heber Jamieson took on the task of making all the necessary dinner arrangements and continued to do so for the next twenty-six years. In 1947, when he was ill in hospital, the Club decided to "relieve him of these onerous duties."

In 1925, the Club changed its name to the Mewburn Reporting Club in honour of Colonel Mewburn. Discussion did not always revolve around the latest medical issues. At a meeting in1936, Sandy Munroe brought a list of ten words said to be the most difficult in the English language to spell, and they had a spelling match. The minutes showed that "the results were really too shocking to record." The membership changed slowly over the years, as some members left the city and new faculty appointments were made. It continued to be by invitation only, however, to ensure compatible people who would not create antagonisms or harbour personality conflicts. Ower, however, went on for ever; but eventually, in January 1958, he asked to be relieved of his duties as secretary, which he had carried ever since the inception of the Club. At the following meeting, Walter Mackenzie brought up the question of membership, as so many had retired or were unable to attend meetings regularly. They decided to "consult Ower who knows all things from the beginning." It seems the Club was not able to continue without him. The 246th and final meeting with fourteen members present, took place on 14 December 1959, thirty-nine years after the Club's inception. Ower, who was diabetic, lost his sight in his later years, and one of the last acts of the Mewburn Club was to present him with an automatic record player for his talking-book records.[54]

This was only one of several "reporting clubs." In 1929, Ower founded the Junior Reporting Club, the charter members of which were all recent graduates of the medical school practising in Edmonton. They included Mark Levey (who later changed his surname to Marshall), Graham Huckell, Percy Sprague, H.E. Rawlinson, Morris Weinlos and Angus McGugan. Individual members gave papers on cases, new treatments of diseases, reviews of books and articles, and discussion followed. They met once a month and followed a few simple rules. The last person to arrive at the meeting was chairman; two successive absences without notification to the secretary (McGugan) would be considered a resignation from the club; meals were not to exceed a cost of 75¢; and the membership should be limited to the number that could be accommodated in a two-hour discussion. In 1933, the Club changed its name to the Ower Club—"in honour of myself," Ower wrote in his diary. He continued,

> Have had an inkling of this for some time from hints—and have resisted on the grounds that I am not old enough in the profession. ... This is a real honor—especially so from this group—which represents the next generation of university professors—and is a real live aggregation.[55]

This club held an annual golf tournament at the Mayfair Golf and Country Club, for which Ower presented a trophy. The first winner, in 1939, was Angus McGugan, who later became the superintendent of the University of Alberta Hospital.[56]

Other clubs included the Harrison Club, named for Dr. J.D. Harrison, a pioneer physician in Edmonton who was Vice-Chancellor of the university for many years, and the Medical Digest Club. The Vango Club, organized by Harold Vango just a year or two before he died, was devoted to pathology. The "5th Reporting Club," organized in 1933 by a group of younger members of the faculty, including Mark Levey, J.W. Macgregor, J. Ross Vant, and M.M. Cantor, later changed its name to the Conn Club in honour of Leighton C. Conn. Finally, as Ower's diary entry for 25 January 1935 announced,

> This will probably be a red letter day in the medical history of Edmonton. Tonight at Heber Jamieson's house—seated amidst a forest of beer bottles—a group of about twenty founded the Jamieson Medical History Club. Heber was elected President and Cantor, Secretary.[57]

The students, too, had their own "reporting club." The Osler Club, named in honour of Sir William Osler, was limited to the students of the graduating year, and it began with the first graduating class in 1924-25. According to its constitution, its object was "to further the interest of its members in medical subjects by means of case reporting, abstracting, historical papers and discussion of scientific questions."[58] Towards the end of its fifth year, the class elected an executive, which invariably met with Ower to organize the programme for the following year. The 1931 class held twelve meetings during the year, as well as an Old Members' Night when graduates of the school attended.[59]

The success and longevity of these various clubs obviously signifies a perceived need for organized discussion sessions to create an awareness of current affairs in the medical profession. Members discussed the latest issues in their own field of medicine and, in some cases, were responsible for reporting on specific magazines. Often they studied cases that would enable them to become familiar with advances in the latest laboratory and clinical methods of treating disease; but over the years, their discussions covered a broad range of subjects, from discussions about rheumatics, bacterial endocarditis, peptic ulcers and radium to the value of cod liver oil, the establishment of the Royal College of Physicians and Surgeons, state health insurance, and even Leonardo da Vinci.

These clubs offered this isolated medical community an opportunity to keep abreast of activities in the profession and also served as a stimulus to individual members to keep up with the literature and activities in their own particular fields. As they generally crossed the boundaries of particular branches of medicine, they also helped to reduce the division between the basic medical scientists and the clinicians.[60] The membership of some of the clubs included both university professors and those in private practice in Edmonton and thus helped to alleviate the town versus gown animosity and to create "understanding and good fellowship between university and non-university practitioners."[61] It was difficult to maintain a close relationship with the centre of medical activities in the twenties and thirties. Travel to central Canada was by train; it took a long time, and the hard economic times prevented regular trips to conferences and courses. Yet, several faculty members did make such trips during these years, often at their own expense, and co-ordinated them with visits en route to other medical schools and teaching hospitals, to colleagues and ex-students, in continuing efforts to upgrade their knowledge in their profession and to enhance their expertise as teachers.

J.B. Collip and the Discovery of Insulin

Not all faculty members were so assiduous, however, and students sometimes complained of faculty members who did not keep up with current knowledge nor offer any variety in their lectures and demonstrations.[62] One of these was Ardrey Downs, whose appointment caused friction between Tory and J.B. Collip, that would continue as long as they both remained at the University of Alberta.[63] Collip had been on the faculty since 1915, and had been responsible for the departments of physiology, biochemistry and pharmacology since Moshier left in 1917. When Downs was brought in as professor of physiology and biochemistry, with Collip as assistant professor, the latter was "cut to the quick...not so much perhaps from the point of view of salary as from the fact that I believed my ability as a teacher and researcher was definitely reflected upon."[64] Collip was an excellent biochemist, a field that had just recently come into its own, and a tireless researcher. He preferred the solitude of his laboratory to the lecture platform, and while not a good teacher, he was an excellent scientist.[65] By 1920, and still a young man, he had already published some sixteen articles describing his various research activities and was becoming well known in his field. Downs, in Collip's opinion, was "old-fashioned and ten years behind the times."[66]

Perhaps to assuage those hurt feelings—and the tensions that undoubtedly existed in the physiology and biochemistry departments—Tory applied to the Rockefeller Foundation for a travelling fellowship for Collip for one year. Collip arranged to visit Toronto, New York and London and work in well-equipped laboratories that would offer him a good training.

He intended to spend several months in each location, and while on this sabbatical he would determine whether he wished to return to the University of Alberta. If he did, he was promised a promotion to the rank of full professor and the headship of the department of biochemistry. The university also agreed to pay Collip an additional $1,000 to supplement the Rockefeller grant, which he had to repay if he did not return to Edmonton.[67]

In May 1921, Collip left Edmonton for what was to become a momentous year, not only in his own life but also for Canadian medicine. His first stop, however, was at the University of Toronto where J.J.R. Macleod, professor of physiology, offered him a one-year appointment in the department of pathological chemistry, beginning on 1 September. Collip wrote to Rankin informing him of this change in his plans and sought an increase in his salary if the University of Alberta wished him to return in September 1922. Both Tory and Rankin expressed disappointment, as they felt he should "go abroad for study to get some experience in an atmosphere wider than Canada [can] give you."[68] But Collip, fortuitously, decided to accept the offer and was, in fact, discussing the university appointment with Macleod when he first met Dr. Frederick Banting (the discoverer of insulin) and learned firsthand of the research project that was to take place that summer. Collip spent the summer at the Woods Hole Marine Laboratory near Boston, Massachusetts,[69] and then returned to Toronto to take up his position at the university. He taught for eight hours a week, while the rest of his time was free for research in the university's pathological chemistry laboratory. During those autumn months, Collip dropped in from time to time to see Banting and his assistant, Charles Best, to enquire about the progress of their research and also to offer his help.[70]

The story of the discovery of insulin, and the animosity that developed between the various members of the team involved in the project, has been told many times and will not be repeated here, except as it relates to Collip and his association with the University of Alberta's medical school.[71] Collip joined the team in December 1921, and "it is my problem to isolate in a form suitable for human administration the principle which has such wondrous powers...."[72] Previous injections had caused abscesses at the point of injection. "The problem seemed almost hopeless," he wrote to Tory,

so you can imagine my delight when about midnight one day last week I discovered a way to get the active principle free from all the 'muck' with which it appeared to be inseparably bound.... I have never had such an absolutely satisfactory experience.... To be associated in an intimate way

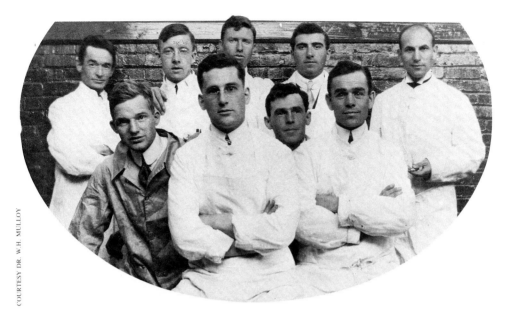

Group of medical students in 1915. *Back row, left to right:* Nat Minish, Wm. H. Hill, Percy Backus, ?? Hanson, G. Novak. *Front row, left to right:* G.D. McBride, A. Webster Bowles, J.K. Mulloy, J.H. Riopel.

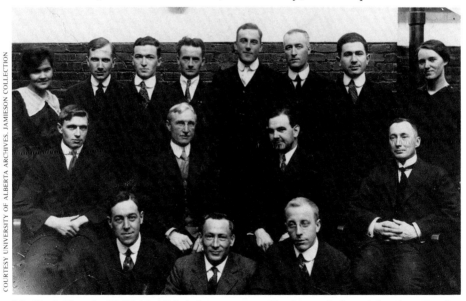

Medical Class in 1917-18. Third class to enter. *Back row, left to right:* Ann Curtin, John W. Scott, L.A. Miller, T.F. Foley, Morley A.R. Young, M. McLeod, D.M. Baltzan, Isabel Teskey Ayer. *Middle row:* Professors J.B. Collip, D.G. Revell, Gordon C. Gray, H.C. Jamieson. *Front row:* F.D. Facey, W.F. Beamish, W.F. Gillespie.

Dr. Heber H. Moshier, professor of physiology and pharmacology, 1915-1917. He organized the 11th Field Ambulance Corps and took it overseas to France, where he was killed in 1918. The Moshier Memorial Award, presented to the top student in the graduating year, is named after him.

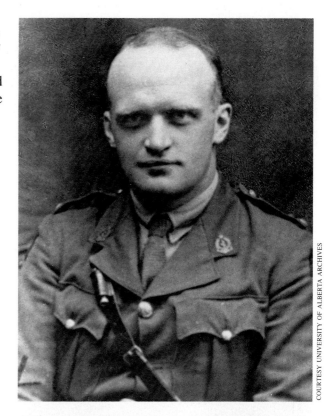

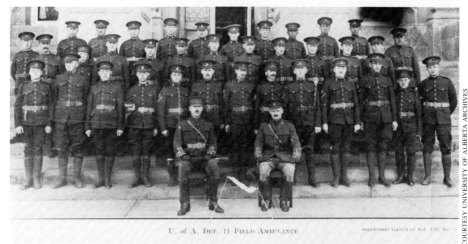

U. of A. Det. 11 Field Ambulance

Supplement Gateway Vol. VII. No. 11

The 11th Field Ambulance Unit in training at the University of Alberta, 1916-17. This unit was composed mainly of medical, dental and pharmacy students.

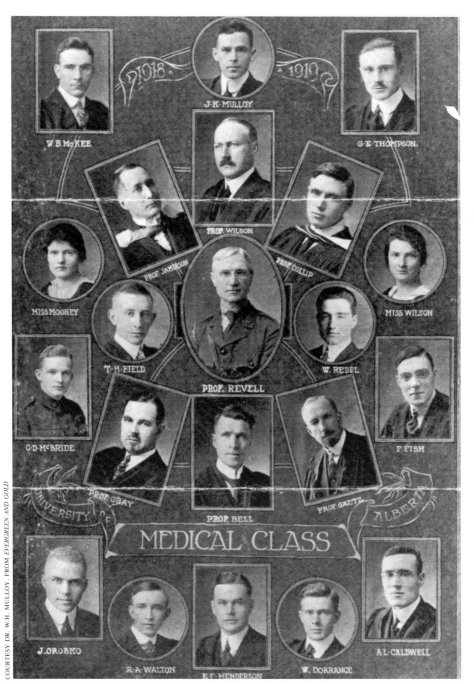

Third-year class, 1919. Students and faculty members, with Professor Revell and one of the students still in military uniform.

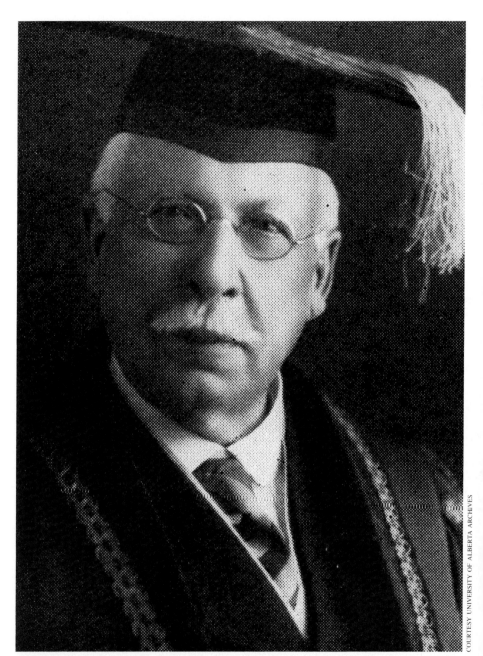

The Honourable Alexander Cameron Rutherford, Premier of the Province of Alberta and Minister of Education, 1905-10 and Chancellor of the University of Alberta, 1927-1941. Rutherford was instrumental in the initial development of the University of Alberta.

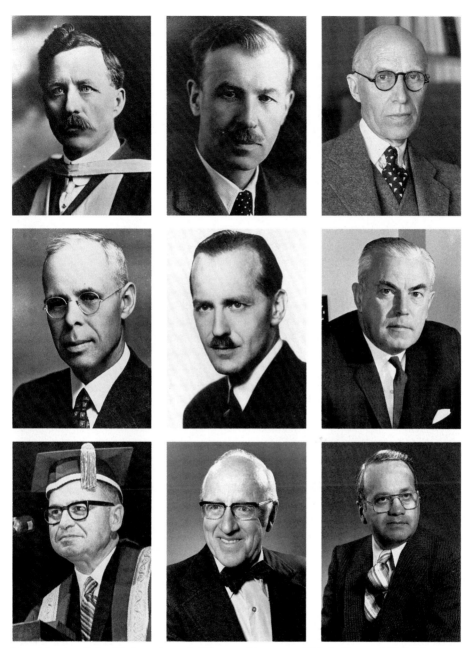

Presidents of the University of Alberta. *Top row:* H.M. Tory, 1908-28; Robert C. Wallace, 1928-36; W.A.R. Kerr, 1936-41; *Second row:* Robert Newton, 1941-50; Andrew Stewart, 1950-59; Walter H. Johns, 1959-69; *Third row:* Max Wyman, 1969-74; Harry Emmett Gunning, 1974-79; Myer Horowitz, 1979-89.

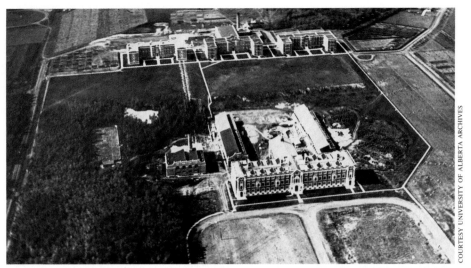

Aerial view of the campus, 1919, looking west, showing the three residences—Pembina, Athabasca and Assiniboia Halls—at the centre back and the Arts Building in the foreground. The tennis court and the native woodland at the lower left of the building is the location of the future Medical Building.

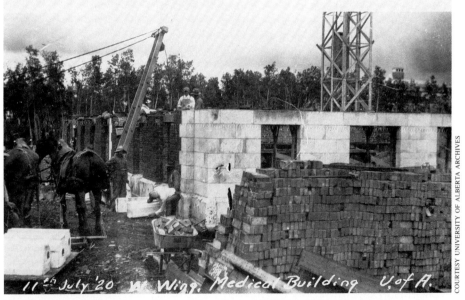

The Medical Building under construction, 1920-21. This photo shows the construction of the west wing in July 1920, and that at the top of the next page shows the building almost complete in 1921.

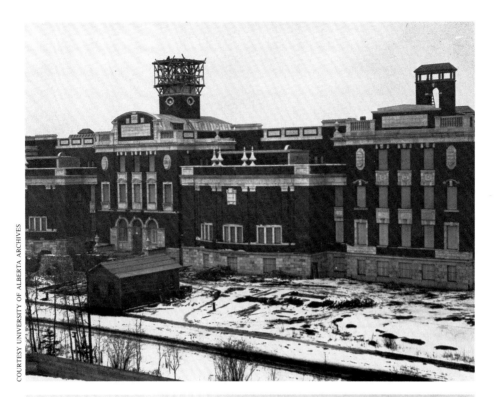

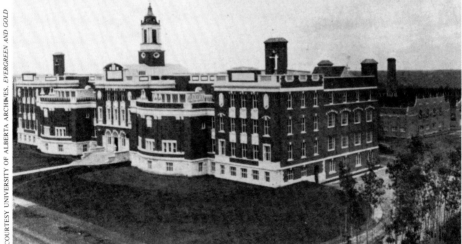

"The Pride of the Campus." The new Medical Building of the University of Alberta, 1921. Shows the Arts Building, centre right, Convocation Hall behind it and the Power Plant behind the Medical Building. Note the native woodland still remaining in the lower right corner and the unpaved roads.

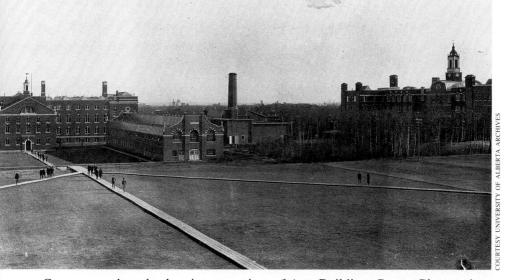

Campus quadrangle showing rear view of Arts Building, Power Plant and Medical Building as seen from the top floor of Athabasca Hall. Note remains of virgin woodland.

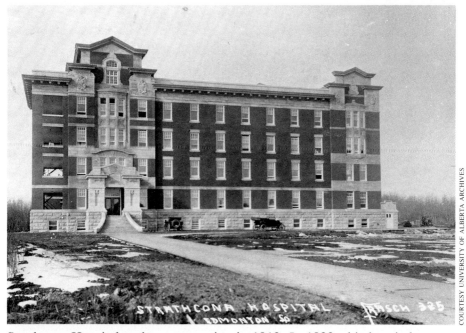

Strathcona Hospital under construction in 1913. In 1922, this hospital was turned over to the university and was renamed the University of Alberta Hospital.

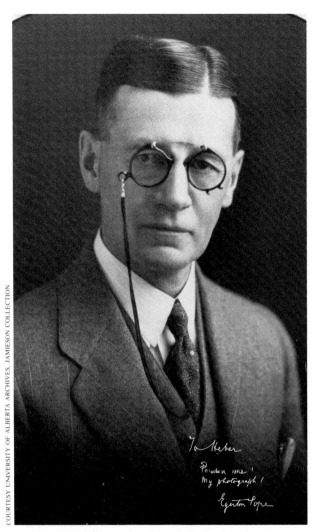

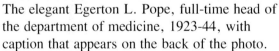

The elegant Egerton L. Pope, full-time head of
the department of medicine, 1923-44, with
caption that appears on the back of the photo.

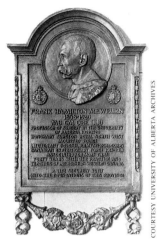

Plaque commemorating
Frank Hamilton
Mewburn, the first full-
time professor of
surgery at the
University of Alberta.

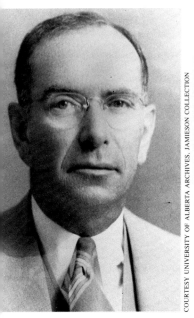

Leighton C. Conn,
first head of the
department of
obstetrics and
gynaecology, 1923-41.

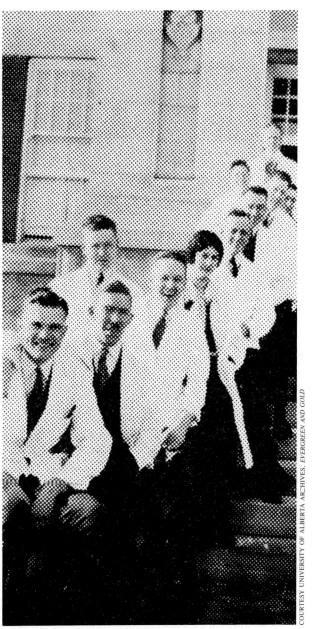

The first graduating class, 1925.
From front to back: Bill Eadie, J.C. Grimson,
Frank Law, Geo. Lewis, Leone McGregor, C.G.
Lee, E.J. Leisemer, Bob Morrow, Don Weston,
Harry Bercov and Johnnie Glenn.

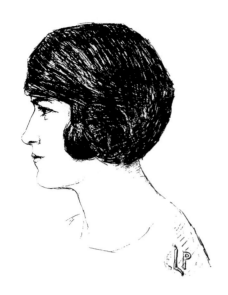

Sketch of Leone McGregor, done by Egerton Pope, 1925.

WEE MACGREEGOR. SHE WILL BE THE FAIRST MAIDICAL DOCTOR FRAE THE UNIVAIRSITY OF ALBAIRTA.

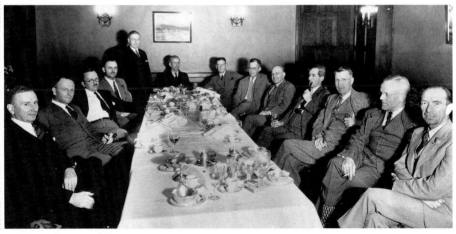

Meeting of the Mewburn Club at the Macdonald Hotel on the occasion of a visit by J.B. Collip in October 1934. *Clockwise around the table:* John J. Ower, Harold Orr, Hastings Mewburn, ??, J.B. Collip (standing), ??, Egerton L. Pope, Douglas Leitch, Dean Allan Rankin, ??, Irving Bell, ??, Leighton C. Conn.

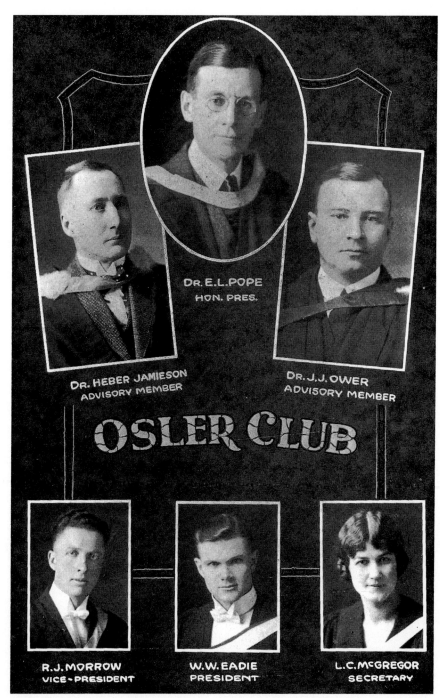

DR. E.L. POPE
HON. PRES.

DR. HEBER JAMIESON
ADVISORY MEMBER

DR. J.J. OWER
ADVISORY MEMBER

OSLER CLUB

R.J. MORROW
VICE-PRESIDENT

W.W. EADIE
PRESIDENT

L.C. MᶜGREGOR
SECRETARY

The first executive of the students' reporting club, the Osler Club, 1924-25.

I planned a series of experiments the results
of which when obtained gave me a direct lead
to the solution of the basic functional derangement
in diabetes. The crucial experiment was tried
out just before the Xmas break and the results
were so striking that even the most skeptical
I think would be convinced. I have never
had such an absolutely satisfactory experience
before namely going in a logical way from
point to point into an unexplored field building
absolutely solid structure all the way. However
to make a long story short we have obtained from
the pancreas of animals a mysterious something
which when injected into totally diabetic
dogs completely removes all the cardinal
symptoms of the disease. Just at the moment it
is my problem to isolate in a form
suitable for human administration the principle
which has such wonderous powers. The existence
of which many have suspected but no one has
hitherto proved. If the substance works on the

Extract from a letter from J.B. Collip to President Tory, dated 8 January
1922, just prior to his successful isolation of insulin fit for administering to
humans.

Cartoon sketch of J.B.
Collip done by Egerton
L. Pope, c. 1925.

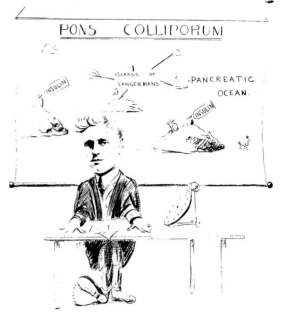

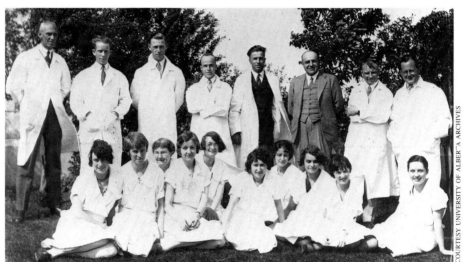

Staff of the Provincial Laboratory, c. 1928. *Standing, left to right:* R.M.
Shaw, F.H. (Fred) Howells, Doug Roxborough, J. MacGregor, John ??,
Dean Allan Rankin, John J. Ower, Harold M. Vango. *Sitting:* Marjorie
Race, Greta Lempson, Anne Hewton, Connie McFarlane, Marge Long,
Dorothy Toofs(?), Lillian Holland, Elizabeth West, Geneva Fanning,
Dorothy Dixon Craig.

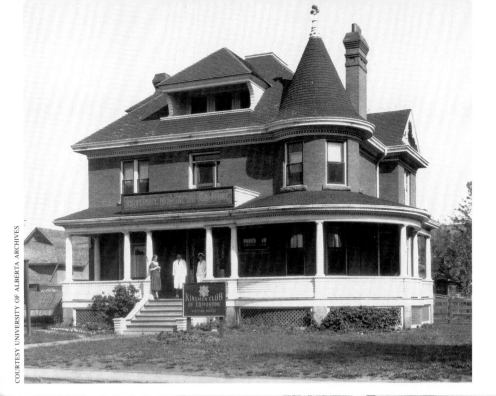

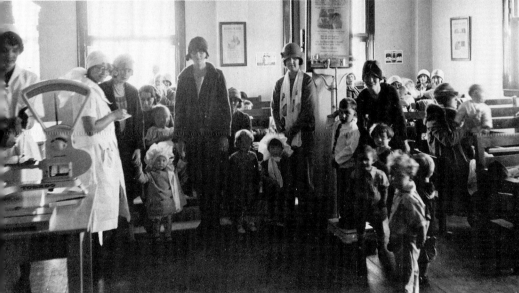

Top: The University Hospital Outdoor Clinic located in downtown Edmonton at 99th Street and 103rd Avenue, where students received some of their clinical training. *Bottom:* Mothers and babies inside the clinic.

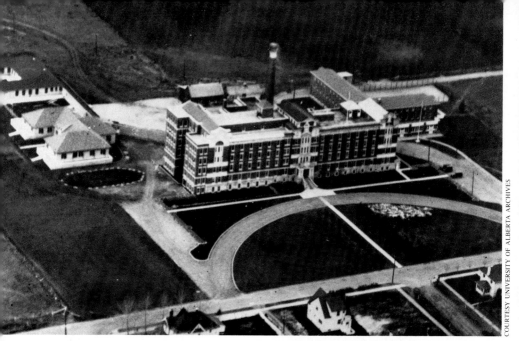

Aerial view, looking west, of the University of Alberta Hospitals, showing the new wing added to the south end of the original hospital; the Soldiers Civil Re-establishment wing to the north and west of the hospital; and two pavilions, the Red Cross Unit and a special unit for polio patients, to the south and west of the main hospital, 1931.

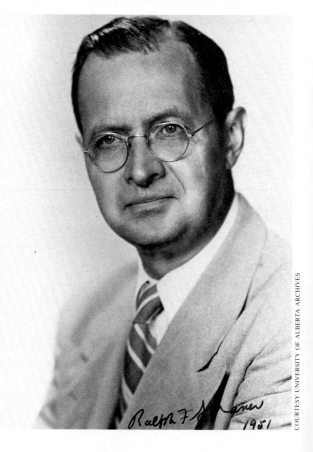

Dr. Ralph Faust Shaner, department of anatomy, 1921-59.

with the solution of a problem which for years has resisted all efforts was something I had never anticipated. I only wish that the various papers which will be published on this work were coming from Alberta rather than Toronto. A whole new field has been thrown open however and I will continue to work along these lines for some time no doubt.[73]

Collip's extract was the first ever made that could be used safely and effectively on humans.[74] He remained with the team as it developed the process for manufacturing the product and was named, along with Banting and Best, in the insulin patent. He shared with them the royalties from the sale of the product, which were, by common consent, turned over to the University of Toronto.[75] However, under the terms of an agreement reached by the University of Toronto and Banting, Best and Collip in 1923, the three each received one-sixth of the royalties, to be used to support their research activities. In Collip's case, the university that employed him received his share.[76] In 1925 the University of Alberta received $8,000 from the royalties on insulin, a sum that was used for research purposes in the department of biochemistry.[77]

The University of Alberta benefited in other ways as well. Collip planned to continue his research on insulin and diabetes, and before returning to Edmonton wired Tory asking for increased funding for the biochemistry laboratory in Edmonton.[78] Money flooded in—the College of Physicians and Surgeons of Alberta contributed $9,000 over the following two years,[79] and the Carnegie Corporation of New York donated a further $10,000.[80] In addition, the Rockefeller Foundation made a grant of $5,000 for the extended use of insulin for those in the hospital who were unable to pay for the treatment.[81]

Collip's participation in the process was an integral part of the success of the entire project, but his role never received the recognition that it deserved. He has been called "the forgotten man" in the discovery of insulin. In 1924, the Nobel Prize in Medicine was awarded to Banting and Macleod, entirely bypassing the other two members of the team, Best and Collip. Promptly, Banting announced that he would share his half of the prize with Best, and Macleod, in an effort to recognize his important contribution to the discovery, shared his half with Collip.[82] Many people, feeling that both Best and Collip had been unfairly treated, made efforts to correct the situation. Best eventually achieved recognition in his native Ontario, but despite letters from the University of Alberta, and representations from the provincial government and the College of Physicians and Surgeons of Alberta, Collip remained the "forgotten man." If he had been from a more established school, representations might have carried more weight, but "far-away Alberta" had little influence in the power struggles that took place.

The University of Alberta did what it could; it awarded him its highest degree, a doctor of science, for his work in the isolation of insulin. When he returned to Edmonton at the end of his sabbatical year, he was a hero in the eyes of Albertans. He was lauded at banquets, by medical associations, the government, and the media as well as the university. In 1924 the provincial government, in a unanimous resolution,

> expressed its gratitude to Dr. J. B. Collip who has rendered such distinguished service to humanity...co-discoverer of the insulin treatment for diabetes, has conferred inestimable benefits on sufferers in all parts of the world, and, by his generous and disinterested action in placing the discovery at the disposal of the public, has placed it within reach of all sufferers at moderate cost.[83]

Collip then went on to other things. First, he decided to get a medical degree and enrolled as a student, an anomalous situation when he was the head of a department. Obviously, he did not need to take any of the medical science courses, but he was required to complete the fifth and sixth years of the programme.[84] He hoped to graduate along with the first class of graduands, but "he had not assisted with the delivery of sufficient babies" to pass in obstetrics and gynaecology.[85] He completed this assignment during the following year, and graduated as an M.D. in 1926.

While his insulin colleagues basked in their new-found fame, Collip experienced the bitterness of neglect. This was, no doubt, one of the reasons why he felt his place was in eastern Canada where his achievements would receive more recognition. As early as 1921, he had remarked that the East would offer him "both academic and financial advantages" not available in Alberta.[86] In June 1927, he left Edmonton rather hurriedly. His wife had been unwell for some time and suddenly became much worse. He took her to the Mayo Clinic for diagnosis and treatment,[87] and from there he wrote a letter of resignation to the university, but gave no reason for this decision. He had, he said, "no feeling of dissatisfaction" and appreciated the "kindly consideration" afforded him by Tory and the Board of Governors.[88] Just two weeks later, he cabled to ask if his position was still open, and the following day sent another telegram saying he would return to Edmonton for the fall term.[89] In December of the same year, he once again submitted a letter of resignation, as he had accepted the position of head of the department of biochemistry at McGill, succeeding his former teacher, A. B. Macallum, who was retiring. The Board of Governors accepted his resignation with "great regret" and expressed their appreciation for his services to the University of Alberta, the enthusiasm he had brought to his work, and the distinction he had brought to the University.[90]

Although Collip never received his due for his contribution to the discovery of insulin, he did receive many honours during his lifetime and achieved several positions of importance. He was, at different times, dean of medicine of the University of Western Ontario in London and director of the Division of Medical Research of the National Research Council. He became a fellow of the Royal Society in 1933, and later an honorary fellow of the Royal College of Physicians and Surgeons of both England and Canada, the American College of Physicians and the Royal Society of Canada. He received the Charles Mickle Fellowship awarded by the University of Toronto and the Starr Medal of the Canadian Medical Association.[91]

Tory anticipated no trouble in finding a high calibre replacement for Collip. His name and reputation were well known in the field of biochemistry, and the grants received from the Carnegie Foundation and the CPSA, as well as the insulin royalties, had helped to improve the equipment in the biochemistry laboratories. They were now up-to-date and should attract people interested in research. The search began in Great Britain. Tory contacted Canadians living and working in Edinburgh and Cambridge, and advertised the position in an English periodical and the Universities Bureau of the British Empire. The position carried a salary of $4,500 a year; yet it attracted little interest overseas. Typical salaries in Britain for a similar position ranged from £600 to £700 (the equivalent of $3,000 to $3,500); yet most felt the salary was not high enough. Location appeared to be the major problem. "Alberta seems to be regarded as rather a long way off...it is rather out of the way... [and]... living is probably more expensive there," were some of the excuses given for lack of interest in the position. Others, in North America, replied that they "needed the stimulus that is only to be found in very large schools."[92] Eventually, only two people applied, and George Hunter of Toronto was hired.[93]

Tory left the University of Alberta in 1928. He had been president of the National Research Council for the previous five years on a part-time basis, but the demands on his time increased so substantially that he could not continue to hold the two positions. After twenty years at the helm,

Tory left to take on another venture that needed someone with his drive and enthusiasm. The new president, Robert C. Wallace, came from the University of Manitoba. He faced many problems. Registration continued to increase each year, but new buildings and new equipment did not keep pace—and worse was yet to come.

Effect of the Great Depression on the Medical School

With the severe downturn in the economy, beginning in 1929, Premier Brownlee informed President Wallace that "drastic reductions in all expenditures [were] inevitable." Towards the end of 1931, President Wallace called a special meeting of all faculty members of the university to inform them that their salaries would be reduced. There was a "moderate amount of discussion, but the general feeling was that there was nothing to be said and we might be in for something worse."[94] Indeed, things did get worse. The first reduction ranged from 2% to 10% for married personnel and 3% to 10% for those who were single, depending upon the rate of pay. In 1933, a further reduction in the budget necessitated further cuts in salaries, which amounted to 7% for those who earned up to $1,000; 12% on a salary up to $2,000; and 15% on a salary over $2,000.[95] The following year the provincial auditor informed the premier that these reductions were not as much as other government employees had received and recommended that the university salaries be reduced further still.[96] Soon after its election in 1935, the Social Credit government created "prosperity certificates," often known as "scrip" and sometimes simply as "funny money." Each certificate, valued at a dollar, was intended to be used to pay for goods and services. Many businesses would not accept these certificates, the government itself would not accept them, yet, 25% of the professors' salaries were paid in this form of "currency."[97] In addition, there were constant requests to salaried staff, through the president of the university, to contribute to agencies assisting the poor and unemployed. The exasperation is evident in a letter to the president from Shaner in 1939, "Enclosed is my contribution...which the university can forward to the proper agency...I have a very strong Anglo-Saxon objection to any further 'voluntary' tampering with my salary."[98]

Meanwhile, Premier Brownlee communicated with his colleagues in the other western provinces to discuss the possibility of amalgamating some of the schools and faculties in the four provincial universities to save money. "There is considerable feeling that the cost of the university is too high," he stated. The premiers agreed that something had to be done to effect economies in the universities, and a committee comprising the presidents of the Universities of Alberta, British Columbia, Manitoba and Saskatchewan met on several occasions during 1932-33 to discuss ways and means of eliminating the duplication of programmes offered in the four western universities. The committee discussed various alternatives, including amalgamating some of the existing professional schools into one or, at most, two.[99]

The University of Manitoba medical school dated back to 1883. The University of Saskatchewan began offering the preclinical years of a medical programme in 1926, and some of its students completed their courses at either Alberta or Manitoba. The University of British Columbia offered a premedical course, and some of these students also came to Alberta or Manitoba. In 1933, there were five hundred students enrolled in medicine in the western provinces, and Toronto and McGill had already placed limits on their enrolment, making it more difficult for western students to attend those universities.[100] The committee eventually agreed that western Canada needed two complete schools of medicine. Neither Manitoba nor Alberta could accommodate five hundred students without considerable capital outlay in buildings, equipment and staff, and it was impossible to raise the fees high enough to meet the costs of an expanded medical school. No amalgamation took place, but there was also no increase in the university's budget.

So, Alberta's Faculty of Medicine survived. Some curriculum changes took place, some obligatory courses were made optional, and others were eliminated entirely.[101] Student registration in medicine remained fairly stagnant during the late 1920s and the early 1930s, but in 1933-34, it began a steady increase that continued throughout the decade. There were no funds to hire more staff or to provide additional space and equipment, and the already crowded conditions, insufficient equipment, inadequate clinical facilities and shortage of staff deteriorated still further. In 1935, A.R. Munroe, head of the surgical department, complained that the classes in surgery were so overcrowded that bedside groups were far too large. He requested more instructors, preferably in different surgical fields, but, he added, ''some remuneration would have to be arranged.''[102]

The only answer was to limit entry into the programme. Admission into the second year of medicine came from the first-year premedical course and from the graduates of the B.A. section of a combined B.A., M.D. programme. For the year 1936-37, entry into the second year was limited to those who had an average of 65% in their previous year's work. This restriction, however, did not reduce the numbers sufficiently; so the Faculty Council established a quota of forty students, with entry based solely on academic standing. In 1937, a total of seventy-one students applied for admission to second year; 102 applied in 1938; and 125 in 1939.[103] Table 2, giving the numbers of students and graduates during the years 1924 to 1940, shows that the number of students in the medical school almost doubled during those years; yet there was no budgetary increase for additional space, equipment, facilities or staff.

TABLE 2: NUMBER OF STUDENTS ENROLLED IN MEDICINE, AND GRADUATES[104] 1924-1940

Year	6-year Medicine Programme	Arts & Medicine Programme	Arts for Medicine Programme	Total	Graduates
1924-25	115	47	10	172	11
1925-26	117	51	10	178	17
1926-27	123	47	10	180	15
1927-28	147	40	11	198	18
1928-29	151	43	—	194	18
1929-30	155	48	—	203	19
1930-31	157	41	—	198	31
1931-32	166	38	—	204	22
1932-33	164	32	—	196	15
1933-34	180	41	—	221	24
1934-35	197	52	—	251	29
1935-36	194	67	—	261	21
1936-37	205	74	—	279	32
1937-38	221	59	—	280	31
1938-39	223	64	—	287	32
1939-40	233	82	—	315	35

Several changes in the membership of the Faculty Council occurred during the thirties. Quite a number of the school's own graduates joined the faculty. They were a young and enthusiastic group, most had been away for postgraduate training and they "kept well abreast of all advances."[105] In 1937, Revell retired and Shaner succeeded him as head of the department of anatomy. A.R. (Sandy) Munroe succeeded Mewburn as head of the department of surgery. He, too, was a McGill graduate and had served under Mewburn at the Canadian military hospital in Taplow, England, during World War I, where he honed his skills as a surgeon. Upon his return to Edmonton. Munroe worked at the Strathcona Hospital, when it was still under the management of the Department of National Defence and began to work with the Faculty of Medicine. Mewburn instituted surgical rounds in the University of Alberta Hospital on Wednesday mornings, and Munroe continued and expanded them. Assisted by Heber Jamieson of the department of medicine, he established the first "ward rounds" that included a visit to each bed in both the surgical and medical wards, and lasted the entire morning. They were highly instructive and soon began to attract physicians from surrounding towns.[106]

The popularity of "ward rounds" eventually led to the annual refresher course offered by the Faculty of Medicine to the general practitioners of the province, to bring them up-to-date with changes and new procedures in the profession—the beginning of formalized continuing medical education in the province. These courses were given at the University of Alberta Hospital and were arranged in conjunction with the Alberta Medical Association. Initially, they were held without charge to the medical practitioners and without remuneration to the instructors.[107] The association covered administration costs, and those who attended could stay in the university residences at a reasonable cost. Sixty-five doctors, many of them from rural districts, attended the first course held in May 1932.[108] It was well received by those who participated, and by popular demand became an annual event. In a similar vein, some of the faculty members went on tours to small towns in Alberta and B.C. to give clinics and lectures and to attend medical meetings.[109]

Changes also took place at the hospital. An addition to the south end of the original hospital was completed in October 1930.[110] It provided an additional 122 beds and afforded space for an expansion of the clinical departments and subdivisions of some of the departments so that a more specialized training could be offered to the students. The addition incorporated a number of technological advances: an automatic elevator; a paging system; a lecture room, complete with a "magic lantern" for visual demonstrations; and an x-ray developing room adjacent to the operating rooms. Two adjacent pavilions, a Red Cross Unit and a special unit for the treatment of polio patients, became a part of the University of Alberta Hospital.[111] The outdoor clinic, however, outgrew its premises in the downtown area and required larger and better accommodation.[112] Also the facilities for teaching obstetrics and gynaecology remained inadequate. The United Farm Women of Alberta, at its annual conference in 1930, passed a resolution requesting additional instruction in practical obstetrics for the undergraduate medical students.[113] Temporary arrangements for teaching at the Misericordia Hospital filled the gap, until a small obstetrical unit of fifteen beds opened at the University Hospital; but this, too, proved inadequate for the teaching needs of the medical school.[114]

As the depression deepened and the government systematically reduced the university budget each year, the university, in turn, cut its grant to the hospital. From 1922 to 1931, the yearly grant was $25,000. This was cut to $21,500 in 1932, and reduced yet further to $17,500 in subsequent years. The Hospital Board did its best to reverse these decisions, complaining that "its services to the university had not been reduced," but "had no option but to accept the reduction."[115] The years of depression affected the hospital even more drastically than the university. As a result, it gave increasing preference to paying patients, thereby reducing the number of beds available for nonpaying patients, those who had traditionally served as teaching patients for the medical school. After the university cut its grant, the hospital could guarantee only seventy-five teaching beds to the medical school, and later reduced the number for indigent patients still further.[116]

The lack of teaching beds combined with increasing registration caused grave concern for the dean and members of the Faculty Council, together with a fear that the A-rating of the medical school was in jeopardy. In 1935, the school applied for membership in the Association of American Medical Colleges (AAMC), an association that "embraced most of the best schools and established standards." Munroe made the initial suggestion, expressing the sentiment that "our extreme isolation will... be counteracted by coming in contact with professors of other medical schools annually." The school would also be classified, and this was necessary for graduates going on to postgraduate education and for American licensing bodies. With the approval of the Faculty Council, Dean Rankin took the proposal to the Board of Governors. "There was," he told the board, "no body in Canada interested in fostering cooperation amongst our medical schools... [and]... we would acquire prestige and protection." Annual dues were $150, not an inconsiderable sum in 1935; but first the school had to be inspected. McGill, Toronto and Manitoba were already members, and Dalhousie had recently applied for membership also. The Board of Governors not only concurred but also agreed to pay the travelling expenses of representatives attending conventions.[117]

The medical school was anxious for an inspection, the results of which would point out the inadequate facilities and the lack of sufficient staff in the school and bring them clearly to the attention of the president, the Board of Governors and the provincial government.[118] The Education Committee of the American Medical Association was the only body qualified to carry out such an inspection, and at the school's request Dr. Fred C. Zappfe, secretary of that committee, conducted an inspection in October 1938. As expected, the report generally regarded the staff and administration favourably, but criticized the physical facilities and the inadequacy of teaching material in the University Hospital.

The report began with encouraging words, "Only words of commendation can be spoken about the organization and administration of the Faculty."[119] Zappfe praised the careful selection of students, encouraged the move towards increasing the academic requirements for admission, and recommended more full-time professors in the basic medical sciences, so that time would be available for research. In the clinical departments, however, there were severe deficiencies "related entirely to inadequate teaching facilities." The obstetric and pediatric services were singled out as being quite insufficient for the needs of the students, but the outdoor clinic was "the outstanding defect.... This department...is a disgrace to the university, the city, the public. The present housing absolutely prohibits doing any teaching...."[120]

Zappfe stressed that "everyone connected with the medical faculty or the hospital is aware" of these deficiencies, and that the "lack is wholly financial." He suggested that the faculty establish teaching units in the other city hospitals, appoint full-time supervisors in the teaching departments, and concluded with the words.

> ...the Province of Alberta has a medical school, a good school, it should be more than willing to support it in the manner in which it should be supported. It should not stint. The wealth of any community is the health of that community.[121]

The report had little immediate effect on the financial support given to the school. In his annual report to the Board of Governors in 1938-39, the dean still complained that the "deficiencies are hardly in keeping with our standing amongst medical schools and can only lead to unfortunate consequences, if some improvement cannot be achieved in the near future."[122] Dean Rankin did begin to negotiate with the other city hospitals. If they were to offer teaching beds, however, they required some financial recompense, and the relationship between the Royal Alexandra and the

University of Alberta hospitals had rarely been cordial. The town-gown dichotomy, the strong McGill tradition at the Faculty of Medicine, and the few doctors from the Royal Alexandra Hospital receiving appointments to the faculty of the medical school had prevented the development of a close relationship.[123] Negotiations continued, however, and Walter Mackenzie and A.H. Maclennan received appointments to teach students at the Royal Alexandra Hospital. The various city hospitals agreed to take final-year students as clinical clerks, the University Hospital developed its own obstetrical unit, and, in 1939, the government made space available in a new provincial building for an outdoor clinic on 101A Avenue at 100th Street.[124]

In the sixteen years after the school began offering the full programme, 370 doctors of medicine graduated. Most became general practitioners, and more than half remained in Alberta. Students from British Columbia and Saskatchewan always constituted a significant minority in the student body, and these two provinces claimed a number of the graduands.[125] While increasing enrolment was, in some measure, a result of the quota system established in eastern universities, it also signified a growing acceptance of a medical school in the far West and an awareness of the quality of instruction offered at the University of Alberta's Faculty of Medicine. By 1939, the school was firmly established and had managed to survive severe budgetary restraints. It had a nucleus of full-time professors in the basic medical sciences and in the department of medicine, and part-time teachers with the rank of full professor in the clinical sciences. Most had been with the school for a long time and were a small and closely knit group, with the inevitable personality conflicts. It was they, however, who constituted the Faculty Council and developed the policy of the medical school. They had shepherded it through the Great Depression and would now be called upon to see it through yet another world war.

* * * * *

CHAPTER 3

World War II and the Beginning of Expansion

The forties and the fifties

CANADA DECLARED war on Germany on 10 September 1939. Almost immediately, Dean Rankin offered his services to the Department of National Defence and was promptly appointed director of hygiene for the military services of Canada, with the rank of Lieutenant-Colonel. Before he left for Ottawa, the university's Board of Governors granted him a leave of absence, gave him an assurance that his position as dean would be protected during his absence and that his pension payments would continue uninterrupted—and appointed John J. Ower as Acting Dean.[1]

When a country goes to war, it has an immediate and pressing need for medical practitioners, and not just for the obvious reason of treatment of the wounded. All service personnel, in army, navy and air force units, wherever they were stationed, required medical care and treatment, enlistment and discharge procedures called for medical examinations, and numerous medical and advisory boards required the active participation of medical practitioners. In the first month of the war, the number who enlisted in Military District No. 13, with headquarters in Calgary, "taxed the capacity of medical boards."[2] The Royal Canadian Army Medical Corps set up general hospitals in Great Britain and in Europe, and field hospitals and casualty ambulance units accompanied all land forces. By the end of November 1944, Canada had established ten general hospitals in Great Britain, with a total capacity of 7,000 beds, and another twelve in Europe.

In addition, the Canadian overseas medical establishment included a 2,000-bed convalescent depot, plastic surgery and neurological hospitals, and a number of other smaller units.[3] At home, the dominion government undertook a construction programme of Department of Veterans' Affairs (DVA) hospitals in various parts of the country, including one in Edmonton. Built on university property, it was ready for occupancy in 1945 and was named the Colonel Mewburn Pavilion after the first professor of surgery of the medical faculty.

In the first year of the war, the presidents of all Canadian universities met with the Department of National Defence in Ottawa to determine the military service that would be required of university students. As a result, all male students within the "call-up" age group were required to take military training during their time at university. To accomplish this, the academic schedule began at 8 a.m. and ended at 4 p.m., so that students could take their military training from 4 p.m. to 6 p.m. each day. In addition, they attended a two-week military camp at the end of the spring session. Initially, all medical students participated in this training, but subsequent arrangements exempted those in their final years. Instead, they attended courses on the most recent developments in "war medicine," including such topics as treatment of military injuries, shock blood transfusion, and prevention and treatment of gas intoxication.[4]

During the same period, the Department of National Defence set up a Medical Procurement and Assignment Board in each province, with a mandate to assess the medical needs of both the armed forces and the civilian population. Dr. Howard H. Hepburn, an Edmonton neurosurgeon and faculty member, chaired Alberta's board, which proceeded to determine the needs of the civilian population so as to establish the minimum number of practitioners required to cope with medical care and education in the province.[5] As a result of such surveys in all provinces, the Department of National Defence concluded that the requirements of the services for medical personnel could not be met from the numbers of qualified physicians in the country. The director general of medical services then called together the deans of all the medical schools in the country. They, too, met in Ottawa to discuss the shortage of medical officers in the services and unanimously agreed to "speed up the graduation of medical students" by offering courses on a continuous basis throughout the year.[6] Various changes or relaxation of regulations were required to implement such a system. Hospitals would have to accept a reduced internship of eight months rather than the usual twelve; provincial licensing bodies would have to accept a modification in the requirements of the curriculum; and students would need financial assistance from the dominion government. Without a long break in the summer, there would be no opportunity to earn the necessary money to finance the following year's tuition and expenses.[7] The resolution remained on hold until the individual universities submitted their estimates of the costs of such an undertaking to the dominion government.

Alberta submitted a ''modest estimate of approximately $2,000.'' Other schools, however, requested much larger sums of money. Manitoba asked for $50,000 a year, and the total amount from all schools was so large that the government found ''it was inadvisable to proceed with the scheme.'' Nevertheless, an emergency meeting of Alberta's medical faculty decided to proceed with its acceleration programme immediately even though no financial aid was assured.[8] The need for more doctors in the services was still pressing, final-year students had already been notified that their course would begin on 2 July, and all arrangements for acceleration were in place.[9] Later in the year, Ralph Shaner proposed that the whole medical school be put into ''continuous operation for the duration of the war.'' He proposed a scheme whereby eligible students would enrol in the services and be assigned to the medical school by the military authorities. Their military pay would cover tuition, and the dominion government should offer loans to cover extra financial requirements. As for those students who were unfit for military service, they ''would have to adapt themselves to conditions as best they could.''[10]

Acceleration of all classes in the medical programme at the University of Alberta began in 1942. Those who completed their year in May, started their next year on 1 June 1942. The following session began on 1 February 1943, and the third session coincided with the regular 1943-44 academic year. Medical students spent eleven months each year in classes. The one-month break afforded insufficient time to earn money for their tuition, but the W.K. Kellogg Foundation and a Dominion-Provincial Youth Training Scholarship Fund provided some financial assistance.[11] In 1943, arrangements with the military authorities provided for the enlistment of students in the Royal Canadian Army Medical Corps, who would then receive military subsistence allowances. Students enrolled as privates and received a commission on graduation. The Faculty Council instructed the Admissions Committee to give preference to male students who were physically fit and willing to enlist in the armed forces, and ''to use their judgement as to the allocation of female and medically unfit male students.''[12]

Acting Dean Ower faced immense problems in guiding the school through this period of acceleration. It was difficult both to maintain the quality of the programme and to find teachers to instruct on a year-round basis. Nineteen Alberta doctors joined up in the first month of the war,[13] and, in addition to Dean Rankin, three other members of the Faculty of Medicine enlisted in the first year. One of them, Dr. R.T. Washburn, superintendent of the University of Alberta Hospital, was placed in charge of the No. 4 Casualty Clearing Station, with officer personnel made up entirely of recent Faculty of Medicine graduates.[14] As more and more physicians, some of them faculty members, joined the services, this reduced not only the number of physicians available to care for the civilian population but also the availability of those able to teach medical students. In addition, the school was adapting to a new curriculum, adopted in 1940-41, that called for increased prerequisite requirements. It added a year to the overall programme, for a total of two years of premedical and five years of medical training. Students spent their fifth and final professional year as interns in a hospital, and graduates of the complete programme earned both a B.Sc. and M.D. degrees.[15]

By the beginning of 1943, Ower reported to his Faculty Council that the staff was at the minimum "which could be considered essential for carrying on." Ower discussed the problem with President Newton, who put the case to the Minister of National Defence. He replied that "the armed forces would not accept essential staff members without the consent of the Dean of the Faculty of Medicine;"[16] yet, it was difficult to refuse those who wished to enlist, and faculty members continued to leave. In July 1943, Mark Levey (Marshall) joined up, and early in the following year the Canadian Red Cross asked Graham Huckell to accept the position of chief surgeon at the Canadian orthopaedic unit at Hairmyre in Scotland. Before the war ended twenty faculty members, about 20% of the instructional staff, answered the "call to the colours." Drastic reduction in the teaching staff and accelerated courses for the student body were the direct and immediate results of the war, but many more would arise in the postwar years.

By the end of 1943, the tide began to turn. Dean Rankin was released from the services and the country's needs for medical practitioners in the services were substantially fulfilled. Many members of the faculty felt that they should begin to taper off the acceleration of the medical course, and stop it altogether as soon as conditions permitted. In his annual report, Ower stated that:

> The process of acceleration is responsible for conditions which have made instruction unsatisfactory from the point of view of both the students and the staff and the procedure has been generally criticized by medical and educational authorities. It has been tried in both Great Britain and the Soviet Union and abandoned.

As these views were shared by all medical schools in the country, with the exception of Toronto, the newly formed Association of Canadian Medical Colleges appealed to the Department of National Defence, which agreed that the first year could revert to the normal academic year.[17] The incoming first-year medical students started classes in September 1944 in the normal university fall session. As the war drew to a close, those in the final years of the accelerated programme interned for twelve months rather than eight, and those in the final accelerated class obtained their release from the army as soon as their internships were complete.[18] An anomaly of this "deceleration" procedure, when the classes gradually settled back into the normal university academic year, was the absence of a fourth-year class in 1945-46 and a graduating class in 1947.

The war ended in 1945, and the medical school welcomed the return of those faculty members who had enlisted. The remaining instructors, many of whom had been too old to serve, had taught almost constantly since July 1942, with only very short breaks, coping as well with the demands of a greatly increased number of patients in their private practices. Egerton Pope, the first professor of medicine, retired in 1944, and two long-time members of the faculty died: L.C. Conn, head of the department of obstetrics, and Charles Hurlburt, professor of cardiology. Medical officers in the armed forces serving in Edmonton had been able to contribute some of their time to assist with teaching in the the clinical departments during those traumatic years. The air force established a clinical investigation unit at what is now Corbett Hall, and members of this unit assisted with clinical teaching from 1942 on.[19] Members of the United States Army Medical Corps, who were posted to Edmonton to care for those American servicemen employed in building the Alaska Highway, conducted bedside teaching clinics for medical students in their corps hospital (later the first Charles Camsell Hospital). They also took medical rounds with students at other city hospitals.

University Survey Committee, 1941

After years of neglect, the provincial government began to take an interest in university affairs in the early 1940s and appointed a Survey Committee to evaluate the place of the university and its function in future development of the province. The mandate of this committee, struck in 1941, included a review of the internal organization and administration, an assessment of the courses offered in relation to the need for them, projected financial and building requirements, and proposed activities of university departments in the area of research. Howard H. Parlee, K.C., who was chairman of the Board of Governors from 1940 to 1950, chaired the Survey Committee, which also included G. Frederick McNally, the provincial Minister of Education, and Robert Newton, the new President of the university. The seven-man committee got to work at once, sought submissions from various groups and individuals, held a public hearing in Edmonton,[20] and the following year produced an analytical report with no fewer than fifty-eight specific recommendations and a ten-year building programme for the expansion of facilities.[21]

The report pointed out that lack of government support had affected the university in three major areas: the facilities themselves, the staff and opportunities for research. In the case of facilities, the report stated that "overcrowding conditions cannot be exaggerated...one class meets regularly in a corridor of the Arts Building...[and]...the Provincial Laboratory is so overcrowded as to constitute a public danger."[22] As for the staff, a salary scale with annual increments was set up in 1930 but never implemented; instead, salaries had been reduced. Moreover, the staff received neither pedagogical training nor assessment of teaching ability when it came to promotion. As for research, "the life blood of an institution," none had taken place except that conducted by individual members of the staff on their own initiatives and either at their own expense or with money raised through their own efforts.[23]

The Faculty of Medicine, which included the schools of dentistry, nursing and pharmacy, as well as the Provincial Laboratory, "represents the largest financial requirement of the university...[and]...warrants special consideration by the government."

In the Faculty proper, the greatest defect is in hospital facilities for clinical instruction. The University Hospital cannot provide enough teaching beds, and the use of other city hospitals to more than a limited extent seems fraught with difficulties. Teaching needs often call for admitting patients to hospital who do not require hospitalization. Such patients must be given free beds.... To give the University the required clinical facilities would involve building a new wing to the University Hospital and increasing the annual grant of the University to the University Hospital from its present level of $17,500 to perhaps $50,000. There seem to be only two alternatives to the forego-ing: (a) to reduce the annual quota of medical students from its present level of 40; or (b) to sacrifice the Grade A rating which the Medical Faculty has enjoyed from the outset, and drop to Grade B.[24]

Looking to the future, the committee pointed out that an influx of students could be expected after the war, which would overtax an already overtaxed institution. The committee proposed the construction of seven buildings over a ten-year period (shown in Table 3), to start immediately. Four of them involved the Faculty of Medicine, including the addition of two wings to the Medical Building, one of which would include space for the Provincial Laboratory, and two additions to the University Hospital.

This warning, by the government-appointed committee, that the medical faculty was in desperate need of improved facilities, only con-firmed the four-year-old report of the accreditation committee of the American Medical Association. Still the government did not act, and it would be another four years before construction finally began on the east wing of the Medical Building. In the meantime, the federal government began construction of a new DVA hospital. The only addition provided by the provincial government was a tuberculosis hospital, the Aberhart Memorial Hospital, which also opened in 1945. These would provide improved teaching facilities; but, until their completion, the faculty had to adapt to the deprivations of wartime conditions in the same inadequate facilities, while training medical students at an accelerated rate.

TABLE 3: TEN-YEAR BUILDING PLAN PROPOSED BY THE SURVEY COMMITTEE[25] 1942

Proposed Building	Year	Cost
1. East wing of Medical Building	1942-43	$100,000
	1943-44	100,000
2. Centre wing of Medical Building	1944-45	100,000
	1945-46	90,000
3. Completion of Normal School to house Faculty of Education	1945-46	10,000
4. New wing at University Hospital	1946-47	100,000
	1947-48	100,000
5. Biological Sciences Building	1948-49	100,000
	1949-50	100,000
6. Chemical and Petroleum Engineering Building	1950-51	100,000
7. Nurses Home at University Hospital	1951-52	100,000

The PostWar Period

Dean Ower's successor, John W. Scott, would later remark that Ower suffered more of the "slings and arrows of outrageous fortune" than seemed fair and reasonable. Indeed, his time as Acting Dean, from 1939 until 1943, when Rankin was released from the services, and as Dean from 1945, when Rankin retired, to 1948, covered a period of continuing difficulties. In the words of President Newton, they were "particularly trying years. They included the second world war and three years of educational dislocation following the war."[26] The war's end did not eliminate problems within the Faculty of Medicine or in the university as a whole. Large numbers of veterans enrolled in the medical school, which was short of teachers and heavily involved in planning new buildings, as well as developing a postgraduate programme for the training of specialists.

Dean Scott did not have an easy time either. Events in the years following World War II tested all his diplomatic skills, as he dealt with pressures both from within and without the university. After years of depression and war, a fast-growing population demanded a "better life." In Alberta, an increasingly urban and sophisticated society became more aware of the great advances in science and medicine and demanded access to higher standards of medical care and expected increased specialized knowledge in those administering that care. In addition, the new postwar generation of medical students expected a more flexible training programme; one that was not fragmented into subjects that lacked integration. Both the philosophy and policy of medical schools had to change to meet these demands, to improve and broaden medical education, and to promote opportunities for research. The medical faculty at the University of Alberta, however, was preoccupied with basic and fundamental problems such as shortage of staff, an inability to compete with lucrative situations in commerce and industry, a shortage of well-qualified medical students, a university requirement that they teach students in other faculties, an ever-present need for more and improved physical facilities, and a growing demand for the introduction of full-time clinical professors.

During these postwar years, the preclinical departments were, in most cases, headed by professors who had been with the school since its early days and were close to or past retirement age. Because replacements were unavailable, however, some were persuaded to remain in their positions. Indeed, for many years, both clinical and preclinical departments had vacancies for which it was difficult to find candidates because medical schools across the continent had discontinued the training of young staff members during the war.[27] In addition, the "lucrative lures of industry, professional practice, and the greener teaching and research fields of the United States" offered strong competition.[28] In 1954, when medical science departments still complained of extremely heavy teaching and administrative loads, leaving no time for research, the university introduced a school of physiotherapy under the jurisdiction of the Faculty of Medicine, which served to increase the teaching load further still. Altogether, medical faculty staff taught twenty-nine courses to students in nine other schools and faculties of the university.[29]

The remainder of this chapter will begin with an overview of the building programme and changes in the administration of the faculty. It will then go on to explore some of the challenges that faced the medical school during the postwar years—some they overcame; others were insurmountable and eventually culminated in an adverse accreditation report from the Liaison Committee on Medical Education in 1956.

Building Programme
Construction finally began on the west wing of the Medical Building in 1946. While plans were in place to start on the east wing the following year, delays caused by strikes and shortages of labour and material— endemic problems immediately following the war—delayed its completion. Both wings were ready for occupancy for the 1948-49 session, and about the same time renovations to the Medical Building brought it up to modern standards. A new Provincial Laboratory building opened in 1950, and together these buildings added much needed extra laboratory space for the increased number of students. That same year, construction began on an addition to the University Hospital, which was completed in 1951 and added another 350 beds and two large lecture rooms.[30] Construction of the John S. McEachran Cancer Research Laboratory in 1952 demonstrated an increasing recognition of the need for medical research. With money made available by the Alberta Division of the Canadian Cancer Society, the university erected a small two-storey structure behind the Medical Building, between the east and west wings. Nevertheless, the building programme never managed to keep pace with the growth of the school and its need for increased facilities.

Changes in the Administration
In 1948, Dean Ower submitted his resignation as dean because of ill health, but continued to teach pathology until his normal retirement date in 1951.

John W. Scott, the first clinician to become dean, succeeded him. Scott began his medical training in 1914 at the University of Alberta's infant medical school when it was a three-year school offering only the preclinical subjects. Before completing his medical degree at McGill, he joined the Tank Corps and served overseas in the first world war. Upon his return to Alberta, Scott set up practice in a rural community, the town of Provost, thus fulfilling the mission of Alberta's medical school to provide doctors for rural communities. Subsequently, he opened a practice in Edmonton and returned to the medical school to teach biochemistry under the aegis of J.B. Collip; in fact, he did most of the teaching in this subject, leaving Collip free to conduct research. Scott showed such a remarkable ability in this area that Collip did his best to persuade him to forsake clinical medicine and continue with biochemistry. After much soul-searching, Scott declined, and went to Great Britain for further study in internal medicine; but his intimate knowledge and interest in this science led to his reputation as the quintessential physician who "brought the laboratory to the bedside."

John Scott was a soft-spoken and gentle man, with incredible energy and a deep love for his profession and for humanity. He was highly respected and revered not only by his peers and students in the medical school but also by the medical profession, locally and nationally. His achievements were prodigious. In addition to his responsibilities as dean, he retained his duties as head of the department of medicine and director of the Student Medical Services, and also conducted his own private practice. He held memberships in most of the local, national and international medical associations, and was president of a number of them, including the Association of Canadian Medical Colleges and the Royal College of Physicians and Surgeons of Canada. Dean Scott's role in the history of the medical school has been commemorated by naming the fine library in the W.C. Mackenzie Health Sciences Centre after him.

In 1954, after a bout of ill health, the workload became too much for him, and he submitted his resignation as dean. Given his reputation in medical circles across the country and his proven abilities, the university was loathe to let him go at a time when so many changes were taking place. He was persuaded to remain as dean, with a substantial increase in salary, and he gave up the position as head of the department of medicine. His position was still part time, however. James S. Thompson, a professor in the department of anatomy, was appointed executive secretary, also on a part-time basis, and provided valuable assistance in the administration of the faculty.

Postwar Registration

As in the years following the first world war, large numbers of veterans swelled the ranks of the student body in universities across the country. These included those who had joined up when, under normal circumstances, they would have entered university, as well as students who had interrupted their studies to join the services. Once again, the University of Alberta faced enormous problems in assimilating large numbers into an institution that had experienced no growth in faculty or facilities. Furthermore, this time a federal government department, the Department of Veterans' Affairs (DVA), and an active and powerful Royal Canadian Legion ensured that veterans received fair treatment. Under the terms of the "Veterans' Charter," they received financial assistance for their training, or retraining, as well as preferential treatment in access to courses of their choice. Despite inadequate facilities, public pressure was brought to bear on all faculties to take more students than they could reasonably accommodate. The Faculty of Medicine felt unable to accept more than the prewar quota of forty, but Dean Ower, a beleaguered man, was pressured on all sides: by large numbers of applicants seeking admission to the Faculty of Medicine, both veterans and civilians; by graduates of the accelerated courses who wanted postgraduate courses to compensate for their abbreviated internships; and by returning practitioners who wanted refresher courses. DVA sponsored refresher courses for "medical rehabilitation," to reintroduce returning physicians into civilian practice.[31]

A few veterans began to appear in the halls of the Medical Building as early as 1944. Registration had fallen off during the war years, but now it began to increase, though slowly at first. Applications came not only from Alberta but also from other parts of Canada, and from the United States and Europe. Given the facilities, particularly for clinical teaching, no more than forty in any one year could be accommodated safely. Despite this, forty-five were admitted in 1946, and no veteran or Alberta resident was refused if they were qualified. The large influx of veterans had not yet hit the professional medical programme, but eighty-eight students, of whom sixty-two were veterans, were in the second year of the B.Sc. M.D. programme, and sixty-seven students, of whom forty-eight were veterans, were registered in the first year.[32]

Obviously, a new policy would have to be determined. The President, the Board of Governors, the provincial government, DVA and the Royal Canadian Legion, all pressured the faculty to increase its quota. It was a delicate and political issue. The President advised faculty council members "to consider very carefully their policy in regard to setting a quota for admission to Medicine," and asked for full information before a final decision was reached.[33] Despite this warning, the Quota Committee recommended that, given the limited hospital facilities for the three clinical years, the quota should remain at forty, and set the absolute maximum number that could be accommodated safely at forty-five. Despite this recommendation, fifty students were admitted, of whom forty-five were veterans and five were "high standing civilians."[34] The committee, headed initially by Professor Downs and later by H.E. Rawlinson, devised a point system (shown in Table 4) based on length of war service, age and academic standing. Every qualified veteran and a few civilians who had high academic standings were admitted under this system in 1947.

TABLE 4: POINT SYSTEM FOR ADMISSION TO FIRST-YEAR MEDICINE 1947-48

Age	Points	War Service (months)	Points	Grade %	Points
27	5	60	10	100	16
26	5	54	9	95-99	14
25	4.5	48	8	90-94	12
24	4	42	7	85-89	10
23	3.5	36	6	80-84	8
22	3	30	5	75-79	6
21	2.5	24	4	70-74	4
20	2	18	3	65-69	2
19	1.5	12	2		
18	1	6	1		

In 1948, 111 applications were received, and President Newton made the decision that academically qualified veterans completing the second year of the B.Sc., M.D. course, and civilians who had completed it the previous year, were to be given first preference and rated according to academic standing only. Again, fifty were admitted. In 1949, the number of applicants reached an unprecedented high. More than 890 applications were received, 122 from Alberta, ninety-one from British Columbia, and almost six hundred from the United States. This was the peak year, as by this time, all veterans had completed their premedical training, and applicants from the entire continent sought places in the relatively few established medical schools. In their efforts to find a place, aspiring medical students sent applications to a large number of universities. Again, preference was given to Alberta veterans and previously deferred civilian candidates.

As new and expanded facilities opened up, particularly in the United States, the number of "out of province" applicants began to decline, and this was the last year in which large numbers of veterans applied for admission. By 1950, one-third of the first-year students were veterans, and the following year only six of fifty. Throughout North America, universities had scrambled to accommodate the large numbers of veterans from a war which, for Canada, had lasted six years. To do so, they had placed regular applicants, for the most part, on deferred lists. Only those civilians with a sufficiently high academic standing were accepted at their first try, and it was virtually impossible for students who lived in provinces that did not have medical schools to get into medicine. Most schools gave preference to applicants from their own provinces and stretched their quotas beyond an acceptable limit to do so. Traditionally Alberta's medical college had taken students from British Columbia, and advanced students from Saskatchewan, following completion of the first two years of a medical programme at the University of Saskatchewan. The President of the University of British Columbia wrote to President Newton, pleading for places for "a few of our best students." In his reply, Newton commented, "you knew when you were writing your letter that you were asking an awfully hard thing." He went on,

> Only yesterday morning I was talking to Dean Ower about our obligation to our neighbouring provinces. He is pretty worried about the whole situation as you know what a row the Canadian Legion can raise. They did it last year while I was away and managed to jam in more Dental students than we can handle properly, with the consequence that we have been in a muddle all year.[35]

The expanded quota in the medical school raised the problem of supervision of a large number of students in their clinical years, and particularly their accommodation in the affiliated Edmonton hospitals for the final, internship year. The programme was designed for forty students, the number that could be adequately accommodated in Edmonton's hospitals. To solve this problem, the faculty decided to drop the final undergraduate internship year, grant the medical degree after the fourth year, and require the newly qualified M.D. to complete a year of graduate internship before receiving an enabling certificate to write the LMCC licensing examinations.

To relieve the pressure on the affiliated hospitals in Edmonton, the graduate internship year could be taken at any approved hospital. The new system was implemented immediately; so, after a year with no graduates, there were two graduating classes in 1948. One had completed a five-year programme, including an undergraduate internship year, and the other had finished a four-year programme, but still required junior graduate internships.[36]

As facilities for teaching improved, both in the laboratory and the hospital, the yearly quota for admissions gradually increased. To accommodate all qualified Albertans, fifty-eight students were accepted in 1951, and sixty the following year. In 1953, however, the tide began to turn, and there were not enough qualified applicants, including non-Albertans, to fill the quota. Furthermore, a number withdrew at the last moment, and the faculty decided to institute a nonrefundable deposit of $25 from each applicant on acceptance, which was applied to first-year tuition fees. The quantity and quality of applicants continued to decline, however, for the rest of the decade and into the 1960s. In 1950, 73% of those admitted to first-year medicine had an average mark of 70% or more; by 1953, only 35% had a similar average. Over the same time period, those who had less than 65% increased from none to 18%.[37]

By 1956, the University of Saskatchewan had extended its medical school to a full degree-granting programme, so no further students from that school would require admission to Alberta with advanced standing. As a consequence, the quota increased to sixty-five, but even when several students with less than the required 65% average were admitted, this number was not reached.[38] Over the next several years, even fewer students applied, and a number of them had only mediocre academic qualifications.[39] The admission of borderline students caused an increase in the number of dropouts and failures, particularly in the first year. In the belief that more highly qualified applicants might be attracted into the medical school if the fees were lower, the Faculty Council sought permission from the Board of Governors to have the fees reduced, at least for the first year. Medical school fees had always been the highest in the university, and student grants and loans were still difficult to obtain. The Board of Governors did not agree to an overall reduction of fees, though it did approve a reduction of first-year fees from $450 to $300. Second-year fees remained the same at $450, and the fees for the third and fourth years increased to $500, so that the total cost for all four years remained at the same figure of $1,750.[40]

Although total enrolment in universities across the country increased sharply during the 1950s, the decline in the number of qualified applicants to medical schools reflected a continent-wide phenomenon that caused great concern in the profession. In the United States, the lowest number of applications and acceptances "in the history of modern medical education" occurred during this period.[41] A large number of doctors from Great Britain and Europe immigrated to Canada during the postwar years, helping to maintain an equable doctor/patient ratio; but when this immigration levelled off, as it was beginning to do, there would be a shortage of qualified practitioners all across the country, and at a time when universal medicare was looming on the horizon and more physicians would be required.

Several factors contributed to this decline, and certainly fees might have been one of them. They were high, and there was little or no financial assistance, whereas students in the physical sciences were eligible for National Research Council grants of $2,200 a year right through to the completion of a Ph.D.[42] The major professions before the war—medicine, law and theology—now had to compete for the brighter students with several other attractive and well-paying careers. Following the war, the media glamourized exciting advances in the fields of science and technology, many of them resulting from the needs of war. Additionally, the oil industry, heralded in Alberta by a major discovery in the Leduc area in February 1947, was beginning to offer influential and lucrative careers to well-qualified science students.

An editorial in the *Canadian Medical Association Journal* in 1958 urged its members to keep an eye open for likely candidates for the profession. In a continuing effort to assist with recruitment, the *Journal* developed a brochure entitled "Doctors of Tomorrow," in which the editor stated that "we must compete for the attention of the brightest boys and girls when they are considering their life's work." The Canadian Medical Association distributed the booklet throughout the school systems of the country, and urged physicians to take part in "Career Days" in their communities.[43] The medical schools themselves conducted recruiting campaigns in high schools and among undergraduates in their own universities, and eventually these activities began to pay off. In 1962-63, deans of medicine across the country reported an increase in applications of 17% over the previous year.[44]

Graduate Training Programme

The introduction of a graduate training programme in 1946 constituted both a major change in philosophy and a first step towards programmed expansion. Hitherto, the curriculum of the school had been geared towards the training of general practitioners, and those who wished to take further specialized training had to go to centres in eastern Canada or the United States. After the war, places in these establishments were difficult to secure, as most were taken by local veteran graduates. Furthermore, many of the Alberta graduates of the accelerated programme, who had entered the services directly after completing a short internship, had given little thought to plans for their future in the profession. As they went from one class to another, and progressed rapidly from one year to the next, there was no time for such speculation—their minds were focused on completing their training and going into the services to do their part in the war effort.[45] Now, with time to consider their future careers, many wanted to go on to graduate specialty training. Dean Ower, together with John Scott, who was then the head of the department of medicine, and Mark Marshall, professor of ophthalmology, spent an evening discussing these problems and ways to resolve them. They decided the time had come to set up a graduate training programme in the medical school. Marshall agreed to investigate procedures and direct the programme, which would follow the outline of training programmes for certification or fellowship in the various specialties recently prepared by the Royal College of Physicians and Surgeons of Canada.[46]

Mark Marshall was a good choice for this project, which would in time change the basic philosophy of the school.[47] In addition to being a well-trained and highly competent ophthalmologist, Marshall's organizational abilities were unexcelled, as was his propensity for meticulous detail. (One of his lectures was on the importance of keeping copies of letters.) When he first arrived at the University of Alberta in 1920, as a freshman in the medical school, he had behind him an illustrious military career. At the outbreak of the first world war he joined the Canadian Machine Gun Corps as a private, and went overseas immediately. He rose to the rank of brigade major, was wounded twice, was awarded the Military Medal, coauthored the official history of the Machine Gun Corps on his return to Canada and wrote a manual concerning the use and maintenance of the machine gun.

Marshall was small in stature, but during his years as a student he became what was termed in those days "a big man on campus." He was an active participant in many clubs, including the French Club, which "he set on its feet," and the Dramatic Club, in whose plays he acted and directed. He was editor-in-chief of the student newspaper, *The Gateway*; and was elected president of the Students' Union by acclamation. In his own faculty, he was both president of his class and of the Med Club, and director of Med Night (the first time that it ever made money). Marshall went on to McGill for his graduating year and took postgraduate training in his specialty in Great Britain and Europe before returning to Edmonton and the Faculty of Medicine.

He was an extremely strong character, with a determined personality, and a political force in the Faculty of Medicine in the years following the war. A manipulative and uncommunicative man, it came as a complete surprise to everyone on campus, including the President and the Dean of Medicine, when he began construction of his own office on university property—as an annex, and with access to, the Mewburn Pavilion. Construction of the office was arranged in private consultation with the provincial government, was built with his own money, and remained there until the Mewburn itself was torn down. Marshall set extremely high standards both for himself and his students. He conducted his rounds with regimental precision. Everyone except the patient had to stand to attention—the bedsheets, however, had to be perfectly aligned—and no one was allowed to speak unless questioned.

Marshall formed a small nucleus committee with Percy Sprague, professor of internal medicine, and Walter Mackenzie,[48] professor of surgery, to discuss ways and means of developing a graduate training programme in Edmonton. The committee met with representatives of the University of Alberta and the Royal Alexandra hospitals as well as the basic science departments of the Faculty of Medicine. They devised a training programme in the medical and clinical sciences that satisfied the requirements of such bodies as the Royal College of Physicians and Surgeons and American specialty boards. Each specialty had its own committee, and a system of committees planned and supervised the programme and training of each individual candidate. The first programme was in surgery; it was submitted to and approved by the Education Committee of the American College of Surgeons.[49] Subsequent programmes were developed in obstetrics and gynaecology, internal medicine and ophthalmology. The postgraduate training programme came to be known as "The Marshall Plan," and Marshall maintained rigid control over it until his retirement in 1961, when he was succeeded by R.E. Rossall.[50]

Successful applicants to the specialty training programme had to be graduates of an approved medical school and had to have completed a year of postgraduate rotating internship in an approved hospital. Training included a year in the basic sciences, followed by a year each as a senior intern, an assistant resident, and a resident in the chosen specialty. Trainees were encouraged to become actively involved in a research project and to strive for excellence—''only those of a high calibre [were] accepted and only those who measured up to the standard [were] allowed to continue.''[51]

In the first eight years of the programme, the majority of the forty-five participants were graduates of the University of Alberta, but some came from the Universities of Manitoba, Toronto, Western Ontario and McGill. Alberta graduates usually completed two or three years in Edmonton and then went elsewhere for their final year. By 1954, twenty-three had completed their training, and seventeen of these were practising in Alberta and twelve were on the teaching staff of the medical school. Over those eight years, ten had withdrawn, mainly for financial reasons, and a number of them went to other centres where fellowships and bursaries were available, and were thus lost to the province.

The programme was of direct benefit to the province and its medical school, and there was no additional cost to the university; yet, participants in the programme were not eligible for payment by the university for their graduate teaching, and faculty members received no credit from the university for the time they spent teaching in the graduate school. It was several years before the Faculty of Graduate Studies recognized the programme; the point of contention being that the degree and the examinations were conducted by a body other than the university. In their first year in the medical sciences, trainees often worked as demonstrators and received an honorarium for this work. In subsequent years, those who were accepted as a resident at the hospital received $100 a month. Many were married and had families and experienced some difficulty financing their training.[52] The faculty and President Stewart began a campaign to obtain donations from business and industry, seeking three or four fellowships each worth $8,000 to provide $2,000 a year for the four years of training.[53] Finally, in 1958, the dean's office received $10,000 to be used in honoraria for trainees.[54]

Full-time versus Part-time Professors
One of the most significant changes to take place during this period was the appointment of full-time professors in the clinical departments. The movement towards full-time clinicians in medical education, strongly recommended by the 1910 Flexner Report, was slow to catch on in

Canadian circles. Since the appointments of Pope and Mewburn in the early 1920s, no full-time clinical professors had been appointed at the University of Alberta's medical college. After World War II, the advantages and disadvantages of full-time clinicians became a hotly debated topic, not only in the medical profession but also with the administrative bodies of the universities. In 1948, the Board of Governors of the University of Alberta became "a little exercised over the seemingly endless procession of part-time medical appointments."[55] The board queried not only the number of part-time teachers but also their qualifications for teaching, selection procedures, and the whole question of the ratio of classes that should be taught by part-time, as opposed to full-time, professors. Dean Scott discussed these concerns with the board, and at the same time President Newton contacted presidents of other Canadian universities regarding the policies in their medical schools with respect to part-time and full-time appointments. The replies were epitomized by F. Cyril James, principal of McGill University, who said: "The problem to which you refer . . . is one that exists in practically every Medical Faculty." While McGill (and most other schools) had full-time appointments for heads of major departments, "most of our clinical departments are staffed by leading physicians and surgeons, who for a modest stipend do a good deal of splendid teaching on a part-time basis." While James acknowledged the difficulties in administering a large part-time staff, he felt that "the relations with the medical profession and the general public that result from eminent clinicians serving as members of the part-time staff, is a very happy one."[56]

Some members of the profession felt strongly that those who taught aspiring physicians should themselves be actively involved in the practice of medicine on a day-to-day basis, and should bring their current knowledge and experience to the classroom. Others argued that patients would, and should, have priority on the time of part-time professors with a private practice, regardless of their dedication to the students. Many felt the introduction of the full-time "academic physician" or "professor physician" would only lead to a widening of the already deep gulf between "town and gown." To keep up with advances in medicine and in medical education, however, the medical school needed faculty members whose first priority was their students. As Alberta was widening its focus from a school solely for training general practitioners, and because the trend towards full-time appointments was gathering momentum across the country, many felt that the medical school should move with the times.

There were, however, several administrative problems to be resolved.

Experience at Alberta had shown that local practitioners generally were not interested in giving up private practice to take on full-time positions at the university. The difference between a professor's salary and one that could be earned in private practice was substantial.[57] To meet the concerns on all sides of the discussion, the university adopted the "geographic full-time" concept that was followed in several other medical schools. Under this system, a full-time professor was allowed to maintain a consulting practice but his office had to be located "geographically" within the university's teaching hospital. The financial arrangements, approved by the Board of Governors in 1959, established a ceiling of $10,000 a year in excess earnings, "with the privilege of retaining 50% of professional earnings above this level, with 25% of the balance going into a departmental fund, and 25% into a Faculty fund."[58] Another problem concerned office space. The superintendent of the University of Alberta Hospital, Angus McGugan, opposed the idea as he was required to find office space at the already overcrowded hospital for geographic full-time professors. Although Pope and Mewburn had both had consulting offices in the hospital, these had long since been taken over for other purposes;[59] however, office space for full-time professors was incorporated into plans for a further addition to the hospital and McGugan's resistance subsided.

The first geographic full-time appointment was the head of the department of medicine in 1954, to succeed Dean Scott. It was also the first administrative position in the Faculty of Medicine to be filled under new regulations requiring the appointment of a President's Advisory Selection Committee. On the recommendation of the Survey Committee of the early 1940s, President Newton instituted regulations concerning the hiring and promotion of professors, and each faculty was required to form an advisory selection committee, which then made recommendations to the president. Eight people applied for the position of head of the department of medicine, but some were immediately disqualified as they were not fellows of the Royal College of Physicians and Surgeons of Canada.[60] The committee based its assessment on four factors: competence in the classroom; executive capabilities; an interest in research; and an ability to get along with fellow workers. The unanimous decision to recommend Donald R. Wilson for the position was accompanied by a suggestion that the appointment should be full-time.[61]

Donald Wilson's father, W.A. Wilson, was one of Edmonton's pioneer doctors and had been an associate professor of surgery in the young medical school. The younger Wilson began his medical training at the University of Alberta and in 1934 won a Rhodes scholarship to Oxford University in England. Upon his return to Canada, he completed his medical degree at McGill, his father's *alma mater*. By this time, the country was at war and Wilson went straight into the Royal Canadian Air Force. He returned to Edmonton and the Faculty of Medicine after the war as a part-time teacher, and later began to develop an endocrine laboratory in the original wing of the University of Alberta Hospital.[62]

Over the next few years, other geographic full-time appointments were made in clinical departments: Robert S. Fraser and J.A.L. Gilbert in internal medicine; Robert A. Macbeth and R. Cameron Harrison in surgery; W.M. Paul in obstetrics and gynaecology;[63] J. K. Martin and W.C. Taylor in pediatrics; and K.A. Yonge in psychiatry.[64] Space for consulting offices was made available in the new addition to the hospital, and money for secretarial assistance was provided through the Faculty of Medicine and the hospital.[65] Foundations began to provide assistance also. The Markle Foundation awarded twenty-one scholarships annually to medical schools in the United States and Canada to provide "both academic security and financial aid to faculty members at the start of their careers in academic medicine." The scholarships covered a five-year period and provided $6,000 a year to assist the university in hiring full-time clinical and research scholars.[66] They were instrumental in promoting the full-time concept, as well as enabling young scholars to fulfil research activities, and played a significant role in the establishment of the full-time system at Alberta.

Drs. Donald A. Wilson, Robert S. Fraser and Lionel E. McLeod each received a five-year Markle Foundation scholarship, and they ran consecutively from the period 1948 to 1963. Following graduation from the University of Alberta in 1946, Robert S. Fraser carried out research work in biochemistry and earned an M.Sc. in 1950. He then took postgraduate training in hospitals in Edmonton and Vancouver and at the University of Minnesota, where he obtained a fellowship to conduct research in the field of cardiology.[67] After his return to Edmonton, he established a cardiovascular unit, and received the first Muttart Research Associate Professorship in Medicine. Fraser later succeeded Donald Wilson as head of the department of medicine, and was closely involved with open-heart surgery at the University of Alberta Hospital. Lionel McLeod, the third recipient of a Markle scholarship, later became dean of the Faculty of Medicine at the University of Calgary, and from there received the appointment of president of the newly established Alberta Heritage Foundation for Medical Research.

Visit of the Liaison Survey Committee, 1956

Despite these full-time appointments, part-time teachers still conducted much of the clinical teaching and often served as heads of departments. There were still too few full-time professors in both the medical and clinical science departments, and they were too busy with their teaching schedules and administrative duties to initiate any changes in a curriculum that had remained static for many years. Aware of changes in curriculum and teaching methods taking place in more progressive schools, certain members of the faculty felt the need for professional guidance in adapting these changes to Alberta's medical school. One way of achieving this was to request a "visitation" by an accreditation team of the Education Committee of the American Medical Association. The team typically consisted of three or four experienced academics, who could not only point out deficiencies and problems in a school but also offer expert advice on how to overcome such problems. Since the formation of the Association of Canadian Medical Colleges in 1943, the team included a Canadian when Canadian colleges were being assessed.[68]

The acccreditation team that visited Alberta consisted of a representative from each of the Association of American Medical Colleges, the Council on Medical Education and Hospitals of the American Medical Association, and the Association of Canadian Medical Colleges. Jointly known as the Liaison Survey Committee, its visit in May 1956 was to accomplish three objectives: first, to assist with solving problems faced by all medical schools; second, to identify areas of concern specific to Alberta; and third, "to evaluate the educational experience of the medical students at the University of Alberta in the light of the aims and standards set forth by the three Associations." The committee's report clearly emphasized the opinion that general practice carried on by individuals in isolation was "incompatible with optimum patient care" as currently viewed by society. As Alberta's Faculty of Medicine had traditionally been a training school for individual practice, it was obvious that major changes in policy, curriculum and methods of teaching would be recommended.[69]

In summary, the Liaison Survey Committee identified areas of strength to support future development, but also pointed out many areas of concern in the medical school and urgently recommended a number of changes. The report assessed each department individually and offered suggestions for changes and improvements. Many of the problems emanated from the medical school's rapid growth during the postwar years, after a long period of limited economic growth, reflecting the general experience in Alberta.[70]

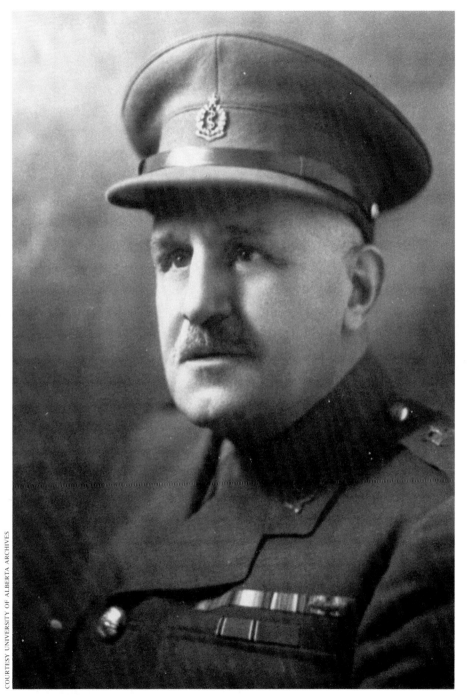

Dean Rankin in military uniform, c. 1940.

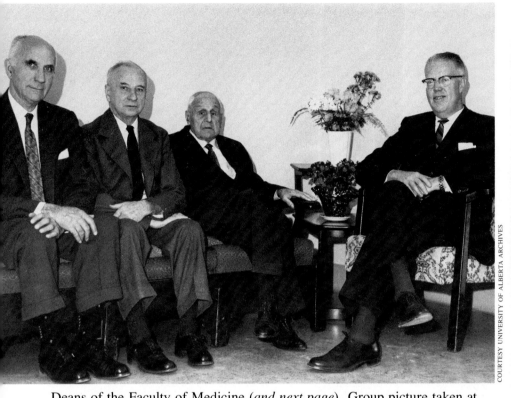

Deans of the Faculty of Medicine (*and next page*). Group picture taken at the time of W.C. Mackenzie's appointment in 1959, and just a few days before Dean Rankin's death. *Left to right:* John W. Scott, 1948-59, John J. Ower, 1944-48, Allan C. Rankin, 1919-44, Walter C. Mackenzie, 1959-74.

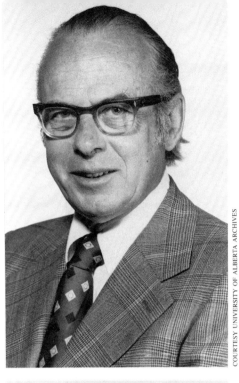

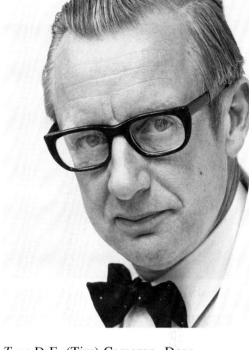

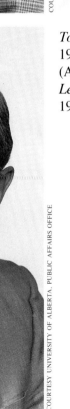

Top: D.F. (Tim) Cameron, Dean, 1974-83; and Robert S. Fraser (Acting), 1983-84.
Left: Douglas R. Wilson, Dean, 1984 to present.

Premier Peter Lougheed opening the W.C. Mackenzie Health Sciences Building. *On platform, left to right:* John Schlosser, Chairman, Board of Governors, University of Alberta; Mrs. Jeanne Lougheed; Peter Owen, Q.C., Chairman, University Hospital Board of Directors; Dr. Bernard Snell, President, University Hospital.

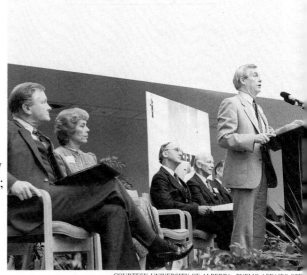

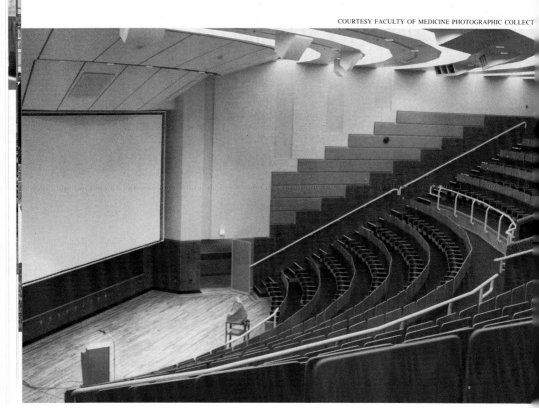

The Bernard Snell Hall in the W.C. Mackenzie Health Sciences Centre.

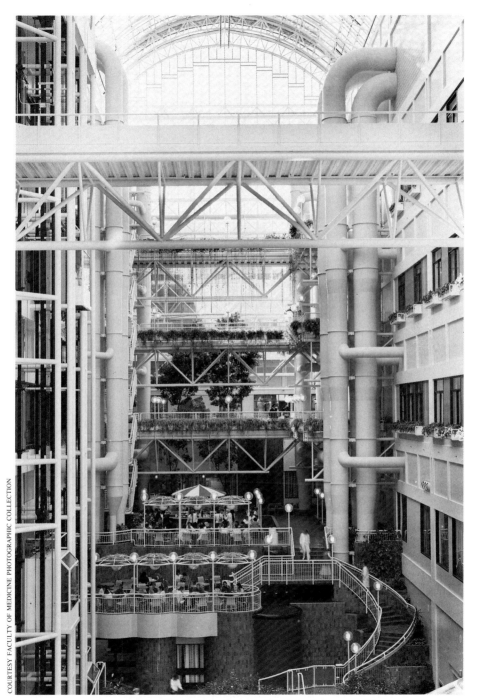

Five-storey atrium in the W.C. Mackenzie Health Sciences Centre.

The John W. Scott
Health Sciences
Library in the W.C.
Mackenzie Health
Sciences Centre.

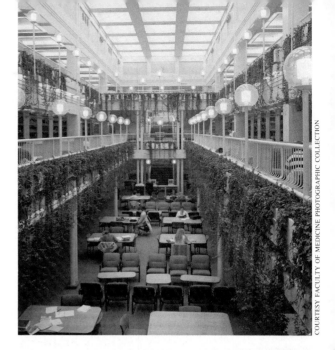

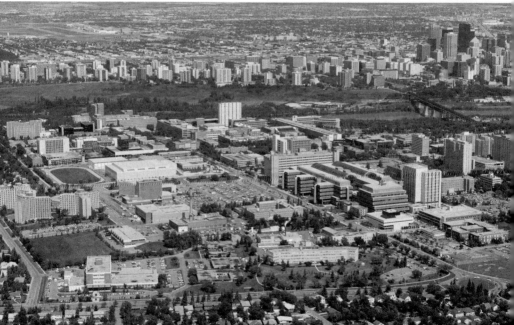

Aerial view of the campus of the University of Alberta, looking northwest towards the High Level Bridge, the legislature buildings and downtown Edmonton. The W.C. Mackenzie Health Sciences Centre is in the right centre, and is flanked by the Clinical and Medical Sciences buildings. The original Medical Building is two blocks due north of this medical complex.

The committee applauded the medical school's adoption of geographic full-time appointments in clinical departments, but recommended the addition of many more staff members. The team felt strongly that the responsibilities of staff members to students other than medical students threatened the primary functions of the medical faculty—the training of physicians and research for the acquisition of new knowledge.[71] The curriculum had not changed and had remained fragmented in a number of unrelated courses because of a shortage of staff in both preclinical and clinical sciences.[72] Didactic lectures were convenient ways of dealing with large numbers in a limited period of time, but current needs required lifetime habits of self-education that could not be encouraged in a lecture format. The team pointed out the "severe limitation of space for the proper development of pre-clinical departments and a critical shortage of space for the clinical departments."[73] It recommended an outpatient department at the University of Alberta Hospital and an immediate increase in staff in all the basic medical science departments and in the clinical departments as well. Given the relative isolation of the school, the team felt travel expenses were inadequate and recommended that staff members be encouraged to visit other schools to study teaching methods and to use this information as background for changes within their own departments.[74] Overall, the recommendations called for an increase in staff, facilities and budget. While the Liaison Committee expressed confidence that the medical school could solve these problems, given the necessary support, it nevertheless recommended a "confidential probation" of two years, followed by another visit to determine its subsequent status.[75]

As can be imagined, the report of the accreditation team was greeted with consternation and concern, though not by those members of the faculty who had been well aware of deficiencies in the school in the areas of both staff and facilities. It did come as a shock to the university's President, Chancellor, and Board of Governors, as well as to the provincial government, all of whom had apparently taken little or no notice of the yearly warnings of the Dean of Medicine. Suddenly, the possible loss of a Grade A rating for their medical school became a matter of great urgency. Its loss would reflect seriously on both the undergraduate and graduate teaching programme, as graduates would not be eligible for further training and advanced standing in the medical profession.

President Stewart and the Chancellor promptly called a meeting of the dean and all department heads on 15 May 1956 to examine the situation thoroughly.[76] These officials struck two committees, one made up of clinical department heads and the other of the heads of the medical science departments, to analyse their respective needs for staff, facilities and curriculum. The clinical departments recommended that all department heads be geographic full-time appointments, that each department have a nucleus of full-time appointments, and that the dean also be full-time, in keeping with the trend in medical schools across the country. While they agreed with the Liaison Committee's recommendations for changes in curriculum and improvements in teaching methods, they emphasized that improvements could not be accomplished without the recommended additional staff.[77]

The basic sciences committee also supported the changes suggested by the accreditation team and recommended that the academic year be increased from twenty-eight to thirty-three weeks, starting immediately, with a revised first-year curriculum that would incorporate small-group teaching. They also emphasized the need for a considerable number of new staff appointments, as well as more space in all departments, to implement improvements in the curriculum and teaching structure. This committee pointed out, however, the necessity for some adjustments to the salary scale to decrease the disparity between academic and industrial salaries for basic scientists. Since the end of the war, it had been extremely difficult to obtain superior applicants for vacancies in the basic science departments.[78]

Such major changes in most areas of a school take a great deal of time and money to implement. Faculty members and university administrators worked together to carry out as many of the recommendations of the accreditation committee as they could. Before the next academic year, the faculty appointed three full-time staff members in the basic medical sciences and two geographic full-time headships on the clinical side. The budget contained provisions for at least another ten appointments, and selection committees were already at work to fill these positions. An addition to the Provincial Laboratory, offering improved teaching facilities, was approved and ready for occupancy in the fall of 1959. The faculty revised its plans for a centre wing, to be constructed between the east and west wings on the north side of the Medical Building, and designed a six-storey T-shaped building incorporating the existing McEachern Cancer Laboratory. A service wing and outpatient facilities at the University of Alberta Hospital were expected to be finished by the summer of 1960.[79] The faculty extended its academic year to thirty-three weeks and greatly reduced lecture time. The new first-year curriculum went into effect immediately, and curriculum changes for subsequent years of the programme took place one year at a time. Some of the departments still taught many students from other faculties, but they all considered the teaching of medical students and medical research to be their prime responsibilities.[80]

One gratifying result of the accreditation report was an increase in the faculty's budget from $394,000 in 1956, the year of the report, to $825,000 in 1959. This substantial increase allowed for not only a number of new full-time positions in both the preclinical and clinical departments but also an increase in salary for all faculty members.[81] Travelling expenses increased markedly as well, and many members of the staff made trips to several medical schools, both in Canada and the United States, to study practices in their own fields.

As the new curriculum was not fully in place until 1959, and most of the additional space was not ready until that time, the accreditation team delayed its return visit until 1959. This time, it was a four-member team, but representative of the same three institutions. The team was impressed by the ''remarkable changes'' that had taken place over the previous three years, and expressed itself as ''gratified'' that the 1956 report had proven a useful vehicle for the medical faculty to obtain greater support for the changes needed to improve conditions at the school. While this was not a time for complacency, such a ''striking degree of improvement had occurred'' that the team was pleased to recommend that the school be returned to ''Full Approval.'' The school retained its Grade A rating.[82]

* * * * *

CHAPTER 4

From Medical School to Health Sciences Centre

The sixties to the present

THE 1960s was a decade of tremendous growth and unprecedented changes in administration and organization within the University of Alberta. "In its entire history, no period reflected greater excitement and organizational turbulence."[1] During this period the first "baby-boomers" reached university age, academic staff began to demand increased participation in the policy and the internal government of their institutions, student unrest emerged as a potent force for change in universities across the country, and in Alberta a new university act called for significant changes in the lines of responsibility and the hierarchy of the institution. After the flood of war veterans had worked their way through the institution, the university had settled down to a much slower growth in the 1950s; but this was the calm before the storm—a prelude to the explosion of the sixties when enrolment almost tripled, from 6,400 to 17,300.[2] To provide buildings, equipment and faculty to cope with this tremendous expansion were problems enough, but the new act created even more.

Under the terms of the new University Act of 1966, although the Board of Governors retained ultimate responsibility, essentially major decisions now rested with the General Faculties Council, as its role expanded to include matters of policy in most aspects of university life. To deal effectively with this considerable expansion of its responsibilities, GFC needed a new and much expanded committee structure. It took several years to implement the statutory requirements of the Act fully, and the effect was to make almost every decision about university life by committee. To make any move, the President had first to deal with a series of committees, usually composed of an elected membership, which slowed down progress considerably.[3] Over the years, professors and, in ever increasing numbers, students gained increased representation in all aspects of the administration and government of the university. In the 1960s, democracy invaded the halls of academe, and it came to stay.

Changes took place in the field of medicine also. In 1961, the federal government appointed a royal commission on health services to look into the existing facilities for health care in Canada. Under its mandate, it was also required to assess future needs as well as to propose methods of ensuring the "best possible health care for all Canadians." Chaired by Mr. Justice Emmett Hall of Saskatchewan, over the next two years the Hall Commission conducted a detailed study of all aspects of medical care in the country, including medical education.[4]

The Hall Commission developed a "Health Charter for Canadians," the essence of which was a comprehensive and universal health services plan for the country. At the same time, however, the commission expressed grave concerns about the ability of the existing medical schools to supply a sufficient number of qualified physicians to meet the increased demands that would result from the implementation of a universal health care system. It found the staffing of Canadian medical schools to be "seriously below accepted standards," and recommended a "great expansion of space, facilities and budget."[5] The commission proposed at least five new schools—one in Calgary—and considerable expansion for all the existing schools.[6] By this time, the enrolment in all medical schools was beginning to increase again, while the number of immigrant doctors continued to decline. The Association of Canadian Medical Colleges and most medical educators agreed that if some form of medical insurance scheme was to be implemented then more medical schools would be required. In addition, those already in existence would need considerably increased funding to acquire suitably qualified teachers, as well as teaching and research facilities in laboratories, lecture rooms and hospitals. Faculties of medicine across the country would face many challenges in the years to come.

While little real change had occurred in the University of Alberta's Faculty of Medicine since its early days, now broadly based changes took place over a relatively few years. They occurred in the dean's office; the structure of the Faculty Council; the curriculum; admission procedures;

methods of examining and evaluating students; selection and promotion of personnel; the objectives of the medical school; the process of administration; and the whole concept of a unified health sciences centre within the confines of the university. Expansion occurred in enrolment figures; the graduate training programme; the size of the faculty; the physical facilities and equipment; research activities; and the exponential growth of departments and divisions within those departments. Although the medical school's budget increased enormously, one thing that did not change was that it was never large enough. Expansion in some areas was rapid, whereas changes, which now required endorsement through the laborious committee structure, took much longer to put into place. Many involved curriculum and student evaluation, research, and student activities—all treated in separate chapters. The broad picture emerging from this overview is the metamorphosis of a parochial medical school in the hinterland of medical activity into a dynamic learning centre with a firmly established national position.

Appointment of Dean Walter Mackenzie

The first change to take place was in the occupancy of the dean's chair. In 1959, after thirty-six years of dedicated service to the medical school, Dean Scott retired, modest and unassuming to the end. His last years as dean were spent dealing with the many problems raised by the accreditation team and the school's successful efforts to retain its Grade A rating. The last four years of Dean Scott's tenure were a prelude to the rapid growth that would take place later, a period in which he sowed the seeds of change. In his letter to President Johns, however, he commented on the "very small contribution which I have made to the University as a member of the staff. The years have been very happy ones and the support of the Administration...have [*sic*] been very helpful in making my problems relatively simple."[7]

Government by committee extended throughout the university into all faculties, and perhaps the first major example in the Faculty of Medicine was the appointment of a committee to select a new dean. Dr. E.P. Scarlett, a Calgary physician who had recently completed his term as chancellor of the University of Alberta, chaired a committee that selected Walter C. Mackenzie from a small group of candidates from both within and without the University of Alberta. "Mackenzie should have first consideration," Scarlett wrote to President Stewart, for, his single-minded interest in the school, thorough knowledge of the faculty, informed knowledge, and his record in respect to research and graduate work...and more than the others, he has a national and international reputation.

While he was also "inclined to be arbitrary, has the so-called surgeon's temperament, and is a bit of a driver," these were all described as "good positive characteristics."[8]

A dynamic individual, Mackenzie was in the dean's chair throughout the sixties to guide and oversee the faculty during those turbulent years. Born in Nova Scotia, and educated at Dalhousie University, Mackenzie received his specialty training in surgery at the Royal Victoria Hospital in Montreal and the Mayo Clinic in Minnesota. He then came to Edmonton, principally on the advice of his father who believed that Canada's future lay in the west, and joined the Baker Clinic in Edmonton. Within a year of his arrival, Canada was at war, and Mackenzie spent the following six years as a surgeon-commander in the Royal Canadian Navy. He then returned to his practice in Edmonton, began teaching at the University of Alberta, and in 1950 succeeded H.H. Hepburn as professor and chairman of the department of surgery. Under his guidance, the department experienced a phenomenal growth. Robert Macbeth, his successor as head of surgery, called it "the golden decade of the department,"[9] and according to the accreditation report of 1959, it was Mackenzie's "vigorous and enthusiastic leadership and keen appreciation of the problems of medical education" that produced a high-quality graduate programme in surgery.[10]

From all accounts, one of Dean Mackenzie's main accomplishments was that he "put Alberta's medical school on the world map."[11] He did this by the force of his personality; by his dedication to his specialty, his school, and to the many surgical and medical organizations to which he belonged; by his friendliness, warmth and charm toward those he met; and by his love of travel. A big, heavyset man—known as "Big Walt" to his colleagues—he commanded loyalty and respect, and sometimes fear; but he had the ability to inspire others to work together as a team. He was also adept at delegating work to others when he found that administrative details took too much time away from teaching and his practice. "I'd never be happy as a full-time administrator," he said, "I let my department heads pretty well run things."[12] He was a "joiner," but those organizations with which he became involved benefited greatly from his enthusiasm and propensity for hard work, and he served as president of many of them, and on advisory boards or executive committees of others. He was, at various times, president of the Royal College of Physicians and Surgeons of Canada, the American College of Surgeons, the Association of Canadian Medical Colleges, and the International Federation of Surgical Colleges, to name but a few. An honour of which he was extremely proud was an honorary fellowship in the Royal College of Surgeons of Edinburgh, a surgical college that dated back to the seventeenth century. He received honorary degrees from Dalhousie, Manitoba and McGill Universities and the F.N.G. Starr Award, the most prestigious award of the Canadian Medical Association.

Even before he was appointed dean, Mackenzie already had an international reputation as a first-class surgeon. He was always ready to pack his bags and go off to attend the conferences and meetings of the many associations to which he belonged in Canada, the United States and abroad. Gregarious by nature, he met many people, had a phenomenal memory for names and personal family details, and had friends worldwide. On the journey home, he would write personal letters to those he had met, and encourage them to visit Edmonton. Many took him up on his invitation, visited the school, spoke to the students, and brought a greater international outlook to the school than it had ever experienced before. He was a gracious host, could develop an instant rapport on a one-to-one basis, and ''worked harder in preparing to be Walter Mackenzie than anyone would believe.''[13]

Before he accepted the position of dean, Mackenzie requested an assistant dean, on a part-time basis, preferably someone from a medical science department.[14] James S. Thompson, who had been executive secretary under John Scott, agreed to take the post of assistant dean, which gave him greater responsibility in the dean's office and left him in charge during Mackenzie's absences. Thompson resigned from this position in 1962 to return to full-time teaching and research in the department of anatomy, and D.F. (Tim) Cameron from the department of anaesthesia took his place. Cameron brought with him a great deal of administrative experience from his years in the army during the war, and a long and mutually agreeable relationship developed between the dean and his assistant. Quite different in nature, they understood each other well and together they fulfilled the onerous duties of the dean's office. Mackenzie was able to go off on his travels and leave Cameron in charge, and Cameron was equally proficient in fulfilling the administrative duties of the dean during his absences.

These absences were frequent and sometimes long. At various times, Mackenzie was the Moynihan Lecturer at the Royal College of Surgeons in England, the Munroe Lecturer at the University of Saskatchewan, the F.G. Thompson Memorial Lecturer at St. Joseph's in Missouri, and the Sommer Memorial Lecturer in Portland, Oregon. In 1962, he was named the Sir Arthur Sims Commonwealth Travelling Professor, when he was away for three months travelling and teaching at the University College of Jamaica in the West Indies, at the medical schools of Ghana and Lagos, Nigeria, and finally at the Royal Infirmary at Bristol in Great Britain. In 1971-72, he took a year's sabbatical to visit and study medical centres around the world, leaving Cameron as acting dean. Walter Mackenzie was well known in medical circles on many continents, and, as a result, so was the University of Alberta's Faculty of Medicine.

Early in his tenure as dean, Mackenzie established an executive committee to expedite procedures within the faculty. The Faculty Council was large and unwieldy, and it was difficult to achieve a consensus or arrive at decisions. The accreditation report had recommended an executive committee, and Dean Scott tried to set one up on several occasions. It was vetoed on each occasion, even though the Faculty Council consisted, in 1959, of forty-nine members. Individual council members expressed the desire to be involved in all faculty discussions and decisions and not to leave them to a select few. Dean Mackenzie did manage to establish one in 1960, however, with a membership that included himself, Thompson and three members each from the medical and the clinical sciences.[15] The Faculty Council then met only twice a year. Over the years, it grew in size, as, under the terms of the 1966 University Act, it included the Dean, the President, all full-time members of the academic staff, and a representative of the professional association. The council itself sought a number of additions: part-time heads of clinical departments; clinical professors and part-time professors; representatives of other part-time staff; Medical Research Council associates and scholars; a representative from each of Dentistry, Pharmacy, Nursing and Rehabilitation Medicine; and the Registrar.[16] It is difficult to imagine how any decisions were ever made.

Nevertheless the concept of an executive committee never sat well with the faculty as a whole. Discussion of its size and composition, its powers and responsibilities, took up a great deal of time at Faculty Council meetings on several occasions. As the committee structure swung into high gear, however, many staff members became involved on other committees, and the executive committee conducted a filtering process for committee reports before they were presented to the Faculty Council as a whole. Almost every aspect of life in the faculty had its own committee; the curriculum, examinations and student evaluation, admissions, research, search and selection committees for new faculty members, review committees, the library, test committees for selecting questions for examination, building committees, and on and on. Each one was carefully structured with equal numbers from the medical and clinical sciences, and from the student body, as well as representation from the dean's office. Most were rotating committees in which a certain number of members would be replaced each year; therefore, a nominating committee became an integral part of the whole system. Committee meetings were extremely time-consuming and demanded a great deal of effort from all those involved.

The Concept of a Health Sciences Centre

Mackenzie brought to the dean's chair a vision of a considerably enlarged medical school, and he began his tenure by taking what he called "an indoctrination tour" of medical schools across the country and in Great Britain. [17] Upon his return, he met with members of the faculty in various study groups to discuss the future of the medical school; to study the school's organization and curriculum and to compare it with that of other schools; to assess the continuing and expanding needs of society; and, finally, to consider what changes were necessary and how they could be implemented. The accreditation report of 1959 had restored full approval to the Grade A rating for the school and praised its many accomplishments, but it had also pointed out that "there was still room for further improvement."

In addition, changes were taking place in society as well as in medical education, changes that required thorough and detailed study. Beyond natural population increase, Alberta grew rapidly as its economy, now based on the oil industry, continued to improve and to attract migration from all parts of Canada as well as from other countries. It was clear that if the school was to fulfil its role of meeting the health needs of the people of Alberta, then considerable expansion would have to take place. In the previous ten years, only 28% of the physicians who registered for practice in Alberta had been graduates of its own medical school. To maintain an adequate supply of physicians for the expanding population of the province, the medical school would have to increase its enrolment substantially. This would require considerable expansion in the faculty and in space requirements for teaching, research and teaching beds in hospitals. As a result of his investigations of other institutions and current limitations on prospects for expansion of the medical school at the University of Alberta, Mackenzie proposed to the president and the Board of Governors that there was a need for a long-term plan to provide for the graduation of the required number of physicians for an expanding population. It was at this time, 1962, that a health sciences centre was first proposed, a centre that would combine all the health-related faculties and a teaching hospital on the same site.[18]

In the ten-year period 1958 to 1968, the number of students admitted to first year exactly doubled, from fifty-four to 108. The number of graduate students increased substantially as well, both those in the medical sciences who were going on to advanced degrees and those in the clinical sciences who were taking specialty training and working towards the certification or fellowship examinations of the Royal College of Physicians and Surgeons of Canada. Not only did more students enrol, but also curriculum changes required that they now spend much more time in the hospital during their clinical years. Consequently, their instructors, both part-time and geographic full-time, also spent considerably more time at the hospital, without any increase in hospital space. In addition, under the terms of the geographic full-time status of clinical teachers, the university agreed to give them office space within the University of Alberta Hospital where they could conduct a consulting practice. For this, each doctor needed examining and waiting rooms, and office space for both doctor and nurse/receptionist. With the increasing enrolment in the mid-sixties, additional geographic full-time personnel would be required, but space in the University of Alberta Hospital was extremely limited, and competition for space was fierce. There were horror stories of people using broom closets and coal sheds! Donald Wilson's first office had originally been the coalbin:

> The two rooms which I was allocated were so hot that they were almost beyond human endurance, and I noted, with somewhat pardonable pride, when I made my second move to somewhat cooler quarters, that my original office was converted into a quick drying room for rubber gloves from the operating room.[19]

The demands on the medical school and the hospital were enormous, in both faculty and space requirements. The size of the faculty did increase, in both full-time and part-time personnel, but there was still a need for more. The first step was to improve the facilities so that well-qualified personnel could be attracted to the medical school.

In 1961, a T-shaped central wing, six storeys high, was added to the back of the Medical Building at a cost of $2,750,000. This incorporated the small existing J.S. McEachern Cancer Research Laboratory, and added

22,000 square feet for the new Surgical Medical Research Institute. When this construction was complete, the remainder of the Medical Building was completely renovated to bring it up to current standards. For the time being, the departments of anatomy, physiology and biochemistry had sufficient space for teaching and for research. Dentistry, physiotherapy, nursing, pharmacy, and nonmedical bacteriology also had space in the building, renamed the Medical Science Building.[20] A special services wing added to the University of Alberta Hospital in 1960 included office space for some geographic full-time clinical staff of the medical school, a common room and locker facilities for the students, and outpatient facilities.[21]

Additional space was still urgently required for clinical teaching and research however, and in 1963 the Board of Governors proposed to renovate the old Education Building (now called Corbett Hall) for use as a clinical teaching and research wing. Even with the completed addition to the Medical Building, and this proposed renovation of the old Education Building, Mackenzie felt that within five years additional space would be required again. When the renovations to the Education Building proved to be too costly, this time frame was reduced substantially.[22] Finally, in 1965, Dean Mackenzie reported to the Faculty Council that a

> co-ordinated plan for all facilities associated with the hospital was being developed, and that steps were being taken to establish a Co-ordinating Committee of Health Science Faculties and facilities under joint sponsorship of the university and university hospital Boards of Governors.''[23]

A proposed new Clinical Sciences Building, with access to the University of Alberta Hospital, was already on the drawing board when the concept of a health sciences centre or medical centre reached this official level of discussion. Both the University of Alberta Hospital and the Faculty of Medicine were acutely short of space, equipment and facilities; but both were also concerned that new buildings and additions would duplicate facilities and create overlapping responsibilities. The concept of a centralized structure incorporating all health-related faculties and schools together with a teaching hospital was under consideration by medical educators across the continent. In 1965, J.D. Wallace, the executive director of the University of Alberta Hospital, attended a seminar on ''Relations between the Medical School and its Teaching Hospital'' organized by the American Association of Medical Colleges. As medicine was being taught more and more at the bedside, a closer relationship and understanding between the medical school and its primary teaching hospital became increasingly important. Administrators at both institutions agreed that planning for expansion of either or both should be co-ordinated. Further discussions at the seminar revolved around the co-ordination of management and budget, and the relationship with the parent university, and concluded that the "best solution lies in the development of medical centres in which faculties of medicine and their teaching hospitals become organized as important units in larger organizations."[24]

The concept of a health sciences centre was to provide a centralized area for both the teaching and practice of "comprehensive medicine—the preventive, diagnostic, therapeutic, and rehabilitative aspects of complete patient care." The ultimate goal was to make all health services available in the one area, including all health-related faculties and schools, so that faculty and students would learn to work together as a team and students would be prepared for a co-ordinated approach to patient care. It would be "a facility for the education and training of all those in the health professions... [and teach them] to relate health care training to health care delivery." Ideally, it would also integrate teaching, research and patient care and offer the opportunity for shared courses, faculty and facilities. Interdisciplinary teaching, research and services to patients would be both more efficient and convenient, make more efficient use of limited staff members, and promote the sharing of facilities.[25]

There was considerable discussion concerning the government of such a centre, and how it would relate to the University of Alberta. The university was, and would remain, the ideal environment for educating all health-care professionals. It was, indeed, the university's responsibility to produce well-qualified personnel in these professions, as it was in all other professions. A university setting provided a variety of resources necessary for both the students and faculty administration, the freedom for both research activities and experimentation with different educational methods. The co-ordinating committee agreed that the centre should be located on campus, be built around the primary teaching hospital, and remain in an academic relationship within the university. The committee, composed of representatives from dentistry, medicine, nursing, pharmacy and rehabilitation medicine, and the hospital, agreed to "support the formation of a Health Sciences Council within the general administrative framework of the university." The responsibilities of this council were to "initiate co-operation and co-ordination among the various health sciences faculties and schools and the hospital" with respect to education, research and patient care programmes.[26]

In 1965, the federal government, responding to a recommendation of the Hall Commission, established a Health Resources Fund of $500 million to be used in the construction of new medical schools and for new building in existing medical schools and teaching hospitals.[27] The government agreed to provide to the provinces, on a per capita basis, up to 50% of the cost of construction for new health science facilities, the funds to be matched by the province.[28] With this financial incentive, representatives of the university administration, the medical school, the hospital board and administration met with the provincial Departments of Public Health and Public Works to discuss the development of a health sciences centre, and subsequently received approval of the plan, to be phased in over a period of time. The first phase would co-ordinate the medical and nursing schools with the hospital, whereas dentistry, pharmacy and rehabilitation medicine would be incorporated at later periods, with the possibility of a psychiatric facility and a children's hospital at a still later stage. Development of the first phase, to be constructed to the south of the then present site of the hospital, included the Clinical Sciences Building and a new Basic Medical Sciences Building. Extensions to the Provincial Laboratory (which would include space for the departments of bacteriology and pathology) were incorporated as part of the development, as were the Central Services Building for the hospital, which would include an auditorium, a library and a cafeteria. The hospital also received "approval in principle" to build a clinical specialty unit.

Under a health sciences centre concept, all these buildings would revolve around a central hospital, and the entire development was planned for the area south of 87th Avenue and west of 112th Street. This necessitated the demolition of some of the older buildings in the area, such as the Mewburn and Wells pavilions. The long-range building programme was enthusiastically received by the faculty, however, as it "put the administration in an enviable position to attract and maintain academic personnel of high calibre. In the competitive field of academic staffing today, this is of vital importance."[29]

The Clinical Sciences Building opened in 1969, the first building within the concept of the new Health Sciences Centre. A thirteen-storey building, it provided much needed space for research and teaching facilities for the clinical departments. That same year, the provincial government approved the construction of a new "Centennial Hospital" which had been approved in principle several years previously and would be constructed in phases between 1971 and 1976.[30] Construction was already under way on the first phase of a new basic medical sciences building (completed in 1972) to house the departments of anatomy, bacteriology, and biochemistry. Located immediately west of the Mewburn Pavilion, it brought the basic medical scientists closer to the medical school/hospital environment and would "overcome some of the difficulties of communication and co-operation which had been aggravated by the physical separation of the Medical Building and the hospital."[31] With the completion of this building, the school was able to increase its enrolment to 118 in the fall of 1972.

An American firm was hired to plan the proposed Health Sciences Centre, which was to include both science buildings and the Centennial Hospital. The new hospital, destined to be a specialty hospital, was to be an eight-storey building, with one specialty on each floor and ambulatory care on the ground floor. It would add new and specialized technology to the hospital complex but was designed as an addition to the existing hospital, which would then be used for community service.[32] The proposal soon ran into financial problems, however, projected costs began to outstrip initial estimates, and in 1968 the government placed a ceiling on the cost of construction. Planning resumed, but costs soon outstripped the ceiling and construction was put on "hold" while the administration made changes to the plans to reduce costs. Finally, the ground was readied for construction to begin, the area was fenced off and the heavy equipment moved in; but coincidentally, a provincial election took place, the thirty-six-year-old Social Credit government went down to defeat and the new Conservative government, led by Peter Lougheed, put the project on "hold" once more. Only this time, the "hold" lasted five years.

It was not until October 1976 that the government announced its approval of a "world class" medical centre. Planning began again and the first phase of a health sciences centre was finally completed in 1984.[33] Different in concept from the Centennial Hospital, this centre, named for W.C. Mackenzie, was designed as an all encompassing medical centre to house the medical and nursing schools, the primary teaching hospital, the John Scott Library, a cafeteria and a food centre. There was no place for the old hospital buildings in this plan; the original hospital and the 1930 addition were demolished, and the 1950s addition was left empty. The faculties of dentistry and pharmacy remained in the old Medical Building, renamed the Dental/Pharmacy Building, and the Faculty of Rehabilitation Medicine occupied Corbett Hall.

From the end of the second world war, building seemed to be continuous: new buildings, additions to older ones or renovations. Departments moved around as they expanded and needed more space. Donald Wilson, as chairman of the department of medicine, moved his office seven times during his fifteen-year tenure.[34] Still construction was not yet complete. Two linked research buildings, one funded by the Alberta Heritage Foundation for Medical Research and one by the Health Sciences Centre project, were the latest additions to the complex. The Heritage Wing of the Heritage Medical Research Centre opened in November 1988, and the adjoining Clinical Wing opened a year later.

Student Enrolment
Recruiting measures by the faculty as well as the Canadian Medical Association resulted in an increase in student enrolment in the early 1960s. The increase gathered momentum during the latter half of the decade as the "baby-boom" generation reached university age. With greater competition for places in the medical school, the educational qualifications of those accepted improved also, and the dropout and failure rate began to decline. First-year enrolment increased to sixty-five in 1960, 18% over the previous year, and to seventy-nine in 1962. In 1964, 293 applied for admission, 199 of them students at the University of Alberta, and 110 were accepted—the first time more than one hundred students enrolled in first-year medicine.[35] Thereafter, the number of applicants always exceeded the available places.

The medical science facilities were barely able to accommodate this increased enrolment, and clinical science facilities were entirely inadequate. Nevertheless, because of the increasingly large number of qualified applicants from Alberta and the need to produce more physicians to facilitate the implementation of universal medical care, the faculty felt pressured to accept more students, and did so over the next several years. As can be seen in Table 5, the number of qualified applicants more than doubled between the years 1966 and 1979. The yearly intake increased to 118 in 1972, and stayed at that number over the next two decades. The vast majority of those accepted were Albertans, and most had taken their premedical studies at Alberta universities. About 6% each year were Canadians from other provinces who had taken their premedical studies at Alberta universities, foreign students on student visas, or landed immigrants. Such an admission policy, common to most Canadian medical schools, created a "provincialism," a lack of diversity in both cultural and geographic backgrounds, that caused some concern among educators.[36] As long as assistance programmes for students were financed by provincial authorities, however,

TABLE 5: APPLICATIONS AND ADMISSIONS TO THE FACULTY OF MEDICINE.[38] 1966-1979

Year	Applications Received	Registered in First Year	Accepted but declined
1966	342	104	24
1967	363	109	13
1968	365	108	22
1969	370	112	13
1970	404	112	20
1971	534	112	21
1972	626	118	29
1973	646	118	17
1974	576	118	17
1975	578	118	12
1976	543	118	16
1977	489	118	38
1978	609	118	19
1979	704	118	22

there seemed to be no easy way to alter this arrangement.[37]

With such an increasingly large number of applications each year, the responsibilities of the Admissions Committee became more demanding. Four elected faculty members, four elected student members, the dean, the assistant dean and the director of student affairs comprised this committee, which was responsible to the Faculty Council. In addition, the assistant registrar of the university and a member of Student Counselling Services always received invitations to attend meetings.[39] The committee met several times during the year, and its responsibilities went beyond determining the eligibility of the applicants and the selection of the requisite number of students. The members reviewed their policies and procedures in the light of the performances of applicants chosen in previous years to attempt to improve selection procedures, and recommended any changes that they felt might improve the process. They visited other Canadian and American schools to investigate their procedures, and took part in ongoing studies of selection procedures conducted by the Association of Canadian Medical Colleges and the Association of American Medical Colleges.

Essentially, admission to the medical school was based on academic standing, although the University of Alberta Calendar has always included the phrase "lack of essential personal qualities in an applicant may be deemed sufficient cause for refusal of admission.'' In the early 1960s a minimum 5.5 grade point average[40] (or 65% under the old grading system) was required to be considered for admission to the medical school. As the number of applicants increased, and the academic standing of those admitted gradually rose each year, so the minimum academic rating required for application increased.[41] By 1977, applicants needed a 6.5 grade point average, and by the 1980s a 7.0 average. The committee looked at several factors in determining the selection; academic performance, Medical College Admission Test (this examination became part of the application process in 1961), attitudes and motivation, extracurricular and student activities, ability to communicate, medical assessment where applicable, and general background. In actual fact, selection was based primarily on academic performance, although committee members made several attempts to broaden the base. It was difficult to assess a candidate's motivation and attitude from an interview, and from time to time they experimented with psychological testing, but found the results of little assistance. They admitted freely that ''only in the most unusual cases'' did any of the other factors change the ranking of the candidates based on overall academic performance.[42]

Those who had taken their entrance requirements at a university in Alberta and students from Alberta in attendance at other universities received priority, and committee members interviewed all these applicants. They discouraged those with little chance of success. With two medical schools in the province since 1971, Alberta enjoyed one of the highest ratios of places to provincial population in the country; yet, in 1977, only 24% of applicants to the University of Alberta's medical school were admitted.[43]

Similarly, the graduate training programme expanded dramatically, both in the number of approved courses and in the number of graduates in residence. Masters and doctoral programmes in the basic medical sciences drew students not only from the medical school but also in ever increasing numbers from other faculties, and in 1978 there were seventy-one graduate students in the preclinical departments. Basic science graduates who were interested in graduate studies in the medical field provided a stimulus for the growth of research activities in all departments and contributed to the increased national, and sometimes international, standing of the school.

Although most undergraduates at the medical school were Albertans, other parts of the world were well represented among the graduate trainees. When it first started, the residency training programme was designed principally for graduates of the University of Alberta medical school, but over the years a gradual change took place in the proportion of Alberta graduates in the training programme. As the stature of the school increased, more graduates from outside the province, and later from outside the country, applied for admission. As shown in Table 6 between 40% and 49% of those in graduate training from 1962 to 1967 came from outside Alberta.

By the 1960s, nineteen specialty courses were approved by the Royal College of Physicians and Surgeons of Canada; anaesthesia, bacteriology, general surgery, internal medicine, neurology, neurosurgery, obstetrics and gynaecology, ophthalmology, orthopaedic surgery, otolaryngology, pediatrics, pathology, physical medicine and rehabilitation, plastic surgery, psychiatry, radiology (diagnostic and therapeutic), thoracic and cardiovascular surgery, and urology. Subspecialties, particularly in the area of internal medicine, were under consideration, and within the next few years the Royal College recognized cardiology, gastroenterology and hematology and approved their training programmes. The Division of Postgraduate Medical Education also offered a programme in family medicine for residents preparing themselves for certification by the College of Family Physicians of Canada.

TABLE 6: COUNTRY OF ORIGIN OF GRADUATES IN RESIDENCY TRAINING[44] 1962-1967

	1962-63	1963-64	1964-65	1965-66	1966-67
Alberta	96	94	111	127	108
Rest of Canada	23	32	33	37	46
USA	1	1	2	2	3
UK	22	18	17	14	30
Commonwealth, South Africa & West Indies	-	2	5	6	3
Europe	12	10	12	2	4
Middle East	8	11	7	6	2
South & Central America	2	1	3	3	2
Pakistan & India	1	5	9	8	7
Philippines, Korea, China, Japan	7	7	12	8	9
Total	**172**	**181**	**211**	**213**	**214**

A long-standing problem in the graduate training programme was inadequate funding for the graduate students—specialty training was not accepted by the university's Faculty of Graduate Studies, as the students were studying for examinations set by another body. They were not then eligible for graduate teaching funds. Residents' programmes lasted for three, four or five years, depending upon the specialty, and some were unable to complete their course because of financial restraints. Eventually the Alberta Hospitals Services Commission, an arm of the provincial government, accepted the responsibility for the payment of residents; it also set a quota on the number of residents in Alberta's hospitals, and at the same time established a salary scale for the trainees. In 1977, 651 graduates applied for a total of only fifty first-year vacancies in the University of Alberta's graduate training programme.

The Royal College changed its procedures for accreditation of graduate training programmes in 1968, and instituted a more formalized and regular survey of specialty programmes and residents. From that time on the RCPSC and the Association of Canadian Medical Colleges co-ordinated their periodic on-site surveys of the residency programmes and the undergraduate schools to take place at the same time, usually every five to seven years. As for the results of the training programmes, sixty-six residents sat the RCPSC examination in 1976 and thirty-three passed both their oral and written examinations. Fifty per cent of candidates from across Canada were successful in the Royal College examinations that year, so Alberta's candidates performed exactly as well as the national average. The RCPSC examinations were designed to ensure a level of competence and satisfactory expertise of specialists. In 1977, Alberta's candidates did considerably better than the national average, as is shown in Table 7. As Assistant Dean Kling remarked, ''the surgical results would mean that this school must be just about number one in Canada on the 1977 examinations.''[45]

Intense competition for the limited spaces in both the undergraduate and graduate programmes of the medical school raised the standards for admission at both levels. To fulfil the demands of the universal medicare system, most medical schools admitted as many students as their facilities and available staff would allow. The University of Alberta increased its intake to 118 in 1972, even though this number stretched the current facilities. Subsequently, the quota did not increase because of uncertainties in the number of medical practitioners required in the country for optimum patient care. As for the graduate programme; interns and residents became

TABLE 7: RCPSC EXAMINATIONS, 1977. SUCCESSFUL CANDIDATES, BY PERCENTAGES, FROM THE UNIVERSITY OF ALBERTA AND THE NATIONAL AVERAGE

	Written Examination		Oral Examination	
	University of Alberta	National Average	University of Alberta	National Average
Medical Specialties	65%	61%	90%	72%
Surgical Specialties	90%	53%	100%	61%

an integral part of the infrastructure of the hospital system, and in Alberta the number was limited by the Alberta Hospitals Commission.

Curriculum, Evaluation and the R.S. McLaughlin Centre

Two of the major changes to take place in the medical school during these later years concerned curriculum and student evaluation. The former involved not only the subjects to be offered but also changing methods of teaching, interdisciplinary concepts, and early introduction of students into the hospital milieu. Vastly increased numbers of both students and instructors prevented personal knowledge and assessment, and the new breed of students opposed the traditional written examination as the sole method of evaluation. Although the University of Alberta's medical school tended to be a "follower" in the area of curriculum innovation, it was a leader in adopting new methods of student evaluation.

Important committees of the faculty were, therefore, the Committee on Research in Medical Education, which later became the Curriculum Advisory Committee, and the Student Evaluation Board, which evolved out of the Committee on Examinations. These two committees worked together closely, so that the objectives of the curriculum could be evaluated properly. Dr. J.A.L. Gilbert chaired the Committee on Research in Medical Education and also its successor, the Curriculum Advisory Committee. J.A.L. Gilbert, who spent many years at the University Hospital before moving over to the Royal Alexandra Hospital, spent a great deal of time studying changes in medical education and the most appropriate methods of changing the curriculum of the University of Alberta. The appointment of the Curriculum Committee in itself constituted a dramatic change in procedure, as traditionally the curriculum was in the hands of individual departments who were allotted a specified amount of time, which they filled with their own subject matter. Now, a committee composed of representatives from various departments, and eventually students as well, instituted integrated programmes, reduced hours in some cases, increased in them in others, and removed from some departments their long-held beliefs in the relative importance of their particular disciplines. A totally integrated curriculum, which co-ordinated basic medical sciences and clinical teaching, proved extremely difficult to implement in schools such as the University of Alberta's, which had a long-entrenched departmental structure; but it did result in each department studying its course content carefully and evaluating it in relation to the entire curriculum.[46]

The committee first set out the new aims and objectives of the Faculty of Medicine:

1. To educate medical students to a level from which, with appropriate further training, they can successfully undertake medical practice, teaching or research.
2. To inculcate in the students the habits of self-education.
3. To foster in the medical student a desirable professional attitude.
4. To fulfil the needs of this province for medical personnel of all types.[47]

The next step was to study the curriculum to determine where it fell short of these objectives, and to find the necessary solutions. The Curriculum Advisory Committee had a revolving membership of professors from both the clinical and medical sciences, as well as students from each phase of the programme. Its continuing efforts and the changes it initiated are dealt with in greater detail in Chapter 6. By the 1980s, the result was a four-year course divided into three phases. In the first year, Phase I offered medical science courses, while Phase II, in the second year, incorporated interdisciplinary teaching on a "systems" approach. Phase III covered the third and fourth years on a continuing basis, with just a four-week break in the middle, and students spent most of this time in hospital on clinical clerkships and elective studies. The recent pattern has featured constant study and review of the curriculum to meet the changing needs of society.

Examination and evaluation of students' progress is closely related to the aims and objectives of a curriculum. When the school was small, professors were able to get to know their students and to assess their capabilities on a personal basis. These assessments, together with written and oral examinations, were the traditional methods of evaluating student performance. The advantage of a personal assessment could also be a disadvantage, given the lack of guidelines and the risk of personality conflicts. It became even less equitable as enrolment increased. In the late 1950s, class pictures were distributed to all departments so that teachers could identify the students in their classes.[48]

One alternative was the adoption of comprehensive, multiple-choice examinations. Although the Faculty Council approved the concept of these ''in principle'' in 1963, it was several years before they adopted the procedure. Multiple-choice questions, already in use in the United States, were introduced only gradually into Canada because many teachers opposed the system. They felt that attitudes and motivation could only be assessed by a personal knowledge of the student, and that written examinations, if well designed and marked with care, were a better method of evaluating a student's knowledge and ability. However, multiple-choice examinations offered reliability in scoring, the elimination of any variance in marking, speed and ease in scoring, and coverage of a wide range of knowledge.[49]

After the dean received several criticisms and complaints about the examination system, including one from the Medical Students' Association, he established a Student Evaluation Board in 1970 to look into the development of a bank of multiple-choice tests. This was the first such board to be established in Canada, and its deliberations were therefore of considerable interest to other schools across the country. Its mandate was to establish a policy on evaluation procedures, including grading and scoring; to co-ordinate the scheduling and timing of examinations; to develop comprehensive examinations, using material submitted by department test committees; to conduct research in new examination techniques; and to conduct periodic reviews of evaluation procedures in relation to curriculum objectives.[50]

Test committees in each of the three phases of the medical school programme received the task of developing an appropriate number of test questions for each discipline or department. Test items included multiple-choice type questions, which contained both graphic and pictorial information, and were designed in such a way that they required a detailed knowledge on the part of the student to answer them correctly. Comprehensive examinations included questions from all departments that had taught students in a particular phase, and a weighting system allocated departmental contributions to the final mark of the student. Within two years, the pool of test items numbered 3,500, ''the largest such pool in the country," and the Student Evaluation Board anticipated an increase of 30% in the forthcoming year. Departments continued to supply examination questions, and in 1972 an exchange programme between universities provided even more. Alberta, Western Ontario and Dalhousie adopted a complete exchange programme at that time, and Memorial, Calgary, Queen's and British Columbia indicated an interest in developing similar exchange programmes. Computer programming stored, retrieved and marked the questions, which were subject to constant review and assessment. Although students were not initially involved in the preparation of test items, in 1971, ten Phase III students helped to prepare, revise and edit test items and "made valuable contributions to the process." As a result, students became involved more closely in the development of test items in other phases as well.[51]

Some faculty members disapproved of this new method of examining and evaluating students; they felt that they had lost control of the evaluation procedures in their particular disciplines. In its second year of operation, some departments requested that they be entirely responsible for final examinations in their discipline for first-year medical students. While some of their colleagues sympathized, it was felt that a "return to departmental control of written examinations would be a retrogressive step."[52]

The medical school was fortunate to have Donald R. Wilson to shepherd these new evaluation procedures into existence. His expertise with multiple-choice examinations began in the early 1960s as a result of his role as an examiner for the RCPSC. At this time, the Royal College examinations consisted of written essays, oral and clinical examinations. With relatively few guidelines on assessing candidates, the validity and reliability of such procedures came under serious questioning by those conducting the examinations. Multiple-choice questions had been used in the United States for the previous ten years, and Wilson agreed to investigate their procedures. He approached the National Board of Medical Examiners in the United States and the American Board of Internal Medicine, and, thanks to their help and assistance, was able to provide three hundred test items to examine scholars in internal medicine. Over the next few years, similar examinations were developed for various other specialties. The Medical Council of Canada, which examined doctors for their licentiate to practise medicine in Canada, asked Wilson to conduct a national survey of its examinations, and as a result changed its procedures and adopted the objective multiple-choice questions.

Most of these questions, however, were still being developed in the

United States, and to produce a Canadian pool of test items the RCPSC sought funding from the R.S. McLaughlin Foundation to develop an evaluation system in the field of graduate studies in Canada. In 1967, the college received a grant of $250,000 that enabled Wilson to establish a unit in Edmonton. With the assistance of Brian Hudson, an Australian physician who received the first J.B. Collip Visiting Professorship in the department of medicine, he set up a computerized base for storage and retrieval of multiple-choice test items. In 1969, Wilson retired from the chairmanship of the department of medicine in order to devote his time fully to directing the R.S. McLaughlin Examination and Research Centre.[53]

The McLaughlin Centre maintained a close relationship with the University of Alberta and had its offices in the medical school complex. A $300,000 donation from the Gladys and Merrill Muttart Foundation in 1973 enabled the centre to develop a totally computerized bank of examinations that could be ''run over a national computer network in both English and French.'' By 1980, it not only produced certifying examinations for the RCPSC and the MCC but also for the Corporation Professionelle des Médecins du Québec, the medical schools of the Universities of Alberta, Laval, McGill, Montreal and Sherbrooke, and the Royal Australian and New Zealand College of Psychiatrists. The ''Research'' in the title indicated investigations designed to improve methods of evaluating physician competence and to develop and evaluate the use of computers in undergraduate and graduate instruction and evaluation.

The centre, a division of the RCPSC, continued to play an integral role in the world of Canadian medicine from its headquarters in Edmonton. It had two divisions, one in Edmonton for English-language activities and the other in Quebec City for translation and French-language activities. In the 1980s the McLaughlin Centre ran afoul of traditional Canadian East-West rivalries. The Royal College was never entirely happy with its evaluation centre being so far away in the West, and moved it to be near its headquarters in Ottawa in 1986.

Community Service in the North

The traditional roles of a medical school are threefold: the training of medical practitioners; research activities that will result in improved patient care; and service to the community. The Faculty of Medicine has participated over a number of years in community health care programmes in northern Canada. From the early 1960s residents and faculty members in pediatrics, psychiatry, medicine, and obstetrics and gynaecology had visited Inuvik, Yellowknife and Hay River for from four days to two weeks every four months, a programme reminiscent of the travelling clinics of the 1920s when health-care workers travelled through the newly settled districts of Alberta. In the 1970s, following negotiations with the director of medical services for the northern region, the medical school agreed to provide health-care and educational opportunities for those living in the north and also to conduct research in the western Arctic in co-operation with the federal government.

The programme provided for visits by graduate students and faculty members, an undergraduate training course and an ambulatory care programme in the Inuvik and Mackenzie zones. Residents in the departments of pediatrics, gynaecology, ENT, ophthalmology and medicine made six visits a year of two weeks each, and faculty members arrived for the second week of each visitation. Both groups assisted in the care of patients at the Inuvik Hospital and its affiliated nursing stations, and they provided teaching programmes for medical, nursing and technical staff. The school offered continuing medical education programmes to practitioners in Yellowknife, Hay River, Fort Smith, Fort Rae and Fort Simpson.

The Faculty of Medicine began as a school to train doctors for the rural communities of Alberta. The shortage of doctors in outlying districts has continued, and the faculty has made efforts to promote an interest in this area. In the 1970s, an undergraduate elective programme enabled four students to take part in northern health care for periods of sixty days each.[54] Several undergraduates selected electives in the field of community and northern medicine, and others took programmes on "northern medicine" at the Charles Camsell Hospital. The school has had a long and close relationship with this hospital, which traditionally provided care for native peoples and other patients from the north.

Expansion of Administration and Departments

Walter Mackenzie retired in 1974, after fifteen years in the dean's chair. He had been the first dean of the faculty to be chosen by a selection committee, in response to the new procedures inaugurated by President Newton following the second world war. The President chose the members of that small selection committee himself. Since that time, the University Act of 1966 had brought about much more democratic, but time-consuming, procedures. The selection committee for Mackenzie's replacement consisted of the university Vice-President (Academic), the Dean of Graduate Studies, three full-time academic members elected by the medical school faculty, three full-time students of the faculty (two undergraduates and one graduate), one person elected by the University General Faculties Council, one person nominated by the professional organization, and a representative of the University of Alberta Hospital. Even this was not enough, apparently, as Dean Mackenzie asked to have representation from the part-time clinical staff added to the committee.[55]

Tim Cameron was selected to succeed Mackenzie. He had served as assistant dean for several years and as acting dean from time to time during Mackenzie's many absences, so he certainly "knew the ropes."[56] Cameron, who took his medical training at the University of Alberta and specialized in anaesthesia, was a born-and-bred Edmontonian whose association with the University of Alberta was of long-standing. His father was the university's first librarian, for whom the Cameron Library on the university campus was named. Cameron served as dean until 1983, and his term covered a period of tremendous growth in the faculty—in its facilities, in increased staff, in the expansion of departments, and in research activities. When he took over, the school was in the five-year hiatus between the cancellation of the Centennial Hospital and approval of the Health Sciences Centre, and inadequate facilities were once again a major problem. It was a difficult period, during which he was involved in a multitude of discussions—with university and hospital administrators, as well as government officials and agencies concerning future developments of the health sciences faculties. It was also a period when no renovations or additions received approval, not even repairs, unless they were absolutely necessary. After the government finally gave its approval for the construction of the Health Sciences Centre, he was closely involved with its planning and construction. During his tenure, administrative duties increased sufficiently that additional administrative positions were necessary in the dean's office, and by the late 1980s there were five assistant and associate deans.

Cameron retired in 1983, the same year that the W.C. Mackenzie Centre opened. Robert Fraser held the position of acting dean for one year, and, in 1984, Douglas Wilson was appointed. He was a graduate of the University of Toronto, was the head of the division of nephrology at that university prior to coming to Edmonton, and was the first dean of medicine of the University of Alberta to come from outside the school.

Expansion took place throughout all departments during these years. All medical science departments experienced considerable growth in and after the 1960s, yet, the departmental organization remained much the same throughout the history of the faculty. Physiology and pharmacology became two distinct departments in 1961, pathology separated from the Provincial Laboratory, and anatomical pathology emerged as a subspecialty. Bacteriology also separated from the Provincial Laboratory to become the department of medical microbiology. Two departments were added: immunology (predominantly a research department) and biomedical engineering. All departments grew considerably in staff and research activities, as well as in masters and doctoral programmes, particularly in the department of biochemistry.

Clinical divisions developed within the department of medicine, and over the years some split off and became departments themselves. Pediatrics, the first to do so, became a department in 1956, under the chairmanship of Kenneth Martin. Keith Yonge headed the new department of psychiatry in 1957, established a graduate training programme, and in 1959 established a division of child psychiatry. In 1960, as rapid developments took place in the field of anaesthesia, that division was elevated to the status of a department under the chairmanship of E.A. Gain. As undergraduate enrolment increased and specialties and graduate specialty programmes developed in the 1960s the department of medicine established major divisions, each of which had a director. In 1984, the department had twelve academic divisions—cardiology, dermatology, endocrinology and metabolism, gastroenterology, general internal medicine, clinical hematology, immunology and nephrology, infectious diseases, neurology, medical oncology, pulmonary medicine, and rheumatology. By the 1980s, new clinical departments included family medicine, public health and preventive medicine, health services administration and community medicine.

The department of surgery was also organized into a number of divisions, each with a divisional director. The eight divisions already established in this department by 1960 continued through to the late 1980s; general surgery, orthopaedic surgery, urology, plastic surgery, neurosurgery, thoracic and cardiovascular surgery, otolaryngology, and experimental surgery. Each division developed its own graduate training programme, and the division of experimental surgery offered a Ph.D. programme.

The rise in specialties within the clinical departments of the medical school led to a commonly held belief that the University of Alberta had become predominantly a "specialty school," in which graduates were encouraged to follow a specialty, leaving few to enter family practice. The results of a 1988 survey belie this theory. The survey covered those 1,443 students who graduated with M.D.s between 1973 and 1985. In 1988, 51%

were in training for or practising a specialty, and 49% were in training for or practising family medicine.[57] Other interesting statistics from the survey revealed that 89% of those graduates remained to practise in Canada, and 62% in Alberta; and that 62% of the graduates practised in metropolitan areas, 17% in medium and small cities, 11% in towns with populations of 5,000 or less, and 10% in villages and rural areas.[58]

* * * * *

Tremendous changes took place in the Faculty of Medicine over a period of close to thirty years, including changes in physical stuctures, concepts of teaching and student evaluation, and, perhaps most importantly, in the basic philosophy of the school and its vastly increased faculty and departmental structure. The sense of isolation that had pervaded the school for so many years diminished as it achieved a national and even international reputation. Other changes took place: in the student body, not only in its size and composition but also in its rising participation in faculty discussions and decisions; in an increasingly urbanized and technology-oriented society; and in the medical profession itself, as the introduction of a universal health-care system created a demand for more physicians and improved health care. Nevertheless, the problems of increased enrolment combined with inadequate facilities made it difficult to attract high calibre instructors. More funding did become available, for the first time from federal government sources, but nevertheless the administration continued to struggle for approval for increased facilities and an expanded full-time faculty to adapt to these changes and to satisfy the needs of society.

* * * * *

PART II

CHAPTER 5

The Meds – and the Co-Meds

Student activities, female medical students and the Medical Alumni Association

TWENTY-SEVEN students registered in the first year of medicine at the University of Alberta in September 1913. They comprised a small percentage (6%) of the total student body of the young university, 434 at that time, but came from a similarly widespread geographic background. Half were from various centres in Alberta, and the remainder hailed from British Columbia, Saskatchewan, Ontario, New Brunswick, and two from England.[1] The members of the first medical class were older than the usual run of students, they were "dependent on their own resources...and... were here for business." An all-male class, they felt they were "the stamp of men the West needs, those whose chief interest is the profession of their choice."[2]

The class lost no time in becoming involved in university and medical activities. Bill Hustler was elected president of the class, they put together a plan to furnish a room in the newly opened South Side Hospital, and J.R. Hammond coached a basketball team whose achievements were "more modest than [their] ambitions."[3] When registration for the second year took place at 8:00 a.m. on 1 October 1914, however, only thirteen of the original class appeared. Over the next few weeks, two more returned, no doubt having to see the harvest in before they had the necessary funds to embark upon their second year.[4] The reason for the serious depletion in numbers can only be surmised, but it probably had much to do with events and the economics of the times. The first world war began in August 1914, and undoubtedly a number joined the services. Several failed their first-year course, and of these some were recent immigrants whose difficulties could be ascribed to an inadequate knowledge of the English language. In addition, Alberta's economy collapsed in 1913, and those who were "dependent on their own resources" might have had trouble finding the necessary money to carry on immediately into their second year.

Subsequent classes continued to attract older students. John Scott, later dean of the faculty, had been out of school for six years when he applied for admittance, and he was advised to take a three-month refresher course at Alberta College. At the conclusion of this, he wrote the Alberta Grade XI examinations and was admitted to first year.[5] Nathaniel James Minish had taught in rural schools and trained in pharmacy at the University of Manitoba before he registered in the second class of medicine at the University of Alberta at the age of thirty-six. He returned to Winnipeg to complete his medical degree at the University of Manitoba, but came back to practise in Edmonton in 1922 and to lecture in the anatomy department, a position he held for many years.[6]

Initially, the fees in medicine were $50 for the first year and $75 for the two subsequent years; and unless students had family or relatives in Edmonton, they were required to live in residence, which cost $26 a month. There was no financial assistance available for students in any of the faculties, except for a few scholarships and awards. In 1915, the College of Physicians and Surgeons of Alberta gave five scholarships to the medical school, each with a value of $50, for which there was strong competition. Entry was restricted therefore to those who had money or could raise it. Over the years, a number of students had to take a year off during their training to earn sufficient money to continue. Angus McGugan, who would later become superintendent of the University of Alberta Hospital, broke his training to teach school so as to able to continue with his course.[7] Herbert Begg, of the Class of '28, took a year off, claiming he "got tired of living with no money in [his] pocket."[8] Some spent a year assisting in the laboratories of the medical school, which, although delaying their training, offered worthwhile experience. Revell offered F.D. Facey a position in the anatomy and physiology departments in 1918, but he turned it down as he expected to make sufficient money during the summer to continue with his medical training without interruption. The crop failure in Saskatchewan that year put paid to that hope, so Facey belatedly accepted the position.[9]

The academic year lasted eight months, and most students worked during the summer months to earn sufficient money to see them through the next year. One of the students in the first year, Walter Morrish, worked on railway construction, with both the Alberta and Great Northern and the Grand Trunk Pacific railways. The following summer, he taught school near Veteran, Alberta, but a killing frost in the middle of August ruined the crop, and it was four months before the local school board was able to come up with the cash to pay his salary. When he went to McGill for his clinical years, wartime contingencies reduced the summer break to two months, so he and Bill Hustler returned to the West by the cheapest and quickest means possible—a "home-seeker's ticket" via Chicago and Winnipeg was only $40 return. Both served "locums," taking on the practices of doctors who wanted to take a holiday. They both realized the risks they were taking but,

> we played it safe, not sticking our necks out, and referring cases we weren't able to handle to other doctors. We learned a lot, particularly about what we would need to know to be successful general practitioners. Neither of us got into any grief, but there were times when we wished that we had those M.D. degrees up our sleeves.[10]

One of the students in the first graduating class, Leone McGregor, also taught school each summer to earn a sufficient amount for the following year, often not arriving back at university until two or three weeks after the term started. During her last couple of summers at the school, she was employed by Chautauqua, a travelling institution that brought cultural programmes to communities in the newly settled west. She travelled around the countryside, making arrangements and taking charge of some of the programmes. Apart from the fascination of the job, it also paid well, and she was able to arrive back at university with more than the minimum amount of money required to cover her fees and room and board.[11] J. Smith (Smitty) Gardner worked each summer at the Cominco smelting plant at Trail, B.C., operating the crane, weighing and pulling zinc.[12] A list of the summer jobs undertaken by medical students in 1923 included bronchobusting, bridge-building, time-keeping, clerking in a drugstore, working with an arctic survey party, acting as a hospital orderly, distributing soap coupons, coal mining, cooking for a survey party, working as a section hand on a railway crew, house painting, acting as a garage attendant, assisting in a V.D. clinic, farming, and serving as a deckhand on an oil tanker.[13]

During the first few years, students were required to wear academic gowns to all lectures and to certain university functions. The gowns were ''of the customary Cambridge shape; i.e. for undergraduates a black stuff gown, not falling below the knee with round sleeve cut above the elbow.'' Hoods were in the Oxford pattern, however, and the faculty colour for medicine was rose.[14] Gradually, the custom of wearing gowns was discontinued. During the years following the first world war, returned soldiers who swelled the ranks of all university classes might have contributed to certain changes in the attitudes and behaviour of students, causing much distress to the administration. Many students were ''restless and impatient of restraint to an extent never before observed in this institution... they challenged authority...creating a situation to be watched with care and handled with tact.''[15] President Tory reported on several occasions that maintaining discipline was a problem, and that the students' ''demand for social life and the lighter side of college life was insistent.'' When scholarship declined, he instituted ''more rigid checking of student activities.''[16] Expectations of a changing order prevailed in all Canadian society after the first world war, particularly among the ex-servicemen, and certainly university students were not immune to it. The new breed of students found such matters as wearing gowns to be unnecessary, resented the cost of purchasing new ones when they became ragged and worn, and were not afraid to let their feelings be known. In a much broader context, a continuation of these attitudes throughout the twenties and the thirties might account for the escalation of some of the more unruly activities of the student body.

In the years between the wars, the University of Alberta's Faculty of Medicine was a small school with an equally small and unchanging faculty. The relationship between student and professor was formal, but with a camaraderie and closeness that would have been impossible in a larger school. Because of the size of the classes and the rigidity of the curriculum, the students were together all the time and not only got to know each other well but also knew and were known by all their teachers.[17] Student and teacher met together socially on a number of occasions. Faculty members attended student parties and celebrations and supported school activities, and students were invited to the homes of faculty members. In May 1932, Ower wrote in his diary,

> Went with Allan Rankin to the home of Trowbridge—graduating class—where final year having a beano. Quite a number of senior members of faculty there—divided into sides and had a spelling match—mostly very complicated medical terms which we could not spell—Conn and Pope were the side leaders.

Even though the school offered the full degree programme from 1924 onwards, a number of students still continued to go to the East for their clinical years. The Class of '30 lost one-third of its members to eastern universities. Six students in the Class of '33 left at the end of their fourth year. The four top students in the Class of '34 left for McGill, as did a number of the Class of '37.[18] The prestige of a degree from an older medical school was a strong drawing card to those who could afford the added costs, and Alberta was still relatively unknown. Faculty members were both disappointed and disapproving when students made this move, for classes were small enough as it was. The number leaving gradually declined as eastern schools instituted quotas in the late 1930s making it more difficult for students to get in.[19]

The Medical Students' Club Established in 1917

The Faculty of Medicine was one of only five faculties on campus during the first world war. Arts and Science, Law, Applied Science (later renamed Engineering), and Agriculture were the other four. Its formative years were not an ideal time for the development of a school, as both staff and students went off to war. The number of registrants did increase slowly, however, and in 1917 they established the Medical Students' Club (MSC), generally referred to as the Med Club. Ann Curtin[20] was its first president, and two students who would later become members of the faculty, W.F. Gillespie and H.M. Vango, were on the executive. The objects and purposes of the club were: to assist in the training of students by means of presentation and discussion of papers by members of the medical and allied professions; to co-operate in advancing the interests of the university and university life; and to promote and encourage social activities.[21] Four lectures were offered that first year—on the medical profession, the history of medicine, the future of medicine, and the practice of medicine in India. The club composed a yell, and designed a pennant (emblazoned with the skull and crossbones) and a pin. The latter did not prove popular and was dropped, and later the symbol of the caduceus replaced the skull and crossbones.[22]

To fulfil the first part of its mandate, the MSC attempted to have a formal meeting with a speaker once a month, but this was not always possible. The timetable was full, and it was difficult to arrange a meeting at a time when all were free to attend. An application to the Faculty Council to free up a time once a month for such meetings was denied.[23] Over the years, however, members of the faculty, local practitioners, and occasionally visiting guest lecturers spoke to club members. In the 1920s they heard lectures on such topics as block anaesthesia, vaccination, goitre, ethics, problems confronting a country physician, and watched a moving picture on the subject of V.D.[24]

Such events were somewhat sporadic, however, so the first graduating class, at the beginning of their final year, formed the Osler Club, under the able direction of Professor Ower, to ''further the interest of its members in medical subjects by means of case reporting, abstracting, historical papers, and discussion of scientific questions.''[25] As membership in the Osler Club was restricted to students in their sixth and final year, it was necessarily reformed each year and the format changed from time to time. Generally, however, meetings were held twice a month, and they usually consisted of one or more of the following: a paper presented by a member of the class; an historical sketch; a pathological treatise; and a case history, followed by a discussion.[26] All class members were required to contribute in some way to the programme, and in this way the Osler Club augmented the academic training of the school. By the 1930s, some sessions concentrated on discussions of problems encountered in their training. Scientific problems, ethical questions and more general topics were threshed out under the guidance of Ower or Professor Cantor.[27]

The MSC also dealt with issues of concern to the students, a number of which concerned the Medical Building and its facilities. In 1920, when it was under construction, a deputation of students appealed, unsuccessfully, to the medical representative on the Board of Governors to include small individual dissecting rooms in the new building, as there were in the Power Plant.[28] Students had several complaints about the anatomy laboratory: the soap usually ran out before the end of the week, and there were no coat hangers, a major problem in a room that invariably had a greasy floor. The new building included space for a common room for the students, but by 1923 it had still not been furnished. The Med Club itemized and priced what they needed for the room—four arm chairs, four plain chairs, two circular tables, a plain oak settee, four blinds, net curtains, overcurtains and valences for the windows, ashtrays, wastebaskets and cuspidors—all of which could be purchased for $250. The club asked the university to pay a portion of this, while MSC members would raise the rest from the proceeds of Med Nite. They also asked for the installation of horse tethers and spur racks at the rear of the Medical Building, as at least three students regularly rode their horses to school.

Other issues dealt with finances and timetabling. The students approached the Senate with a request to institute an instalment method of paying fees. The full payment required at the beginning of each school year caused "considerable hardship to those who are dependent, directly or indirectly, on the sale of crops for sessional fees, as in a number of instances this money cannot be obtained until the session is well advanced."[29] A committee of the MSC met with Edmonton civic authorities to request special rates on the streetcars going to and from hospitals and clinics. A request to the Faculty Council sought a change in the timetable, so that medical students could have a session on their own in the biochemistry laboratory, and also asked for extended hours in the library.[30]

The club was also active in other areas. When the clinical years were added to the programme, the students designed a medical diploma for the first Alberta M.D.s and proposed its acceptance by the Senate.[31] In 1931, following the death of Colonel Mewburn, the first professor of surgery, the MSC presented a gold medal, to be known as the Mewburn Memorial Gold Medal, to be awarded to the student who obtained the highest standing in surgery in the two final years.[32] After Harold Vango's death, the club made several contributions to his memorial, a pathological museum. The MSC also promoted participation in various interfaculty leagues, both in sports and such activities as debating. Depending upon the talents and accomplishments of the current student body, its members enjoyed varying degrees of success.

In those early years, membership in the Med Club was not compulsory, but many of the students lived on campus and actively participated in its events. It was not until 1923, however, that some of the positions on the executive were contested. Candidates presented their platforms at a lively election meeting. Many of those medical students who lived on or near campus also took part in some of the other student clubs and organizations, and a few were active in the Students' Union. Mark Levey [Marshall] was elected president of the Students' Union in 1923, and Anna Wilson achieved the same position in 1929.[33]

One of the first social activities sponsored by the MSC was an annual banquet to bid farewell to those who had completed their preclinical years and were leaving to attend an eastern university. From 1925 on, it honoured the graduating class. It was usually held at the Macdonald Hotel and followed a standard format; a guest speaker representing the medical profession or the university, and several other speeches and toasts, during which faculty members usually came in for some gentle roasting. "Great excitement" occurred at the annual banquet in 1931 when, due to a mix-up in arrangements, R.K. Thompson "the football captain," was called on at the last minute to propose the toast to the faculty, and his roasting was far from gentle. Having imbibed rather freely, he "proceeded instead to bawl out the faculty for having some members who were not up to date in their work. He kept harping on this as the theme of the speech and never got to anything else."[34] By this time, the annual banquet, from which women were excluded, had become a rather drunken affair and the Macdonald Hotel increased its prices to cover the cost of damages incurred. Some faculty members came to the rescue and offered a guarantee, while the executive of the MSC met with Ower to discuss proposals for a change in the proceedings. They designed a more organized programme, incorporating musical solos, a skit or two, and continued "mild roasting" of the faculty, but liquor was sold only at the table, and not in a separate bar.[35]

Activities in the Interwar Years
Undoubtedly, one of the most visible activities of the Med Club was the annual Med Nite. The first performance took place on 11 January 1918 when the main presentation of the evening was a play entitled "A Doctor's Ghost," written, directed and produced by medical students. It was followed by a farce called "The Surgeon's Dream" that featured Gordon Thompson as a blonde "vamp" and Harold Vango as Ethyl Chloride, "a cute(?) brunette." A newly composed "Med Club Yell" had its premier public performance at the end of the programme. Both the participants and the audience had a thoroughly enjoyable time, and the evening concluded with a reception at the home of Dr. and Mrs. Revell.[36] The whole performance was so successful that it became an annual event going by several names over the years: the Med Knights, Med Nite, the Merry Meds, and the Med Show.

Each faculty took its turn to organize the annual undergraduate ball. The medical faculty's turn came in 1918-19, but the influenza epidemic forced the cancellation of the ball, along with all classes and activities at the university for several weeks during the fall term. Although the academic year was disrupted severely, the meds won the hockey interfaculty sports championship, held an annual banquet and dance, heard several guest speakers, and staged Med Nite as arranged previously. "The Tick Dolorous," a two-act play by student A.L. Caldwell, and a skit entitled "A Clinicalamity" were the featured items of the evening.[37] There was a change of pace in 1921 when a Molière play, "Médecin Malgrè Lui," was presented with such style and accomplishment that it went down in history as the best Med Nite of the decade. By 1926, however, complaints began to surface that some of the skits were "coarse, common and vulgar...slap-stick of the low vaudeville theatre variety."[38] The criticism was apparently taken to heart, for the skit of the following year was acclaimed as "clean, snappy and well-acted; it was very much better than its predecessors of former years." A play, "The Society Rebel," and a xylophone solo by J.A. Campbell, one of the students, received similar plaudits.[39]

Med Nite became a popular annual event not only for the meds but also for all students. The question was often raised as to why other faculties did not put on a similar "nite," but, in fact, students of other faculties had a role to play in Med Nite. Students attended as faculty groups, sat in the balcony and had their own cheerleaders, chants, yells and songs. Each faculty decorated its section of the gallery; the students were resplendent in their faculty colours, waved their own flags, sang their own songs and chanted their yells, each one trying to outdo the others in noise and enthusiasm. The words of the songs were thrown up on a screen and everyone joined in the singing, during an evening of spirited interfaculty competition and good-natured rivalry and jousting. "It is one night in the year on which all the faculties get together and have an evening full of fun and good-fellowship, and its popularity can be judged from the capacity houses which always attend the performances."[40]

And somewhere in this early period, the annual fracas between the medical and engineering students developed, either as a result of or in addition to Med Nite. There are various stories about how it all began. According to some, it originated with a clash in the dining hall in Athabasca in 1921, when the meds entered the hall in a body, chanting their yell, and calling on everyone to attend the 4th annual Med Nite. The science (engineering) students counterattacked.[41] A good-natured brawl ensued, and, as each side laid claim to victory, the following year they attempted to steal each other's flags from the roofs of the Medical and Science buildings. It developed into an annual feud, grew in intensity and became a campus institution. In describing the mèlée in 1925, *The Gateway* headline read "Beer Men and Saw Knifers War in Afternoon." The battle raged fiercely for more than an hour, said the reporter, but there were no serious casualties. Ammunition included rotten eggs, water from firehoses, and sharp knives or scissors, which were used to remove buttons and suspenders that held together trousers and other items of apparel.

There was a specific day for the "battle" to take place—it was always on the afternoon of the Med Nite performance, and it usually began with the engineers "storming" their adversaries' building. The event became a great spectator sport for other students on campus, and about 2:00 p.m. on the day of Med Nite, lecture rooms emptied as everyone gathered around the Medical Building. It gradually dawned on the meds and engineers that they were providing an annual free show, and, in 1927, after some preliminary skirmishing had drawn a sufficient number of onlookers, the meds and engineers joined forces and turned on the other students, with particular emphasis on the law students. "Buttons, dignity and suspenders disappeared in a moment" as the erstwhile foes ganged up on the unsuspecting onlookers.[42] This resulted in a certain amount of bitterness among those who had been so accosted, a feeling that was reflected in an altered tone in the usually friendly rivalry of the balcony crowd that Med Nite, and it was not repeated.[43] Accustomed to the results of the annual bout, meds and engineers were appropriately garbed in their oldest clothes, but on this occasion the onlookers who were attacked were taken by surprise and "good suits were absolutely ruined ... no joke in these hard times."[44]

As time went by, the annual event began to cause more and more damage, broken windows and drainpipes, water pouring down halls and corridors, not to mention extreme wear and tear on clothing. Occasionally, an injury or two dampened the enthusiasm somewhat, but all was forgotten by the next year when it was time to continue the strife. The students involved were charged for the damage they caused, and in 1937 this amounted to $500—a large sum of money in those depression years. That same year several casualties were treated in the new infirmary, and the administration decided to take more severe measures.[45] This turned out to be the last hurrah. The engineers involved were hauled on the carpet for breaking and entering and causing damage with firehoses and axes, and the university administration forebade a repeat peformance. In his annual report, the following year, Acting Dean Ower stated that, "the Medico-Science feud seems to have attained its nadir. No dripping ceilings, nor fragmented window panes, nor other results of hyperactivity contributed to the annual depletion of the medical students caution money this year."[46]

The end of the med/engineering feud also brought an end to Med Nite. During the 1930s, it had changed its format. The play had been dropped and each individual class of the medical school produced its own skit. This resulted in less control by the producer and the Med Club, and a continuing recurrence of complaints of vulgarity, bad taste and obscenities. Each year, the provost expressed his concern to the Med Club and laid down a few rules for productions that were presented on campus. Several methods were tried out to accommodate both the medical students and the sensitivities of some of those in the audience. For a couple of years, the audience was restricted to students of the health sciences and the medical fraternity; however, as the med/engineering feud was interwoven so closely with Med Nite, and both were getting out of hand, the university administration put a stop to both. Despite many petitions, from students and faculty as well as some local Edmonton physicians, the administration remained adamant. The second world war broke out a couple of years later, and it would be another fourteen years before Med Nite was revived.

The 1930s also saw the end of the yearly initiation activities. In common with most universities at the time, freshmen at the University of Alberta went through initiation ceremonies, usually perpetrated by the sophomore class, perhaps in revenge for what they had gone through the previous year. Initially, initiation rites took the form of shaven heads, or hair cut in strange patterns, painted faces and a forced ride down a chute into a tank of cold water. Activities varied each year. Sometimes freshmen were grabbed from their beds about 4:30 a.m., tied hand and foot, and then carried to the gymnasium, where their hair was cut, they were force fed strange-looking liquids and foods, sent down a chute into cold water, and then forced to walk between rows of students armed with sandbags. Those in favour of initiation ceremonies reasoned that it was a traditional method of instilling allegiance to the university and an appropriate way to teach freshmen that they had much to learn as they moved from a superior position in high school to an inferior one at university.[47]

As they became more dangerous to life and limb, initiation procedures generated growing opposition in the province. The university was urged to stop them or at least keep them within reasonable limits. Responding to several formal complaints concerning the severity of initiation ceremonies, the university administration did make attempts to curtail them. Nevertheless, they continued until, in 1932, two serious incidents occurred, one of them involving a medical student. That year freshmen were thrown down from the balcony of the gymnasium onto a fireman's net held by a group of sophomores. Walter Johns was a small man, and those who threw him misjudged the throw. As a result, he went too far, landed on the hard rim of the net and suffered a broken shoulder, which necessitated a six-week stay in the University of Alberta Hospital. Had he not been able to complete his first year successfully, the university offered to give him a repeat year free, but this did not prove to be necessary.[48] The second case was much more serious; prolonged assaults and persecutions led to the complete mental breakdown of a student, who was subsequently admitted to a mental institution. This resulted in a successful lawsuit by the parent of the student. From that time on freshmen initiation ceremonies became "social" activities.

They did continue, however, in the fraternities that began to appear on campus at this time. There were no fraternities or sororities on campus during President Tory's tenure, as he was completely opposed to them. After he left in 1928, a few were established, and some medical students tried to start a professional medical fraternity, the Alpha Kappa Kappa (AKK). A number of Edmonton physicians and several faculty members were AKK alumni, and they rallied behind the students in their efforts to form a chapter in Edmonton. President Wallace, however, the Senate and the Committee on Fraternities were all opposed to professional fraternities, as they preferred to see students make broader interfaculty contacts rather than narrow intraprofessional ones.[49] The medical students involved formed the Aesculapian Club and petitioned the university authorities formally to recognize the fraternity on a number of occasions, but without success. They did, nevertheless, obtain a house near campus and called it, unofficially, an AKK house.[50] It had some support from the students, and a few lived there; but without official university recognition, it gradually petered out.

A new breed of students started the process once more in the 1950s, and applied to the Senate Committee on Fraternities and Residential Clubs for permission to establish a branch of the AKK on the campus. Now that more graduates were continuing their education at medical centres across Canada and in the United States, they found it to be an advantage to have a membership in a medical fraternity.[51] The Committee reported to the Senate, however, that it held "no brief for professional fraternities.... If one benefit of fraternity life was the intermingling in fraternities of students from all faculties, the admission of professional fraternities would operate against such an objective ... and narrow still further the interests of students in the professional schools." The Senate, already strongly opposed to professional fraternities, concurred, and refused any further petition for a period of five years.[52]

That was the last application for the admission of the AKK fraternity on campus; but, in 1953, both pharmacy and medicine applied for the admission of an "honour" society. This was not a professional fraternity, there was no pledging or initiation, and membership was based solely on academic achievement. Its major purpose was to hear and present lectures. This too was turned down, as it was felt that faculty clubs should provide these opportunities. Walter Mackenzie and Donald R. Wilson, both strong promoters of this society, pointed out that while the Alpha Omega Alpha (AOA) was known by Greek letters, it was not secret and therefore not subject to the jurisdiction of the Fraternities Committee.[53] They continued to make application for its acceptance each year, and eventually a chapter of the Alpha Omega Alpha Honour Medical Society was established on campus. Induction ceremonies took place on 27 November 1958 when charter memberships were extended to Dean Scott and the department heads in the clinical departments.[54]

Originally established on this continent in 1902, its motto read "To be worthy to serve the suffering," and its members were "dedicated to improving standards in medical training and practice." Members presented clinical cases and scientific papers for discussion at regular meetings though-out the year. The first scientific paper, given by Lawrence Harker, dealt with "Ionizing Radiation." The society was active for some ten years, until its elitism and exclusivity came under question by the students of the 1960s as they went through a period of unswerving allegiance to democratic principles. The chapter was completely inactive during the 1970s until two faculty members, Ted Shnitka and Edward Johnson, reactivated the society in the early 1980's. It has since sponsored yearly lectures by distinguished members of the profession.[55]

Another student activity during the interwar years that attracted some medical students was the Canadian Officers' Training Corps (COTC). Established during the first world war, it maintained a presence on campus until its dissolution in 1968, another victim of the "student uprising." In 1926, it inaugurated a medical corps, composed of about twenty members. Those who joined worked toward an "A" and a "B" certificate, granted by the Department of National Defence. The programme, established by the War Office in London, England, covered infantry training, as well as instruction in first aid, bandaging and stretcher drill.[56] Dean Rankin gave a number of the lectures, on such topics as fractures, shell shock, camp sanitation, prevention of disease, and military medical organizations. In 1927, twelve students received their "A" certificate and gave a display of fieldwork "behind the lines" on inspection day.[57] The Medical Corps continued throughout the interwar years, and many students received their certificates. On the successful completion of both the military training programme and the medical course, graduates received a commission in the Royal Canadian Army Medical Corps (RCAMC). With the onset of World War II, COTC training intensified of course, many students wore uniforms, and the campus took on a distinctly military appearance. In 1944, of the 138 students enrolled in the medical school, more than ninety had enlisted in the RCAMC or CWAC (Canadian Women's Army Corps), and they took one hour a week of basic infantry drill.[58]

The War Years

During the interwar years, membership in the Medical Students Club was not compulsory, and frequently first- and second-year students did not join, particularly if they did not live on campus. It could not, therefore, speak for all medical students. In 1940, the Board of Governors approved a request to have the MSC fee ($2.50) collected from all students at the time of registration, thus making the club representative of all medical students.[59] The MSC adopted a new constitution and a new crest, changed its name to the Medical Undergraduate Society (MUS), and for the first time began to publish a quarterly magazine. One of its first activities was to transform the Common Room in the Medical Building into a Memorial Reading Room honouring L.C. Conn, professor of obstetrics and gynaecology, who had died recently.

Now that it had more money, MUS was able to send a delegate to the annual conferences of the Canadian Association of Medical Students and Internes (CAMSI) and to become involved in national issues. Formed in 1935, this association aimed to "further the welfare and interests of Canadian medical students and interns and encourage and supervise studies of student health, internships and curriculum." CAMSI sponsored a number of projects, and the Alberta medical students received the task of conducting a survey of conditions for interns in Canadian hospitals.[60] Later, the association developed a Canadian Interne Placement Service, which arranged an integrated and systematic method of intern appointments across the country. At a time when the incidence of tuberculosis among medical students had been as high as 25%, another CAMSI project promoted an annual compulsory examination of all medical students for evidence of the disease.[61] As a result, in 1945, Dr. Frank Elliott instituted an examination programme at Alberta that considerably reduced the incidence of tuberculosis in Alberta's medical school.[62] During the war years, the medical directors of all three branches of the military services addressed one of the CAMSI conferences, and delegates also heard accounts of Soviet medicine and participated in a discussion on national health insurance. Alberta hosted the annual conference in 1958, and MUS asked the university to contribute financially to assist students with the extra travel costs they would entail by coming "so far west." By this time, the projects of CAMSI concerned medical education, student finances and remuneration for interns.[63]

With accelerated classes, a shortage of staff, and war-effort activities taking priority, many traditional events ceased during the war years. For the first time in nineteen years, the Medical Ball was not held; however, some activities did take place. Medical students were at university continuously through the summer, and the MUS organized individual class parties and several sports tournaments and leagues, obtained instructional medical films, and arranged for guest speakers on various topics. Students also became involved in such activities as Red Cross blood drives and raising money to buy an ambulance. The executives of both the medical and dental student associations formed the "Summer Students' Union," as during that time these two faculties constituted the student body of the university during the summer months.[64]

Student assistance programmes made their first appearance in the school during the war years, as medical students had no time off to work and supplement their income. The W.K. Kellogg Foundation of Battle Creek, Michigan, set up a fund from which students could apply for emergency loans, and dominion-provincial grants were also available. The 1941 University Survey Committee stressed the need for financial assistance to needy students. "Comparative affluence is one of the pre-requisites of a university education," they reported, which was "student wastage on a grand scale."[65] Following the war, grants and loans did gradually become more available from federal, provincial and institutional sources. The University Women's Club granted small loans to women students, and the Canadian Women's Medical Society established a grant and loan system for female medical students. In addition, the class that graduated in medicine in1941 established a loan fund, which later became an Alumni Loan Fund.[66] The school received some new awards and graduate fellowships. In 1949, the Alberta Tuberculosis Association awarded a graduate fellowship and two undergraduate prizes for the purpose of furthering the study of tuberculosis.[67] About 25% of medical students applied for financial assistance in 1951; and in the 1953-54 academic year thirty-six students received loans or grants ranging from $35 to $500, amounting to a total of $9,400.[68] It was not easy to get assistance, however. First-year students were ineligible, except in cases of grave emergency, and grants were awarded invariably on the basis of scholastic ability.[69]

Postwar Activities

Following the war, veterans once again swelled the ranks of the medical school classes and exerted a lasting influence. Not only were they older and with the experience of war behind them, but also many of them were married and had families. Veterans allowances covered their fees and living expenses. They had overcome stiff competition to get into medical school, were appreciative of the opportunity to study medicine, and were serious about their studies.[70] They were also aware of proposed changes in medical education, and looked critically at the curriculum and teaching practices. A survey of student opinion on the curriculum in 1950, followed by a panel discussion in 1952 at which students discussed their views on medical education, would eventually prove to be the start of a growing pattern of student participation.[71] All faculty members were invited to attend, many did, and a good discussion took place.

The next step was the organization of a Medical Undergraduate Committee on Student Affairs, which later became known as the Liaison Committee. Initially, its aims were to offer constructive criticism of student training, and to encourage closer co-operation and liaison between clinicians and students. The committee was composed of four students from the fourth-year class, three from the third, two from the second, one from the first-year class, and included the dean and honorary president of MUS.[72] The Liaison Committee met monthly and was active for a number of years. It served as a useful vehicle, wherein staff and students met and discussed complaints, suggestions and recommendations for improvements in the medical course.[73] By 1966, it had two main functions: it dealt with day-to-day problems and grievances relating to teaching, and it assessed student opinion on such matters as course content, curriculum changes, teaching techniques, textbooks, and examination and grading procedures.[74] As student representation on faculty committees increased in the late 1960s and early 1970s, the Liaison Committee lost its function and ceased to exist.

MUS also concerned itself with facilities and presented a brief to Dean Scott regarding students' needs at the hospitals. Although third- and fourth-year students were now spending most of their time at the hospitals, there were no lockers for their laboratory coats, stethoscopes, textbooks, and so on, and the only study areas were three small rooms with six chairs— hardly enough for 120 students. The brief requested 120 lockers, a room, or rooms, which would hold at least thirty people; and an adequate library in the proposed University of Alberta Hospital expansion programme. Dean Scott sympathized, ''The needs are obvious,'' he replied, but ''money is the problem.''[75]

The student association continued holding regular meetings, high-lighting lectures by faculty members, other professionals, and sometimes the students themselves. Patricia Simonds of the Class of '57 revived and edited the *MUS Bulletin* as an outlet for student research papers. Panel discussions became popular. Two of the topics were ''The Specialist and the G.P'' and ''Drug addiction.'' Instructional films were often shown, with such titles as ''The Surgical Anatomy of the Femoral Triangle'' and ''Inguinal Hernia.'' At that time Alberta's Board of Censors viewed all films shown in the province. Winthrop-Stearns of Canada Ltd., which marketed medical films to institutions, became somewhat alarmed that their films might be cut,

> This being a medical film for showing to scientific personnel and not for showing to the lay public we fail to see why it should be subjected to review . . . we must insist that this film not be cut or censored by removal of any portion of it . . . if the Board of Censors insist, then we must ask that it be returned to us and not shown.[76]

Social and recreational activities were not ignored. MUS sponsored dances, dinners, smokers, the Med Ball, interfaculty sports, class parties, and also continued to sponsor the annual campus blood drive. Two trophies went along with the blood drive. The Corpuscle Cup went to the faculty with the largest percentage turnout, and the meds and engineers vied for the Ash Trophy, a pale remnant of the prewar med/engineer feuding. It was in 1956 that the annual golf tournament began. Held at the beginning of the fall term, initially it preceded a smoker, but later this was dropped in favour of a barbecue. Its purpose was to stimulate interest and partici-pation in MUS, and to introduce first-year students to those in the other three years and to faculty members—and to the traditional sport of the medical profession! It was obviously a fun tournament and required no ''pre-requisite'': the record score was 149 over nine holes!

In 1950, Med Nite made its reappearance under the new title the Med Show, sometimes called the Merry Meds Show. As before, each class was responsible for its own skit. It achieved immediate popularity with its audiences and within three years extended its run to two nights—the two immediately preceding the annual Banquet and Ball. The Med Show quickly ran into the same problems as its prewar predecessor when complaints about the coarse nature of its contents began to surface. Now it was the Dean's Council that ruled on such university activities, and as before they

restricted admission to students in the health sciences and those connected
with the medical profession. Nevertheless, the 1959 show received approval
from the Dean's Council only provided it "maintain a standard of decency
appropriate to a university performance."[77] Apparently it did not achieve
this standard, as the Dean's Council advised that the show "would have
to be altered and improved if permission was to be granted for its continu-
ance."[78] MUS received permission to produce the show the following year,
but with the proviso that if the quality was not improved permission would
be refused in future years. MUS made a concerted effort to "clean up the
Med Show" that year, and the provost and Dean's Council expressed their
appreciation of this effort, but it seems to have been short-lived. In 1963,
reaction against the Med Show reached an all-time high—from the Dean's
Council, the provost, the dean of medicine and many of the students themselves. The headline of the editorial in the *MUS Bulletin* read: "Resolved:
That the Med Show in its present format is a blight to the Faculty of Medicine."[79] Another student publication, *Mediscope*, pointed out quite bluntly
that the Med Show was the society's main source of income:

> In the past it has not been of a quality which people would expect—in a
> word, it's been too dirty. So dirty in fact that the Dean threatens to call
> it off after the dress rehearsal unless it is more acceptable. Such a move
> would be disastrous.

The Merry Meds of 1964 "proved that an upgraded, much cleaner, but
still funny Med Show is possible whether motivated by unpopular sentiment or by gentle external pressure."[80] Whether a "cleaner" Med Show
has continued is debatable, but the annual performances survived and
thrived. The Med Show still played to soldout audiences (mostly students),
had a four-night run, and was a good moneymaker.[81] The Med Show itself
was an institution on campus, and so was the controversy surrounding its
content.

Demographics of the Student Body

In the 1950s medical schools across the continent experienced difficulty
attracting a sufficient number of qualified students. In an effort to ascertain the reasons for this decline and to encourage qualified students to enter
medicine, medical students were subject to several surveys. J.S. Thompson, who was executive secretary of the Faculty of Medicine and also secretary of the Association of Canadian Medical Colleges in the 1950s,

conducted an extensive survey of the medical students at the University of Alberta and contributed some interesting background and statistical information from this period.

Financial difficulties were often assumed to be a major problem, and the chief reason for student hesitation to enter medicine; yet, the survey showed that the majority of the medical students at the University of Alberta came from medium-to-low-income homes. At a time when the average personal income for an Albertan was $5,082 a year, 11% of students declared their parents' income as less than $2,000, 50% between $2,000 and $5,000, and 39% over $5,000. Sixty-one per cent, therefore, came from families with average to below average incomes.[82] The occupations of the parents of students admitted to the medical school between the years 1952 and 1956 are shown in Table 8. Two hundred and four out of a registration of 218 students answered the questionnaire, and of these twenty-three were putting themselves through school unassisted, while nine more were doing so with small loans or grants from the government's students' assistance programme. Fifty-seven students were married, and thirty-one of these depended upon their wives' income.[84] Thirty-one received assistance from their parents, 127 worked during the summer, and sixty-one found it necessary to work during the term as well to finance their education. Of these, only one quarter felt it interfered with their academic standing. Most expected to be in debt by the time they graduated.[85]

TABLE 8: OCCUPATIONS OF THE PARENTS OF MEDICAL STUDENTS ADMITTED TO THE UNIVERSITY OF ALBERTA[83] 1952-1956

Type of Occupation	Number and Percentage of Students	
Employees in:		
Business enterprises........................ 63	22.1%	
Government 11	3.8%	
Educational institutions..................... 9	3.1%	
Business proprietors........................ 64	22.4%	
Farmers.................................. 63	22.1%	
Professional.............................. 39	13.7%	
(18 of these were physicians)		
Pension income........................... 29	10.2%	
Deceased................................ 4	1.4%	

The Annual Report of the University of Alberta for 1958-59 included a table identifying the distribution of medical students by their home addresses. These are shown in Table 9. Thompson's survey showed, however, that almost half of those who gave Edmonton as their home address had moved there when they started attending university, and overall the students represented fairly the urban/rural split in the province.[86] In summary, Thompson concluded that "residence in the city in which the university is located increases one's chances of attending medical school," and that "twice as many of our students come from the professional or business-proprietor classes as would be expected from the actual size of these categories in the general population."[87]

TABLE 9: DISTRIBUTION OF MEDICAL STUDENTS BY HOME ADDRESS[88] 1958-1959

99	Edmonton	4	Eastern provinces
37	Communities north of Township 38	3	Camrose
29	Calgary	2	Cardston
28	Communities south of Township 38	2	Medicine Hat
10	Other three western provinces	2	USA
6	Lethbridge	1	Vegreville
4	Red Deer	1	Other foreigh country

Increase of Student Activity in Faculty Affairs

In the 1960s, due to the postwar population explosion as well as a wider access to university education, enrolment in medical schools began to increase; and so did student unrest. In 1969, *Evergreen and Gold*, the university's yearbook, declared that "This University Belongs to the Student." Throughout the campus, student representatives took their places on various university committees and councils—on the Board of Governors, the General Faculty Council, the Academic Appeals Board, the Senate, Academic Planning committees and Campus Development boards.[89] Medical students took their seats on the Council of the Faculty of Medicine, the Curriculum Advisory Committee, the Admissions Committee, the Student Evaluation Board, and met with the Executive Committee of the Faculty Council on a regular basis.

In 1971, the student association proposed to the Medical Faculty Council that students be granted representation equal to that of elected faculty members on the Curriculum Advisory Committee, the Admissions

Committee, and the Student Evaluation Board. Faculty Council approved the first two, but tabled the latter for further consideration.[90] As a result, the Curriculum Advisory Committee had a membership of nine ex-officio faculty members appointed by the dean, six elected faculty members (three from medical sciences and three from the clinical sciences), and six elected students (one each from the first and second years, and two from each of the third and fourth years). The Student Evaluation Board had eight faculty members and four students.[91] In 1974, the students' association asked for representation on the Academic Standings committees, because it was "essential that students have complete confidence in the fairness and objectivity of decisions made by these Committees." In the submission, the students commended the faculty for its response to student representation on decision-making bodies, and felt that students had responded "with mature and responsible actions on these committees."[92] Faculty Council agreed to allow one student from Phase IIIa to sit on the Academic Standings committees on a trial basis.[93]

With its increased participation in faculty affairs, and a large student body (the yearly quota increased to 118 in 1972), the executive committee of the students' association increased substantially in both size and responsibilities. In 1969, it had changed its name again, to the Medical Students' Association (MSA), and, even though it was still a voluntary association, most students belonged. The expanded executive now included a vice-president responsible for academic affairs, as well as a representative to the Alberta Medical Association. The association also participated actively in the Canadian Federation of Medical Students, which, together with the Canadian Association of Internes and Residents, was a successor to CAMSI. The MSA publication, which began in 1963, was called the *Mediscope* and was intended to include notices, humorous anecdotes, profiles, editorials and medical/research articles by both students and faculty members. By the 1980s, representatives of the MSA met with the dean of medicine and his assistant on a regular monthly basis, where matters of mutual concern were discussed. Students felt confident that their contributions and opinions were solicited actively and played an important part in faculty decisions.

A major function of the MSA was its academic concerns, and it hosted guest speakers and held noon-hour seminars. It was, however, responsible also for social and sporting events, for both interfaculty and interclass sporting activities, for class parties, the traditional annual events such as the Medical Ball, the Med Show, the graduation banquet, and, for a time, participation in the annual Western Canadian Medical Student Exchange weekend, which involved students from B.C., Saskatchewan and Manitoba. Various other awards and activities were sponsored by the MSA during the seventies and the eighties. In 1971, it introduced the Outstanding Teacher Awards, in which an award was presented annually for excellence as an educator to one teacher in each of three phases of the programme and also to one of the residents. The Shaner Award went to a graduating student for exceptional contributions to the work of the MSA; the Mackenzie Award was for the graduating student judged most proficient in clinical skills; and the Fried Award to the Phase III student who prepared the best written case presentation in Pediatrics. The association also developed a "faculty advisor programme," in which first-year students were matched up with a faculty member in a mentor relationship.[94]

The MSA also developed new projects. Soon after the new Walter Mackenzie Health Sciences Centre opened, the students raised $15,000 to purchase a grand piano. They donated it to the hospital and sponsored the Courtyard Concert Series. Each Thursday noon, an audience of patients, staff and students congregated on the fourth floor atrium to enjoy a concert of classical music, sponsored by the MSA. The Poison Prevention and Control Program, the brainchild of Louis Francescutti, president of MSA in 1987, marketed an informational kit to assist parents in the home. The students participated actively in the annual Shinerama, which raised money for research in cystic fibrosis, and the student journal, *IATROS*, funded by the Medical Alumni Association, published student articles and promoted increased communication between students and alumni.

Women in the Medical School

From its first year of existence, the University of Alberta's doors have been open to women, and on an equal footing with men. While there were no women in the first medical class, there were two in the second, and since then most classes have included at least one female medical student. Until the mid-1930s when a quota was established, there appears to have been no difficulty for qualified students of either gender to be accepted. If they had the required academic prerequisites, they were admitted; but in an era when women were not encouraged to take sciences in high school and, in fact, were probably discouraged, few qualified. Prior to World War II, a number of women went into medicine through the B.A., M.D. programme, probably to obtain the necessary scientific prerequisites.

From the mid-1930s to the1950s, however, even if there was not an actual quota imposed, women were actively discouraged from entering the Faculty of Medicine. The problem first arose when a change in the curriculum included a year of undergraduate internship, and city hospitals refused to take women interns, stating that they could not provide accommodation for them.[95] The university's Board of Governors "did not feel that this was their responsibility," even though it countermanded effectively the philosophy of the university that courses of study were open equally to men and women. The faculty then approached the board of the University of Alberta Hospital, which agreed to accept three women interns. The medical staff at the hospital, however, were unhappy with this decision, as none of the departments wanted women on their service. A "special type of service was arranged," which, though not delineated, was not as thorough as that offered to their male counterparts.[96] Rather than exert any pressure on the hospitals to accommodate female interns, if more than three women were accepted in a class, the Admissions Committee informed them that "there may be problems during your intern year."[97] This, in effect, imposed a quota of three women in each class.

In 1941, the General Faculty Council accused the Faculty of Medicine of discriminating against women and thereby contravening the University Act. The faculty responded with the information that while four women had been eligible that year, three had been accepted and the fourth was not denied admittance but simply "deferred."[98] In 1943, one qualified woman was placed on a waiting list "to be admitted only if one of the women drops out,"[99] which also indicates a quota. A.W. Downs, chairman of the Admissions Committee, conducted a study of all the women who had graduated from the Faculty of Medicine and reported that "the wastage was heavy, principally because of marriage and that at least 30% of the women graduates are not practising." He advised, therefore, that "in case of doubt preference should be given to the men."[100] Downs's study included a list of fifty-seven women who had been accepted in the medical faculty since its inception "as far as I have been able to discover." According to his list, twenty-one (37%) were in practice, sixteen (28%) were still undergraduates, thirteen (23%) were married, and six (10.5%) had withdrawn.[101] He made the assumption that those who had married were not in practice, and, given the mores of the time this might well have been true, but at least one, Leone McGregor Hellstedt, was both married and practising medicine, and there might well have been others.

With accelerated courses during the war, and the need to graduate doctors for military service, women found it even more difficult to get into medicine. After the war, the large number of veterans, mostly male, took precedence over both women and all but the most highly qualified civilian male applicants. In 1949, the Admissions Committee selected fifty applicants from a total of 122. Selection was based on age, time in the services, and scholarship, and five women were admitted. Although those who were selected had the same qualifications as the men, the committee recommended, nevertheless, that "a study be made of the advisability of imposing a definite quota on the number of women students to be accepted in future years."[102] Before any action was taken on this proposal, however, the number of applicants to medical school began to decline, and both the profession and the faculty began to solicit women actively.

Discrimination against women is not confined, however, to admittance to medical school. Those few who were admitted; how were they accepted? The attitude could perhaps be described best as "veiled hostility." Both the faculty and the profession felt that women taking medicine were wasting their own and everyone else's time, as they would inevitably marry, stay at home to raise a family and not use their training.[103] There was a feeling that women medical students were somehow "not feminine," were not popular with men, and, indeed, that they were in medical school partly for that very reason.

As far as their classmates were concerned, women were accepted in the classroom, but they were also patronized, protected and ignored. Male medical students did not view the women in their classes as serious competition for high marks, prizes and awards, although they were often surprised in this respect as women in medicine were often highly qualified and did well academically. In the Class of 1934, there were five women, and one of their fellow students said of them, "We looked at them askance. What the hell were they doing here? We thought they were stupid at the beginning, but they made good marks."[104] The few all-male classes "plumed themselves on their freedom from women."[105] Some of the classes that had only one female student were exceedingly protective—"she is 'our Mary' ... [and] ... helped reconcile the men students to the advent of women in medicine."[106] They were referred to as co-meds, medicalettes, femedicals, ladies, girls, but never just plain medical students. Their participation in the Med Club did not include social or recreational activities, and women's roles in the Med Show were taken more frequently by students from the School of Nursing than by female medical students.

The early banquets to honour the graduating classes were attended solely by men. There was some concern when the top student of the first graduating class turned out to be female, but the women medical students overcame the resulting impasse by holding their own banquet to honour the lone female graduate. This was the beginning of a tradition, as they formed a Women's Medical Students' Club and held their own yearly banquet. In 1931, it was, according to Ower, ''a grand affair and included wives of heads of departments and lady doctors from far and wide. The punch was sweetly (?) scriptural.''[107] A separate banquet continued until 1950 when two of the women students, Frances Richards and Lois MacKenzie, moved that ''women medical students be invited to attend the Medical Graduation Banquet in future''—and the motion passed.[108]

As for the faculty, Leone McGregor Hellstedt said ''there was no favouritism for boys whatever''[109] and after graduation, Professor Ower offered her an internship in pathology. She accepted with delight, but when she wanted to go elsewhere to do postgraduate work she appealed to Egerton Pope for guidance, a man whom she had ''adored'' when a student. ''He was kind and charming but of another generation,'' and said he was unable to advise a woman in furthering her career in the practice of medicine, which was a great disappointment to her. She went to see President Tory, and it was through him that she received a three-year fellowship at the University of Minnesota.[110] Perhaps the feeling of the faculty towards their female students can best be deduced by the words of H.H. Hepburn who concluded an inspiring article to the first graduating class with the words:

> The writer has, through this article, avoided the use of the feminine gender. Not that he has failed to note, nor wished to show any disapproval of the advent of the lady doctor, but rather that he shrinks from the task of attempting to guide the destinies of young ladies.[111]

The hospital, the university and society as a whole exerted their own rules for all women, including medical students. Hospitals did not allow nurses or female medical students to ''bob their hair'' according to the fashionable haircut for women of the twenties. It was regarded as unhygienic. The first thing Leone McGregor did when she graduated was to have her hair cut, which she felt was a first step of ''freedom from stupid rules.'' For many years, the female students in the professional faculties were treated differently and separately. President and Mrs. Tory entertained the female medical students at their home each year, when supper was ''served around the fireplace, and followed by music and conversation.''[112] Mrs. Ower entertained the ''lady medical students'' at tea on a regular basis, often in conjunction with the wives of the members of one or other of the reporting clubs, or "some of the lab girls."[113] Until the 1950s the dean of women held an annual tea for "women graduates in engineering, medicine, dentistry, pharmacy, law, commerce and honour students in Arts and Science."[114]

In the 1950s and early 1960s, when medical schools across the continent experienced difficulty in attracting a sufficient number of qualified applicants into medicine, the profession campaigned actively for both women and men to enter medical school, and when applications began to increase it was "due entirely to the registration of more women."[115] The increase in the percentage of women applicants rose dramatically, and it has continued to increase steadily. In the 1958-59 session, the percentage of women in the fourth year at the University of Alberta was 1.9%; in the third year, 4%; in the second year, 9.6%; and in the first year, 12.5%.[116] The proportion of women graduates in all Canadian medical schools doubled from 5.2% in 1958 to 10.1% in 1962.[117] There is little evidence that there has been a quota since that time. Fewer women than men apply, and in consequence fewer women than men are accepted. Table 10 shows the percentage of female medical students in Canadian universities from 1960 to 1980.

By 1969, 20% of the first-year class at the University of Alberta were women, and, significantly perhaps, it had the highest average of any first-year class.

Consequently there has been tradition-breaking feminine participation in the formerly all-male Med Show. The first year girls have also initiated the formulation of a women's intramural sports unit, as well as lending an able hand with the year book and other MUS activities.[118]

TABLE 10: FIRST YEAR ENROLMENT IN CANADIAN MEDICAL SCHOOLS BY SEX[119] 1960-1980

Year	Total Registration	% Women
1960-61	970	10.3
1965-66	1128	12.7
1970-71	1452	20.2
1975-76	1807	33.0
1980-81	1887	40.0

The percentage of women in the University of Alberta's medical school continued to increase and reached about 35% in the 1980s. Representation of women in the faculty, however, was significantly less.

The Medical Alumni Association

Until the second world war the Faculty of Medicine alumni association showed little interest in university affairs. In 1941, however, graduates of the medical school formed the Medical Alumni Association (MAA), whose objects were to promote and support the Faculty of Medicine, to maintain social contacts between alumni, and to provide financial assistance wherever possible to undergraduates and interns.[120] The MAA became an active organization, sponsoring a number of projects in aid of the medical school. In 1961, the association instituted a breakfast to welcome new graduates and their families on the morning of convocation, and has co-operated in, and sometimes financed, various projects within the faculty. It funded several awards—the John W. Scott Honor Award Fund, the R.F. Shaner Trust and the J.J. Ower Gold Medal and Scholarship for graduating students.[121]

One of the MAA's major activities has been the selection of a graduate for the Outstanding Achievement Award. Of the more than four thousand doctors who graduated between 1925 and 1988, a great many achieved prominence and fame in their particular fields of endeavour in medical centres across the continent and overseas. A large number returned to their *alma mater* to contribute significantly as members of the faculty. The Out-standing Achievement Award has been presented annually since 1963, and a list of the recipients is included in the appendices at the end of this book.

It is impossible even to begin to name the many who deserve recognition. The contributions of only two graduates will be highlighted here; one because she was the first female graduate of the school, and the other because he was one of the first to bring honour to the school. Both received honorary doctorates from the University of Alberta. After graduation, Leone McGregor went to the University of Minnesota where she did research on "histological changes in kidneys in health and disease, especially in essential hypertension."[122] She received an M.Sc. and a Ph.D. for her work. McGregor continued this work under a National Research fellowship at Harvard, in the Boston City Hospital,[123] and then received a Rockefeller scholarship for work in Fahr's Institute of Pathology at Hamburg, Germany. After her marriage to a Swedish businessman, she lived in Sweden and she was astonished to discover that neither her M.D. from Alberta nor her Ph.D. from Minnesota qualified her to practise or continue her research in Sweden. Eventually, the two degrees were accepted as prerequisites, and following two years of medical school, she received a Swedish medical degree in 1937. She took specialty training in a field that had always interested her, psychoanalysis and therapy, and began a psychoanalytic practice, a field in which she made great contributions during nearly forty years of practice. Always interested in women in medicine, she was active in the Medical Women's International Association, served as its president, and wrote a book entitled *Women Physicians of the World*.[124]

Stanley Hartroft was the first student to take advantage of the opportunity to take a break in his medical training and work towards an M.Sc. While in his final year, in January 1941, before he had even graduated with an M.D., the school received a request from Sir Frederick Banting, then chairman of the Medical Research Committee, requesting Hartroft's immediate release to work on special investigations being carried out at the University of Western Ontario. There was some urgency to the request, as the project dealt with war-related problems—the effect of high-altitude flying on the human lung. Hartroft was selected for this project, sponsored by the National Research Council and the Department of National Defence, because of his special qualifications in the field of anatomy. Major Hartroft served overseas later as a pathologist in the RCAMC, and then returned to the University of Toronto as a research associate in the Banting and Best Institute, where he "revolutionized their outlook on the morphological sciences."[125] He received a research medal from the Royal College of Physicians and Surgeons of Canada, and became well known for his extensive work on kidneys. In 1961, when he received an honorary doctorate from his own *alma mater*, he was head of the department of pathology at Washington University in St. Louis and "an internationally recognised expert in the field of experimental pathology."[126]

* * * * *

Changes in the student body at the University of Alberta's Faculty of Medicine are reflected in the changes that took place in Alberta over seventy-five years. In 1913, Alberta's population was largely rural, and, though it had expanded rapidly, the province was still sparsely populated. Alberta was close to the frontier, barely out of the settlement period, and isolated from the more populous parts of the country. Many of the medical students came from farming communities, and a number were newcomers to the province. For many years, the rural influence permeated the philosophy of the university. Because of the school's rigid curriculum, as well as its isolation, the students were a closely knit group who knew each other and their teachers well, it was almost a "family" relationship. The school was small, and so was the university. The Medical Building was within the confines of a quadrangle of university buildings, and medical students maintained a close involvment with the university and all its activities.

After the second world war Alberta became increasingly urbanized, industrial developments attracted a wide immigration to the province, and advances in technology reduced the sense of isolation inherent in its geographic setting. The number of medical students also increased, and most came from urban communities, as the rural influence declined. With a student body of over 450 in the 1980s, and third- and fourth-year students spread out among all the Edmonton hospitals, the students' association had to work hard simply to keep in contact with all the students. Rather than the close relationships enjoyed by students in the early years, by the 1980s communication among students and faculty was on a much more formalized basis. Since the days of "student unrest" in the 1960s, students have become increasingly involved with the university's committee structure, making their relationship with faculty a much more structured one. The medical student body in 1988 was greater than the entire university registration had been in 1913. The medical school complex in 1988 was sufficient unto to itself, and on the perimeter of the university campus, there seemed little communication between medical students and university students in other faculties.

* * * * *

CHAPTER 6

Medical Education

History of medical education in Canada: undergraduate, graduate and continuing medical education at the University of Alberta

IN 1968, a symposium on the history of medical education took place at the University of California in Los Angeles. Even though it was a time of intense scrutiny and revision for medical education, the first conclusion reached by the symposium was that "the present concern with medical education ... and methods of teaching do not represent a solely modern phenomenon. The problem has existed from the time of medicine's origin."[1] More recent controversies can be traced in certain key analyses. Philippe Pinel wrote an essay in 1793 on the clinical training of physicians in France, where medical education was undergoing radical changes.[2] Sir William Osler addressed the medical faculty at McGill University in 1895 on the subject "Teaching and Thinking: The Two Functions of a Medical School," and discussed the dramatic changes taking place, including incorporation of medical education into university programmes.[3] In 1920, J.J.R. Macleod, of insulin fame, wrote: "there has been for some years a feeling among the medical profession that all is not well with the stereotyped medical college curriculum."[4] An editorial in the January 1933 issue of the *Canadian Medical Association Journal*, bearing the title "The Problem of Medical Education," represented similar titles found in any given year in this or any other medical journal of the period. This particular editorial referred to a series of contemporary articles published in *The Lancet*, the publication of the British Medical Association, under the general heading

"What is the Matter with the Medical Curriculum," and announced that the *Journal* proposed a similar series in its own pages in the weeks to come.

In the proliferation of articles, books and essays on the subject, the concepts discussed over these years displayed a remarkable consistency. Frequently they included a preference for small bedside or laboratory groups over didactic lectures; the introduction of the student to the patient early in the educational process; the benefits of the humanities in both prerequisite requirements and the medical course itself for, according to Sir William Osler, "though science permeates and influences the whole, it is not the whole of medicine;"[5] a timetable leaving some free time for the student to follow individual interests and pursuits; and a curriculum designed to teach the students to think for themselves and to instill in them an understanding that medical education is a lifelong procedure. In 1909, the president of the AAMC declared "the greatest deficiency in the conduct of the medical course today" to be "the failure to train the student to think and reason out matters for himself."[6] To quote Osler again; "the hardest conviction to get into the mind of a beginner is that the education upon which he is engaged is not a college course, not a medical course but a life course, of which the work of a few years under teachers is but a preparation."[7]

The Beginning of Medical Education in Canada
Medical education in Canada has followed, to a marked degree, that offered in the United States. In the early days, the apprenticeship system provided the only entry into the profession. The student apprenticed to a practising physician and accompanied him on his house calls, in the hospital and in his examining room, depending completely upon his "master" for quality training—some was good and comprehensive, some was adequate, and some might have included little more than cleaning the office and making sure that the doctor's horse was fed, adequately stabled, and ready at the door when needed. At some point, the apprentice was considered trained sufficiently to offer his services to the public. There were no examinations and no licensing regulations. The affluent student, however, could, and usually did, follow his apprenticeship with clinical training in Great Britain, France or Germany.

In the proprietary school that developed out of the apprenticeship system, particularly in larger centres, rather than offer individual instruction, a group of local practitioners would band together to present medical instruction in a school setting. Students needed no prerequisites beyond an ability to read and write and, provided that they attended the classes and could pay the fees, they were assured of receiving a diploma. This, in most places, entitled them to practise. Initially, the courses lasted little more than three or four months and consisted solely of lectures and demonstrations of anatomical dissections. Few expenses arose from this method of teaching and the lecturers in these commercial enterprises divided the fees among themselves. They depended upon a profit, and individual schools achieved a varied degree of success and longevity.[8] The lengthy settlement period in North America created a need for doctors in new areas long before there were any facilities there for teaching them. Graduates from commercial proprietary schools filled this need. They were much more prevalent in the more populous United States than in Canada.[9] According to the Flexner Report,

> In Canada conditions have never become so badly demoralized as in the United States. There the best features of English clinical teaching had never been wholly forgotten. Convalescence from a relatively mild over-indulgence in commercial medical schools set in earlier and is more nearly completed.[10]

Some of the more successful Canadian schools formed a rather loose relationship with local universities, but in most cases they received little or no assistance with their financial or building requirements, and the universities exerted no control over course content or diploma requirements.

Because the road to Europe for further training continued to be a much travelled one, North American medical education evolved from an amalgam of that developed in Great Britain, France and Germany. In Great Britain and France, medical education grew out of the hospital, where initially the apprentice accompanied his preceptor on his rounds. Traditional group bedside teaching developed out of this process, epitomized by that given at Edinburgh, taken up by McGill in 1845, and subsequently followed by most Canadian medical schools.

While the first half of the nineteenth century belonged to French medicine and its emphasis on the clinical side, the German approach gained ground steadily later in the century. German medical training developed in the universities, emphasizing research as well as teaching. Professors were scientists, and medical philosophy was deeply committed to the scientific aspect of medicine. This tendency followed the inroads made in the first half of the nineteenth century by the natural sciences into the traditional classics-oriented "gentleman's education."[11] Nowhere was the victory of science more evident than in the field of medical education.

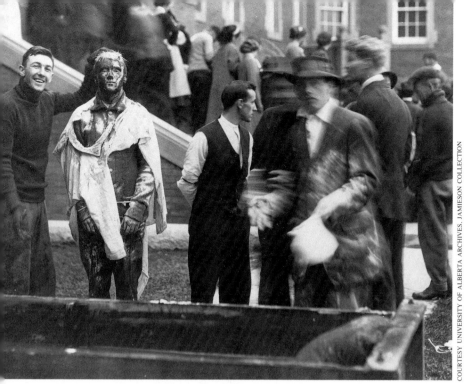

Initiation ceremonies for freshmen class in medicine in October 1913.

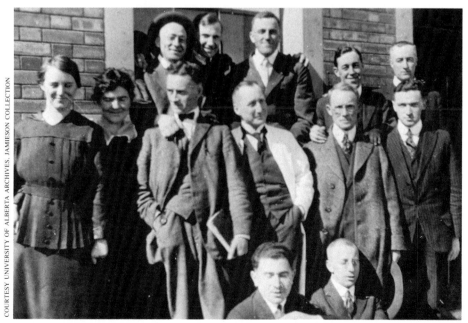

Heber Jamieson (centre, in a white coat) with a group of medical students, c. 1914. The two women students are Isabel Teskey Ayer and Ann Curtin.

Departing Year

J. H. Brodie	E. C. McLeod
W. F. Carscallen	E. J. Millar
W. M. Chesney	Miss E. Nesbitt
E. M. Cooper	H. A. Pearse
F. E. Corbett	J. A. Parker
E. D. Emery	W. A. Redel
R. S. Grimmett	C. J. Rienhorn
C. Gunderson	E. S. Sarvis
Miss G. V. Holmes	S. F. Service
J. C. Jackson	H. M. Vango
F. W. Jones	J. G. Wells
A. F. Kibzey	S. M. Wershof
P. E. Logan	W. Wilkin
P. M. Lyster	G. F. Young
Miss M. E. McLean	

Med. Club Annual Banquet

Athabasca Hall
University of Alberta
March 31st, 1920

Praescriptio

R⟩

Succus Fructuum in Poculis	50 cc.	
Extractum Liquidum Tomatinis	6 fl. oz.	
Cum Panibus Parvis.		
Aves Agrestes Super Foco Semiustae...	200 gr.	
Tubera Humi Vulgaria	100 "	
Pisa Viridia Gallica	50 "	
Concoctio Sine Nomine	150 "	
Cremor Gelatus Vaccae	250 "	
Placentae Dulces et Potis Arabica	Q.S.	

Sig.

Sumat Caute Secundum Naturam Adde Sod. Chlor.
et Condimenta Alia.

"Ad Vivendum Edendum, non ad Edendum
Vivendum est."

Toast List

KING
Dr. J. B. Collip

Address by President of Med. Club

UNIVERSITY
H. G. Garrioch   Dean Howes

PROFESSION
J. A. Parker   Dean Rankin

LADIES
J. W. Lang   Miss M. McLean

DEPARTING GUESTS
Dr. D. G. Revell   H. A. Pearse

Programme of the Med. Club Annual Banquet held for the class of 1920, who were leaving for the completion of their training elsewhere.

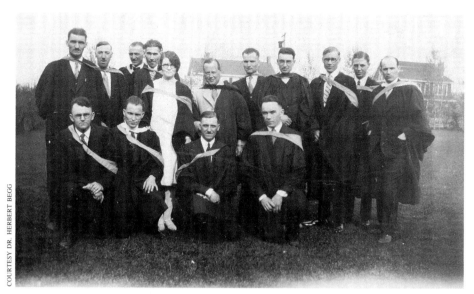

Graduating class of 1928.

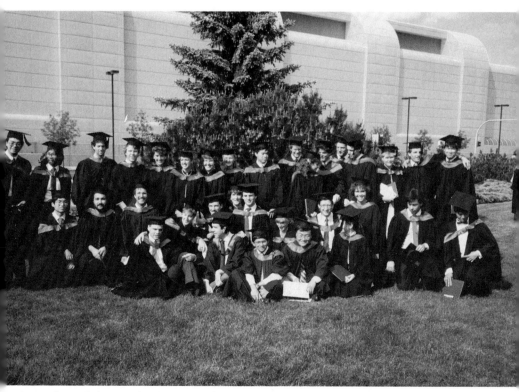

A portion of the graduating class of 1987.

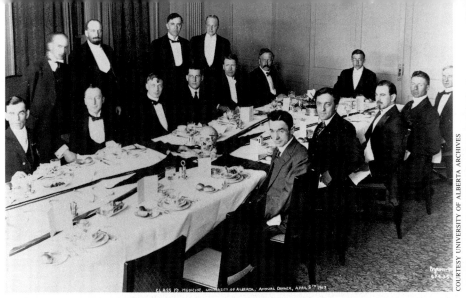

Third-year Class, 1917. Annual dinner, April 5 1917. *Seated, clockwise around the table:* J.H. Riopel, Dr. Heber Jamieson, J.B. Collip, A.W. Bowles, Dr. Irving Bell, President Tory, W.H. Hill, Dr. D.G. Revell, Percy Backus, Dr. Gordon Gray, H.S. Empey, Nat Minish. *Standing, left to right:* G. Novak, Professor Gaetz, Dr. Macpherson, C.H. Hankinson.

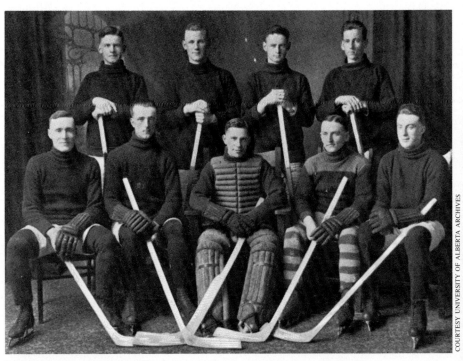

Medical team, interfaculty league winners in hockey, 1918-19.

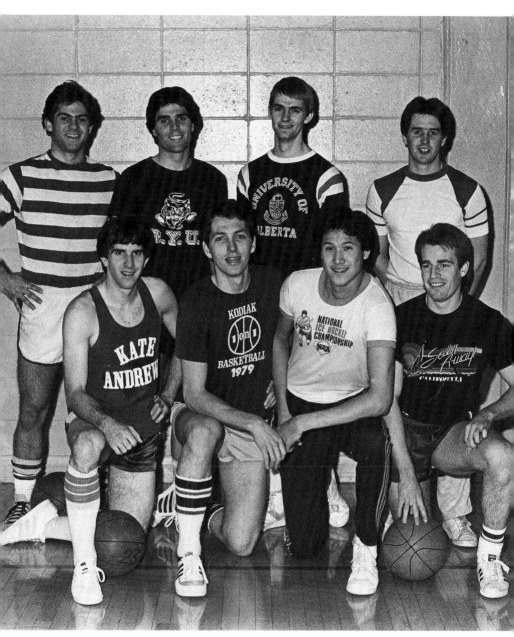

Intramural basketball team - Medicine A team, runners-up, 1983-84.
Back row, left to right: Peter Oleson, Mike Steed, Ron Low, Lamont Leavitt.
Front row: Steve Low, Wade Steed, William Hu, Joe Foster.

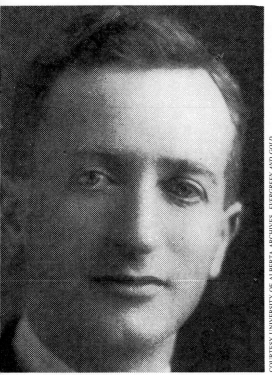
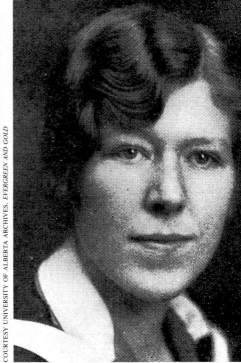

Mark Levey, 1924-25   Anna Wilson, 1928-29

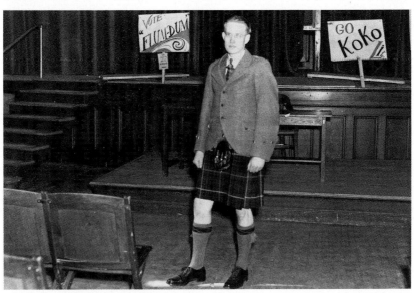

Robert A. Macbeth, 1941-42

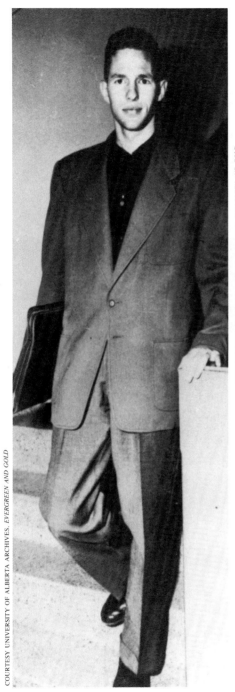

John Chappel, 1956-57

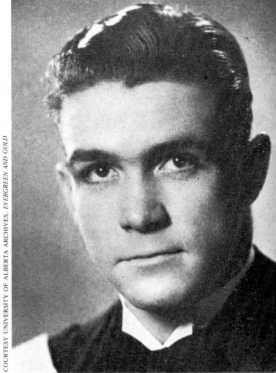

L.C. Grisdale, 1943-44

Five medical students have been elected President of the University's Student Union.

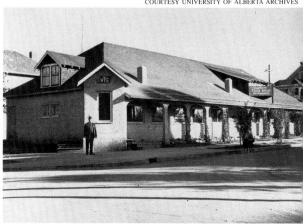

The Tuck Shop, on the corner of 112th Street and 88th Avenue. A popular meeting place for generations of university students, it was demolished in 1970 to make way for The Hub. This picture was taken in 1931.

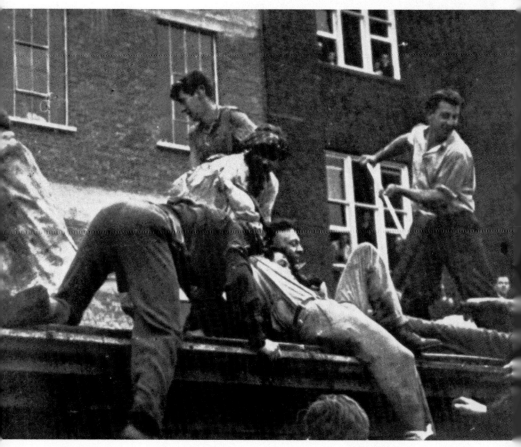

"They're up . . . they're down . . . windows are smashed and tch. tch. tch., that twenty-dollars-a-foot drainpipe is bent again."

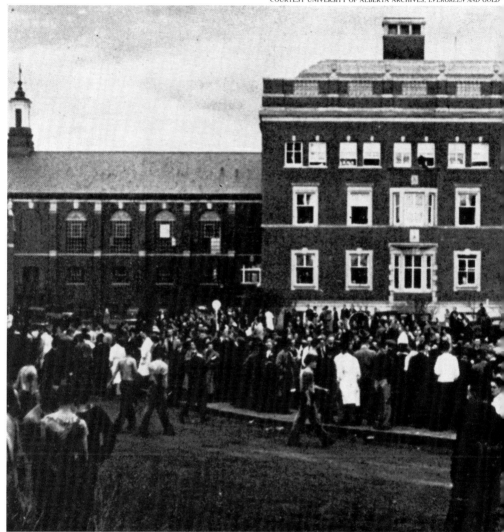

Some scenes from the last of the annual med/engineering battles, 1938.
"The weary attackers withdraw for a brief recess, and by this time lectures
and labs have been temporarily abandoned while onlookers from all the rest
of the faculties watch the proceedings."

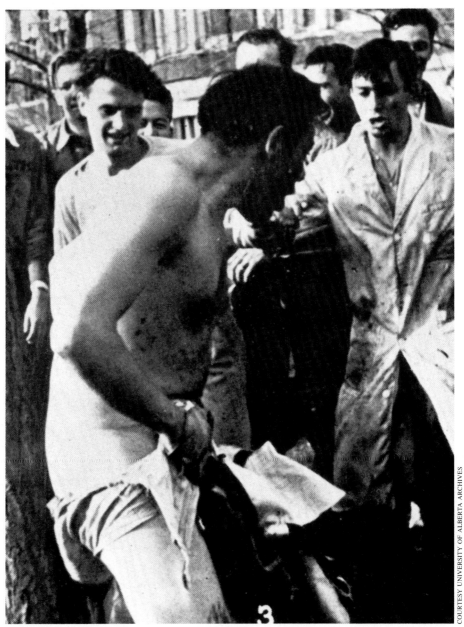

''There ensued a battle royal when the two opposing forces met in a hand-to-hand struggle in which the horrified Sammy Epstein was disrobed.''

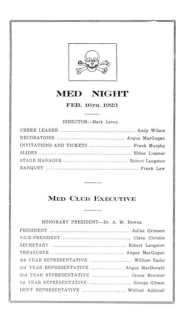
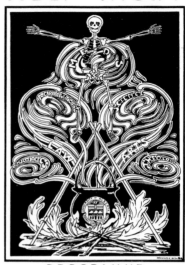
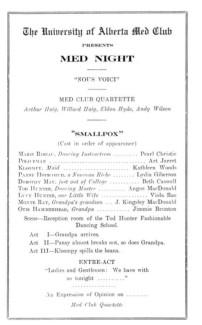
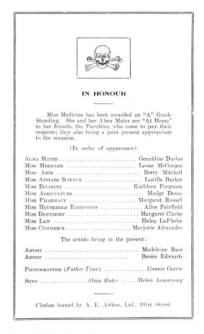

The programme for the annual Med-Night, 1922-23. The cover design incorporates all the other faculties, who were active participants in the festivities of the evening.

52

FACULTY YELL

We run a bluff,
We treat you rough
Aint that enough?
Us PROFS
Alberta.

53

WAUNEITA YELL

Ki-yi itiki, ki, yi yip,
Wauneita, Wauneita, zip, zip, zip,
War-paint, Battle-axe, Peace-pipe,
    gore,
Wauneita, Wauneita, Evermore.

54

ARTS

Fae, facul, factus,
Fac, faculty,
Arts in general,
    Ph.D.
That's the way we yell it,
This is the way we spell it—
    A-R-T-S.
Arts.

55

ENGINEERS

We are, We are,
We are the Engineers;
We can, We can,
We can drink forty beers;
Drink rum, Drink rum,
Drink rum and come with us;
For we don't give a damn
For any damn man
Who don't give a damn for us.

56

AGRICULTURE YELL

Agriculture–Agriculture---Var-si-ty
Agrico, Biblico, Zip ,Zap, Zee,
Griticum, Labrium, Bulbican, Bac
Incus, Humus, Igneous, Lac,
Varsity, Varstiy, U. of A.
Aggies, Aggies, Hip Hur---ray.

57

. **MEDICAL YELL**

The knife—the saw—the saw—the
    knife (slow)
Sit down—lie down—we want your
    life (faster)
We sing—you cry—we live—you
    die. (very fast)
    MEDICALS

58

DENTS

Good teeth, bad teeth,
What's the diff?
Pull 'em out, yank 'em out,
Biff, Biff, Biff!
Tooth Ache, Dentures, Blood, oh, Yea,
Strong arm Dentists, U. of A.

59

PHARMACY YELL

Lotions, Potions, fiat chart
We know 'em all Secundum Art,
Watch the spell binders,
We are the pill grinders
Hydrolzing, carbolizing, olea
PHARMACY--PHARMACY--U. of A.

60

COMMERCE YELL

Money—Money—Money (slow)
Cash—Cash—Cash (faster)
Kale—Kale—Kale (very fast)
COMMERCE.

61

LAW YELL

Treason, Graft or Fraudulence,
Bigamy, Theft or Negligence,
First offence, or Innocence
You get the clink
We get the chink.
LAAAWWW

62

Cluck, cluck, cluck,
Cluck, cluck, cluck,
Hen coop, hen coop,
    Rah, Rah, Rah,
Hen coop, hen coop,
    Pembina
Cock-a-doodle-do.

63

On them—On them—On them—BO
Are you ready,
Let 'er go.

64

YIP—I—ADDY

YIP-I-ADDY, I ay, I ay, YIP-I-Addy,
    I-ay
I don't care what becomes of me
When we're fighting for Varsity.
YIP-I-addy, I-ay, I-ay, I just want to
    shout out HURRAH!
Sing of joy, sing of Bliss, home was
    never like this
YIP-I-addy, I-ay.

65

"I know where the flies go

I know where the profs go in the
    winter time,
Early in September up the stairs they
    climb
Lay their plans and lay them deep,
Keep us from our beauty sleep;
Pile the work on like a Turk,
There's no bluffing, we can't shirk.
Then they say, "We've done our best
To pluck you now we need a rest;
So now you know you where profs go
In the good old winter time!

I know where the profs. go in the
    summer time.
After Convocation, to a foreign clime.
Have their fling, spend all they earn,
Come back on the first of term;
Meet their classes, oh, what joy!
First a girl and then a boy.
Then they sing, we've travelled far,
But found no place like Alberta."
So now you know where profs. go
In the good old summer time!

66

(Tune: "Mademoiselle From Armen-
    tieres.")

Palmer leads the Varsity team,
    Parlez-vous.
Palmer leads the Varsity team,
    Parlez-vous.
The boy's a wonder at half on the line,
    And we're going to back him all
        the time,
Hinky, Pinky, parlez-vous.

V-A-R-S-I-T-Y,
    Score a touch,

V-A-R-S-I-T-Y,
    Score a touch,

V-A-R-S-I-T-Y,
    Tackle low and kick 'em high,

V-A-R-S-I-T-Y.

67

GREEN AND GOLD

Green and Gold, Green and Gold,
    We'd like you to hold that line
    We'd like you to buck that line
Green and Gold, Gold and Green
    Flip 'em, flop 'em
    Flap 'em, flip 'em
    Green and Gold.

The Varsity Cheers for the same year. Each faculty had its own "yell," as did
the University itself.

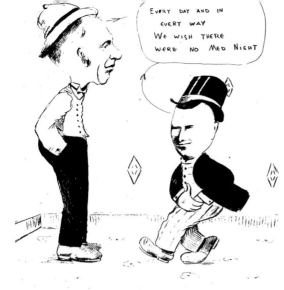

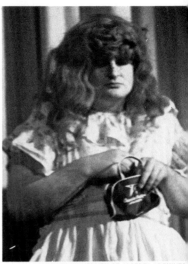

"The Medical Queen,"
1964.

A cartoon by Egerton Pope graphically portrays
what has probably been the feeling of faculty
towards the Med Show over the entire 75 years!
Dr. J.J. Ower is the figure on the left.

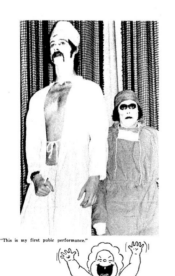

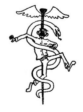

THE MEDICAL STUDENTS' ASSOCIATION
of
THE UNIVERSITY OF ALBERTA

presents

The Med Show
of '74

SILVER ANNIVERSARY
TWENTY-FIFTH ANNUAL MED SHOW

•

Produced by the Students of
THE FACULTY OF MEDICINE
THE UNIVERSITY OF ALBERTA

Staged at
STUDENTS' UNION THEATRE
FEBRUARY 7 and 8, 1974
7:30 P.M.

Programme cover of the 1974 Med Show.

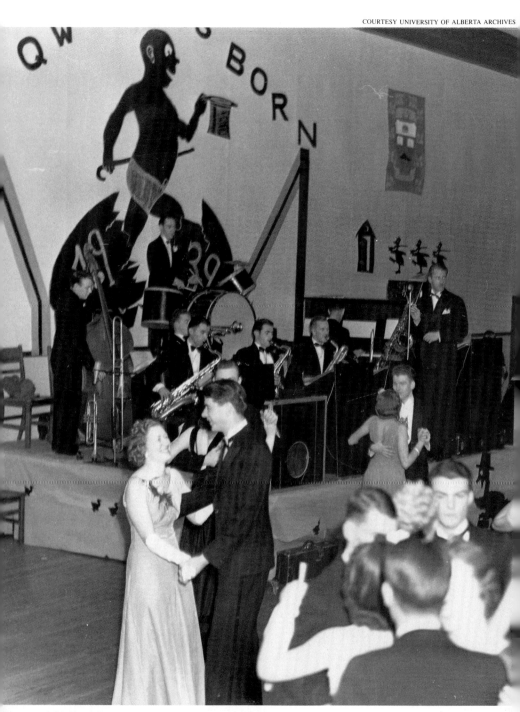

Medical Students dance, January 1939.

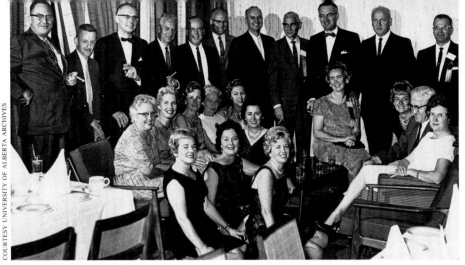

The Class of '38 at their silver anniversary reunion in 1963, with their wives. (This was an all-male class.) *Standing, left to right:* Steve Parlee, Walter Johns, Jack Goddard, Harvey Armitage, Ross Kelly, Hector "Bub" Duggan, Rupert Clare, Fred Conroy, Leonard Bradley, Harley Phillips, Sam Hanson. *Seated, middle row:* Mrs. E. White, Mona Bradley, Norah Kelly, Dagne Lees, Willa Parlee, Mrs. Harley Phillips, Eleanor Clare, Ed White, Sadie Duggan. *Seated on the floor:* Mrs. Harvey Armitage, Rene Conroy, Louise Johns, Mary Hanson. This was a distinguished class - no fewer than five of its members have received the Outstanding Achievement Award. H.A. Arnold, 1972; R.M. Clare, 1982; L.O. Bradley, 1983; H.E. Duggan, 1986; and J.S. Lewis, 1988.

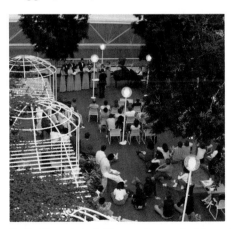 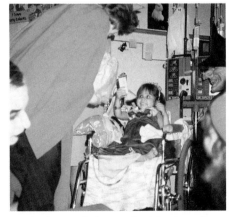

Left: Courtyard Concerts are held on the 4th floor of the W.C. Mackenzie Health Sciences Centre every Thursday during the lunch hour. They are sponsored by the Medical Students' Association, who purchased the grand piano. *Right:* Medical Students entertain in the children's ward on All Hallow's Eve.

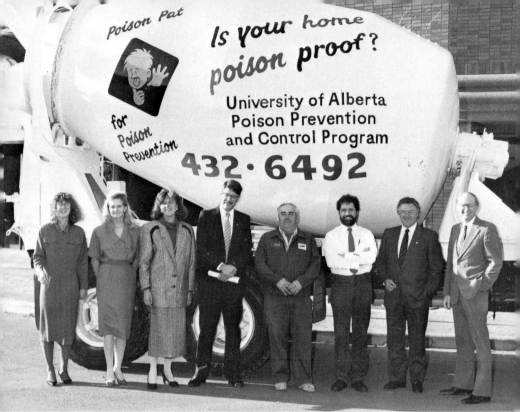

Poison Pat

Is your home poison proof?

for Poison Prevention

University of Alberta
Poison Prevention
and Control Program
432·6492

The Poison Prevention and Control Program was developed by the Medical Students' Association. Designed to help prevent poisoning in the home, it was the brainchild of Louis Francescutti, who is shown here (third from the right) at the launch of the programme in 1987. Dean Douglas R. Wilson is on the far right. COURTESY UNIVERSITY OF ALBERTA

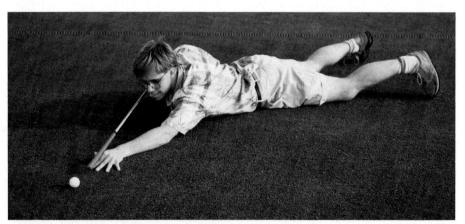

"There's more than one way to sink a putt." Students' annual golf tournament, 1987.

Thomas Henry Huxley, a British scientist, humanist and educator, who had also trained as a physician, was a strong advocate of science in medicine. A dominant figure in the development of medical education on both sides of the Atlantic, Huxley endorsed a study of the sciences, but only insofar as they applied to medicine.[12] A much greater emphasis on the pure sciences, however, developed in the major American medical schools in the late decades of the nineteenth century.[13]

During the latter half of the nineteenth century, in both Canada and the United States, some medical schools gradually achieved a closer relationship with their parent universities. In other cases, notably Harvard, Johns Hopkins and the University of Michigan, major universities established or adopted their own professional medical faculties, following the scientific curricula of the German schools. In the last decade of the nineteenth century, Johns Hopkins emerged as the dominant medical school. On the other hand, Canada, with its strong British background, was influenced more by British schools, particularly Edinburgh, and their emphasis on clinical teaching. When Sir William Osler went from McGill to Johns Hopkins, he took with him the traditional clinical teaching of that school and introduced bedside teaching into the United States.[14]

In the meantime, the proliferation of proprietary schools, and the increasing number of inadequately trained practitioners, caused concern among the medical practitioners of the day. The American Medical Association and the Association of American Medical Colleges, formed respectively in 1847 and 1876, attempted to set licensing regulations and standards for medical colleges.[15] They achieved some successes, and though the end of the proprietary school system has often been credited to a report commissioned by the Carnegie Foundation in 1910, these schools were already on the decline by then. By the turn of the century, the basic medical sciences were firmly entrenched in medical education, and as a result the teaching of medicine became more expensive. It now required laboratories, equipment, hospital affiliations and full-time professional staff; it could no longer generate a profit.[16]

The major foundations of the day, such as Carnegie and Rockefeller, began to take an interest, and the former hired Abraham Flexner, an educationist, to conduct a study of medical education in the United States and Canada. A graduate of Johns Hopkins University, Flexner spent some eighteen months visiting medical schools across the continent and produced what has come to be known as the Flexner Report. In this, he condemned the proprietary schools and recommended an "ideal" programme for the training of medical practitioners similar to the one that had been developed by his *alma mater*. Essentially, his report advocated that every medical school be an integral part of a university, that admission requirements be one or two years of university training in the sciences, and that a four-year medical course include two years of study in basic medical sciences followed by two years in clinical sciences.

The Flexner Report also made it quite clear that an adequate medical college was an expensive proposition. While university schools across the continent scrambled to adopt the recommendations of the report, in many cases they were hampered by lack of funds. Again the foundations stepped in, and while their interference was not overt, medical schools were persuaded to conform to the standards set by the Flexner Report and the Association of American Medical Colleges if they wished to receive financial assistance. Universities competed vigorously with one another for foundation funding. The schools that survived introduced longer and more exacting courses, built laboratories for basic science teaching, affiliated with hospitals for the teaching of clinical sciences, and, to obtain students who were competent to take such training, introduced prerequisites.[17]

By 1925, the year that the University of Alberta graduated its first medical practitioners, the Canadian curriculum was still in transition. An extra year had been added, but this was mainly to ensure an adequate standard in the premedical courses. Canadian medical schools established certain prerequisites for entry into the premedical programme, but high school science courses had generally not achieved an advanced standard sufficient to enable students to obtain these prerequisites. The first two years of university study were devoted, therefore, to basic sciences and other general subjects, which included both dead and living languages, and were a prerequisite for the basic medical sciences given in the first two years of the professional degree programme. The premedical course was highly structured—each subject had to be mastered before the student could advance to the next year and attendance at class was both compulsory and recorded.[18]

As a result of these changes, the medical schools achieved credibility, both within the profession and among the citizenry, who became increasingly aware of the need for educational qualifications in their local practitioners. The poorly trained, the "quacks and charlatans," and the "irregular" medical practitioners were gradually eased out, as universities not only took over the training of physicians but also, in some cases, became involved in examining practitioners for licensure. Alberta was one of these. In many jurisdictions, and Alberta was one of these also, upon successful completion of the university medical programme, the graduate was licensed to commence practice.[19] Following graduation, some chose to intern in a hospital for six months or a year, but this meant extra time and extra money. Hospitals of the day viewed internship as a learning experience and did not pay interns for their work on the wards. A rotating internship through several departments of the hospital was what the new young doctor needed, but few staff members could or would give any time to instruct an intern.[20] Furthermore, as hospital administrators generally did not view either teaching or research as part of their responsibilities, there were few internships available.[21] In 1925, therefore, only about half of Canadian graduates interned.[22] In time, hospital administrators gradually realized the value of having interns in residence, people who could assist the house staff by performing routine tasks, and internships became an integral part of the hospital infrastructure. They are now a requirement for a licence to practise, and are paid positions. But it has continued to be a contentious issue to reach a balance between the responsibilities of the intern to the hospital, and the hospital's responsibility to give instruction and supervision.[23]

The basic lockstep system of two years studying basic medical sciences followed by two years in the clinical sciences advocated by Flexner continued for many years, undergoing only relatively minor tinkering with methodology, content, length of courses, and the occasional change of approach. The sharp division between medical and clinical sciences enabled the "half-school" to operate at institutions such as the University of Alberta, where initially the medical school offered only the first two years of basic medical sciences and its students went on to other schools for the clinical years. It also accentuated the division between the medical and clinical science instructors, who operated in virtual isolation from each other, and frequently failed to define the relationship between their subject areas. The medical sciences were often taught as rigorous scientific subjects, with little attention to their adaptation to the practice of medicine. Anatomy, traditionally the essence of any medical training, remained the major ingredient. Four hours of anatomy each day of the week for the first two years was the norm at many medical schools in the early years of this century, and students did not see a live patient until their third year.[24] Professors in the basic medical science departments traditionally had been full-time employees of the university, and they built up strong empires. Most of the research was conducted in these departments, some of which were run by Ph.D.s and had a number on staff as well. Ph.D./M.D. antagonisms developed, and from the 1950s to the 1980s, when full-time clinicians made their appearance in the halls of medical schools in larger numbers, a power struggle often evolved.[25] The effort to integrate the medical sciences with each other and with the clinical sciences has been an ongoing struggle in medical curriculum and development.

Early Medical Education at the University of Alberta

The University of Alberta opened the doors of its medical school in 1913, just three years after the publication of the Flexner Report, and was thus in a position to try to arrange its curriculum according to the recommendations outlined in that document. A new university in a newly settled part of the country, it was in no position to demand two years of premedical university training in the sciences. In fact, many of the high schools in the province lacked the teaching personnel and equipment to be able to offer advanced courses in either the sciences or the humanities at the Grade XII level. For this reason, admittance to the university required only a Grade XI standing, or junior matriculation, and the first year at university was a preliminary one that offered the Grade XII courses required in the discipline of the student's choice. Thus, the first year in the medical programme was a premedical course in which students studied physics, chemistry, botany, zoology and French or German. Successful completion of these courses gave the students a senior matriculation standing, and they could then go on to the first professional year of studies in anatomy, histology, splanchnology,[26] embryology, physiology, biochemistry and bacteriology. Students devoted three hours of lectures and twenty hours in the laboratory each week to anatomy, combining "dissection of the human body" with "lectures, demonstrations and recitations."[27] In the third year, or second professional year, offered for the first time in 1915-16, slightly fewer hours were spent on anatomy: three hours of lectures and fifteen hours in the laboratory each week. Students received further instruction in neurology, physiology, clinical physiology, general pathology, bacteriology, pathological chemistry, surgery, psychology and pharmacology. On the successful completion of these three years, each student went on to an eastern university, usually Toronto, McGill or Manitoba, for clinical training.

Academic regulations at the university were strict. For a number of years, attendance at classes was compulsory and instructors conducted roll calls. This was a regulation of the university itself, and attendance was required at no fewer than seven-eighths of the lectures in any one course or the student was not permitted to write the final examination. There were two terms, and final examinations were held in January and May. Two-thirds of the final mark was from the final examination and one-third from term work, which was assessed by two tests during each term. In this way, it was "impossible for a person to idle away his term...and chances of failure for the steady and faithful [were] reduced."[28] Professor Revell objected to taking a roll call and proposed that this procedure be dropped in the medical school, but while a lively discussion ensued, it was decided to continue the practice.[29]

As Canada was at war, and a number of teachers and students had left for overseas, few changes were made to the curriculum over the next few years, except for the addition of history to the premedical year. The curriculum was required to follow a pattern approved by the University of Toronto and McGill University, so it can be assumed that they offered similar courses in the first three years. In 1916, both schools extended their medical programmes by adding an extra year, and Alberta followed suit. The additional year basically extended the science years, adding a few extra subjects, such as mathematics and physical education, but the new fourth year now included introductory courses in medicine and surgery. Admittance to the premedical year was still from Grade XI, but as high school standards began to improve in the province, those who had Grade XII could enter directly into second year.

As the school extended its curriculum to the full degree programme, it added clinical subjects in the fifth and sixth years: medicine, surgery, obstetrics and gynaecology. Clinical instruction consisted of lectures, held in the Medical Building, while clinics were conducted at the University Hospital. In their final year, students were "expected to help in routine clinical laboratory work in the hospital, in writing histories and keeping up progress notes." Instructors gave bedside lectures in therapeutics, and conducted clinical and pathological conferences once a week.[30] Other subjects included pathology, hygiene, medical jurisprudence, toxicology, psychopathology, psychiatry, radiology and the history of medicine.

After World War I, the faculty offered a combined course leading to the degrees of B.A. and M.D. Essentially, this added two years to the entire programme. After the first three years of sciences, social sciences and humanities, the student entered the second year of medicine and received a B.A. degree upon the successful completion of that year. The student then continued with the last four years of the medical programme. A similar combined B.Sc. and M.D. programme differed only in the third year, when more science subjects were required.[31] In 1928, after some discussion about providing a combined course in dentistry and medicine, the faculty forwarded a proposal outlining the curriculum requirements and timetabling to the university Board of Governors. Although the programme received approval and was announced in the university calendar, it aroused little interest in the student body. This option arose for discussion again in 1949, but no agreement was reached.[32]

The passing grade in all subjects was set at 50%, and honours required 75%. A student who failed the majority of courses in any one year had to repeat the whole year, but a failure in a minority of subjects provided the alternative of supplemental examinations. All subjects had to be "cleared" before a student could continue into the next year of the programme. All students paid a "caution fee" to cover any breakages, and had to pay any outstanding charges before writing the final examinations.[33] The timetable was full throughout the six years. Classes started at 8:35 a.m. and, with an hour break for lunch, continued to 4:35 or 5:35 from Monday to Friday. On Saturdays, they finished at noon, except for sixth-year students who attended obstetrics and gynaecology clinics on Saturday afternoons.[34]

Few changes appeared in the curriculum prior to the second world war, aside from rearranging the order from time to time. The question of Latin and/or Greek as prerequisites frequently arose for discussion, as a knowledge of Latin was required by some of the licensing bodies.[35] In 1942, the classics department offered a course on Latin and Greek forms and roots with special reference to medical terminology that was made compulsory in the premedical year.[36] A unit on professional ethics, based upon the code of ethics of the Canadian Medical Association, was introduced in 1928 and included in the history of medicine course.[37] This latter subject lasted in Alberta's curriculum longer than at many other medical schools, probably because of faculty member Heber Jamieson's abiding interest in the topic. A special department was established in 1924, and Jamieson was appointed professor of the history of medicine in 1929. He presented a required thirty-two hour course in the fourth and fifth years of the programme. By 1952, this had been reduced to a one hour a week elective taught by Dean Scott, and later still was included only in the orientation programme offered to medical students at the beginning of their first year as a presentation by R.A. Macbeth, professor of surgery. The reason given for this decline was that "students at Alberta are technically oriented and mainly interested in practical matters, paying little attention to subjects that they do not feel are required.''[38] The first move towards a decrease in the number of didactic lectures took place as early as 1926 when a committee was struck to identify the changes necessary in the curriculum if all didactic lectures in the sixth and final year were eliminated. The committee concluded that lectures could be eliminated in the sixth year, but only if they were presented in the fifth year instead.[39]

A New Curriculum is Incorporated, 1940-41

The first major change in the curriculum took place in 1940-41 as a result of adjustments to the prerequisites and premedical programme. In 1935, for the first time, a quota was placed on the admission of students into medicine, brought on by the exigencies of the depressed state of the economy and inadequate facilities. As a result, students in the first year of medicine and those in the third year of arts and medicine could only continue on in the faculty if they completed their year's work with an average of 65% or more. In 1938, fourteen of those accepted had baccalaureates and thirteen were in the combined course. The time appeared to be ripe to increase entrance requirements to two years of university training after Grade XII. Entry would then come via a combined B.Sc., M.D. course. At this juncture, the B.A., M.D. course was dropped; it was similar in content to the B.Sc., M.D. and had proved unsatisfactory for those who did not continue into medicine. The Grade XII senior matriculation requirements now included English, social studies, algebra, geometry, trigonometry, physics, chemistry, and French or German or Latin. The subjects prescribed in the new B.Sc., M.D. course were English, a foreign language, physics, chemistry, zoology and physical education in the first year, and a continuation of the foreign language, psychology, zoology and mathematics, chemistry, and one more course selected from chemistry, physics, entomology or zoology in the second year.[40]

The faculty surveyed recent graduates for their views on the curriculum and suggestions for improvements. Recommendations included; fewer hours in anatomy, more emphasis on the action of drugs on living systems in the pharmacology course, a greater and earlier emphasis on preventive medicine, more practical and hands-on experience given earlier in the course, fewer lectures, and more bedside teaching. Most respondents also complained of the loss of time in getting clinics under way.[41]

The new curriculum, incorporating some of these suggestions, was introduced year by year during the war and was in place by 1945-46. The two years of premedical training were followed by five years in the professional programme, in which the first two years were devoted to basic medical sciences, the third and fourth years to the clinical sciences, and the fifth was extended to a full twelve months in the hospitals on rotating internships. Interns lived at one or another of the city hospitals and rotated through the different services. Final examinations followed the internship year and the newly graduated doctor could then take a senior or graduate internship or go directly into practice.

Change from a Five-year to a Four-year programme
Increased registration following the second world war caused severe over-crowding conditions in the hospitals during the undergraduate internship year. Edmonton's hospitals were unable to accommodate or teach the larger numbers, so the fifth or intern year was dropped in 1948. Students earned their M.D. after the fourth year, and then took a graduate internship in any approved hospital. On the successful completion of this year, they became eligible for an enabling certificate from the College of Physicians and Surgeons of Alberta to write the licensing examinations of the Medical Council of Canada.[42] At the same time, each year of the course was extended in length, a few clinical subjects were introduced in the first and second years, and some applied basic sciences were given in the third and fourth years, making a break from the rigid two-and-two division.[43]

In 1950-51 the faculty discontinued its combined B.Sc., M.D. course along with any formalized and prescribed premedical training. The prerequisite for medicine was set at two full years at a university, with specified courses in physics, organic and inorganic chemistry and zoology. This was an endeavour to make the undergraduate training a more liberal one and to give the students those extra two years in which to make their final decision before entering medicine. The formal premedical course implied that the student was already in the medical programme and was often perceived as an obligation on the part of the Faculty of Medicine to accept into first-year medicine all those who passed the course. It also caused confusion and disappointment when a student, qualified academically through the premedical course, subsequently was not accepted into the professional programme. For those who were either not able to get into medicine or found that it was not really their choice, the new arrangement enabled them to fit into another programme with greater ease, and not to lose those two years of university studies.[44]

In the years following the war, when large classes and a shortage of both space and staff were the order of the day, faculty members were hard pressed to keep up with their teaching and administrative responsibilities. They had little time or energy left to deal with changes in curriculum and to explore new concepts of medical education. Some, nevertheless, became increasingly aware that changes would have to take place. One innovation in 1948 involved a series of orientation lectures and clinics given at the beginning of the first year by staff from various departments, to introduce students to life in the medical school. Shortly after this, Dean Scott proposed a trimester system in the fourth and final year, so that students could be assigned to teaching hospitals as clinical clerks and gain some experience of the conditions that they would face in their intern year. At about the same time, some students began working with the College of Physicians and Surgeons of Alberta on a preceptor programme, allowing them to work with selected general practitioners during the summer and learn first-hand the kinds of experiences they could expect in private practice. In addition, Dr. M.R. Bow, who was the Alberta deputy minister of health and also an associate professor of public health, developed a short course on social medicine to give the students some insight into the sociological problems they would meet in their practice.

Changing Concepts in Medical Education Following World War II
Prior to World War II, the medical school curriculum was designed to produce general practitioners, and given the ratio of rural to urban population in both Canada and the United States, most general practitioners worked in isolation in rural or semirural communities. Most schools, however, were in large urban centres, and the clinical teachers had little or no experience as "country doctors."[45] Other complaints were heard from time to time about various aspects of medical education and, according to Flexner, who advocated full-time professors in both the clinical and medical sciences, too much clinical teaching in both Canada and the United States was still in the hands of "busy local practitioners who had been trained under the old regime," and supervision was, therefore, "loose and inadequate."[46] It was not until after the second world war, however, that recognition of "the problems with medical education" reached its peak. This coincided with a rapid rise in the country's population, both from immigration and a marked increase in the birthrate, creating a need for more physicians. In addition, the number of specialized branches of medicine began to increase rapidly in the 1950s and as each new specialty surfaced, it demanded a place on the curriculum. The result was an overloaded and inflexible curriculum in which subjects were taught as a series of isolated disciplines, rather than

as integrated branches of a whole. While fragmentation of the curriculum had raised complaints for years, the advent of specialization brought the problem to a crisis point.[47] The amount of material a student was expected to cover, and remember, to pass examinations, became overwhelming.

It has been said that advances in medical technology double every ten years. For the 1980s, this might be a conservative estimate. It is impossible to impart so much knowledge to medical students in a short span of four years. Educators were faced with deciding what was most important and what could safely be left out, based on some measure of the intrinsic value of the new knowledge.[48] Over the years, there have been numerous conferences, symposia, studies and discussions on the subject of medical education. From these came a variety of suggestions for overcoming the problems faced by medical schools. First, since the student could not learn everything there was to know, it was the university's task to encourage self-study, to teach the concepts and philosophy, and to promote in the student the personal commitment to search out critical information as needed by study in the library, the laboratory or on the ward. The way to teach this was not by didactic lecturing but by small-group seminars, bedside teaching or even one-on-one experiences. Second, to obtain time for such self-motivated study, the student needed a curriculum that offered free time for selective studies. Third, dramatic scientific advances had not only created improved methods for diagnosis and treatment, they had also introduced ethical conflicts for both the medical profession and society as a whole, conflicts that could not be dealt with in a purely scientific manner. Now more than ever, there was a place for the study of the humanities, both as a prerequisite and in the medical course itself. Fourth, the marked increase of specialties and subspecialties had made it more difficult for the doctor to see and know the patient as an individual. These circumstances called for courses in humanities and the introduction of community medicine and social medicine programmes, courses that dealt with the ''individual and personal'' as opposed to the ''general and impersonal.''[49]

In 1961, the federal government appointed a royal commission on health services in Canada. A group of six doctors, chaired by J.A. Mac-Farlane, undertook a study of medical education in Canada and submitted its findings to this commission. In a thorough and wide-ranging report, the recommendations included social sciences as a prerequisite for medical school; a reduction in didactic lectures and the introduction of methods that involved student participation and involvement; clinical clerkship in a teaching hospital during the final year that would include some responsibility to patients; in view of the growth of specialization, the establishment of departments of general practice; a review of evaluating procedures to dispense with the formal final examinations; more full-time clinicians; and a grouping of all schools and faculties into a health sciences centre. Finally, the group recommended a full-time dean in every medical faculty, "who should be medically qualified, have the training and experience necessary to hold an even balance between [sic] the basic sciences, the clinical fields and the development of research."[50]

But how were these changing concepts to be realized in the existing medical schools? It has frequently been said that it is easier to move a cemetery than change the curriculum in a medical school.[51] Curriculum committees included representatives of the various departments of the faculty, each inevitably looking at the curriculum from a single disciplinary perspective. Only since the 1960s, have students had representation on faculty committees, but curriculum committees were still dominated by educators of one generation formulating the curriculum for students of a succeeding generation who would practise in yet another generation—a problem faced by educators in all disciplines. A further imponderable is the ultimate measurement of effectiveness—how well students perform in their subsequent careers.

The Introduction of Interdisciplinary Teaching

One way to reduce specialized training in each of the individual sciences was to introduce interdisciplinary teaching in the basic medical sciences. Of the numerous experiments in medical schools across North America, the most famous came in the early 1950s at the Case Western Reserve School in Cleveland, Ohio. There, what has come to be known as the "systems" method was first put into practice, with a curriculum designed horizontally rather than vertically. Students studied different body systems—for example the cardiovascular system, the nervous system, the gastrointestinal system, and so on—and were presented with the relevant sciences, both medical and clinical, as they applied to that system. Instructors in basic science and clinical departments taught an integrated analysis of each body system. For instance, they presented the anatomy, physiology, biochemistry, bacteriology and pathology of the cardiovascular system along with diseases of the heart, and surgical and other methods of treatment. Systems followed one another in a logical sequence and all teaching took place in a seminar format. In addition, the curriculum committee rather than the departments controlled the curriculum.[52]

According to some, however, a major disadvantage was that nothing was learned beyond what was required immediately.[53] Another drawback was that the systems method needed a large and full-time faculty to accomplish so much small-group teaching; much larger than many schools had or could afford. For the faculty members, moreover, it involved a great deal of repetition. In a variation of this approach, known as the "block" system, two or three basic medical sciences, or two or three clinical sciences, were taught on an interdisciplinary basis. Most schools attempted some form of interdisciplinary teaching and integrated courses, particularly some of the newer schools, with varying degrees of success. Traditionalists were unhappy at throwing out the "tried and true" in favour of what had yet to be proven useful, however, and for older schools with strongly entrenched departments, integration was difficult to achieve.[54]

Any significant change in the medical school curriculum required at least a core of full-time clinical instructors, a change that began in Canada in the 1950s. In time, as specialty programmes and research demanded more and more time, it became necessary for medical schools to engage more clinicians who were willing and able to devote most of their time to the needs of the school. Traditionally, clinical teaching had been carried out by local practitioners on a part-time basis, and many were loathe to give up a lucrative private practice and enter the "ivory tower" of academic medicine. The "geographic full-time" system of appointments developed gradually to permit clinical professors to maintain private practices, but only within the "geographic" confines of the medical school and its teaching hospital.[55]

Changes in curriculum, either in content or presentation, were not the only answers to improved medical education; student selection and evaluation also came under intense scrutiny, following the concept that the "art of medicine ... lies in the careful selection of students for their personal qualities."[56] It was easy to agree that those with "qualities of independence and critical capacity," with interests in the affairs of the community and cultural activities, and not simply those with high grades in scientific subjects, should be chosen for entrance into medical school. But such attributes proved difficult to recognize and assess.

Changes occurred also in the evaluation of student performance. For many years, the only yardstick was the formal examination, and students were ranked in order of academic achievement. As this standing played some part in the assessment of candidates for graduate training schools, this emphasis tended to create a competitive, rather than the preferred co-operative, relationship among students. In 1933, Egerton Pope, head of the faculty's department of medicine, wrote an article extolling the virtues of examinations. A career in medicine, he contended, was a series of examinations, and the best place to get used to them was in medical school.[57] Small-group teaching allowed personal assessment by instructors to be included in student evaluation, however, and a movement toward a pass/fail or honours/pass/fail system gradually won approval in many medical schools.

In 1984, the extensive and searching report of a panel of medical practitioners on the General Professional Education of the Physician (GPEP) and College Preparation for Medicine was published as a supplement to the *Journal of Medical Education*. Commissioned by the Association of American Medical Colleges and known as the GPEP Report, it was expected to become a benchmark for future developments in medical education on this continent.[58] A far-reaching report, it made many recommendations for changes in medical education that would, ideally, produce a "physician of tomorrow " who would be "caring, compassionate and dedicated to patients ... committed to work, to learning, to rationality, to science and to serving the greater society." It argued for education in the skills and attitudes that would enable a doctor to adapt to, and assess, new procedures and practices as they became available—a more important attribute than the straight acquisition of modern technical knowledge.[59]

The numerous recommendations included an emphasis on "health promotion and disease prevention;" a reduction in scheduled timetabling and lecture periods and increased time for the pursuit of elective subjects; "broad study in the natural and the social sciences and in the humanities;" the development of effective writing skills; a change in evaluation procedures; integration of basic medical and clinical sciences; the establishment of a "mentor relationship" between a faculty member and individual students; and improved communication between the medical and other university faculties.[60] In addition, the report advocated increased opportunities for qualified students to aspire to a career in medicine, regardless of "sex, race, ethnic origin or financial status."[61]

Science has had a stranglehold on medical education for a century or more; yet, the concept of medicine as a social art, for humanities in the medical curriculum, has always had its supporters. If the GPEP Report was to have the effect on medical education predicted at the outset, then the pool of students from which the medical schools would draw their entrants would be larger and more diverse in background and interests. In 1983-84, the major undergraduate subjects studied by 68% of the accepted applicants in United States medical schools was in the biological or physical sciences; for only 10% was it in nonscience areas.[62]

The report had at least one warning in common with the Flexner Report—that medical education in the twenty-first century would be much more expensive. The emphasis on small-group teaching, the mentor relationship, supervision of electives, all require a large full-time faculty. In 1982-83, most Canadian medical schools had a ratio of less than two students to one full-time professor. At McMaster University in Hamilton, Ontario, the ratio was less than one to one yet at the University of Alberta it was slightly more than two students to one full-time professor.[63] To fulfill the demands made for the future of medical education, this ratio would no doubt have to be reduced even further.

Achieving the ideal medical education is a never-ending pursuit. The Josiah Macy Jr. Foundation undertook to finance a series of studies on medical education, the first of which was released in November 1988. Its findings supported the general thesis of the GPEP Report.[64] All Canadian medical schools have been visited on a regular basis by accreditation teams representing the Royal College of Physicians and Surgeons of Canada, the Association of Canadian Medical Colleges and the Association of American Medical Colleges. These visitations not only assessed the standards of each school but also offered professional assistance to faculty members in their efforts to meet the shifting demands of the profession, the public and the student body.

Postwar Changes in Medical Education at the University of Alberta
In the early 1950s, the Association of American Medical Colleges offered short courses in the teaching of medical sciences, and some members of the faculty attended. They brought back information about new methods of teaching: integrated courses in three or more sciences, the value of small-group teaching, and the dangers of rigid standardization in the medical curriculum. H.V. Rice, professor of physiology, who attended one of these courses, suggested that less emphasis be placed on the scientific techniques of the basic medical sciences and more on their application to medical procedures. Although most agreed that the whole subject of teaching and the curriculum should be discussed by the entire teaching staff, before this happened the accreditation team report of 1956 catalyzed the process, making major changes in the curriculum an urgent necessity.

The accreditation team reported that 4,640 hours of instruction were offered over the four-year programme, of which nearly one-fifth (870 hours) was devoted to anatomy. Forty per cent of the total time was spent in lectures, and the curriculum was severely overloaded and fragmented into a number of unrelated courses. The curriculum consisted of fifteen different subjects in the second year, fourteen in the third, and twelve in the fourth; and at the end of each, students were evaluated by a final, formal examination. The team recommended an extension of the school year, fewer lectures and more small teaching groups, less anatomy, more integrated courses, and more free time both for electives and for the observance of the course of an illness in the hospital wards.

It would have been well-nigh impossible for the University of Alberta's Faculty of Medicine to make any sweeping changes given its limited number of full-time staff and its inadequate facilities. In addition, some of the staff, while they agreed with the attempt to adopt newer teaching techniques, felt that the traditional system had much of value that should be retained.[65] The faculty did make certain immediate changes, however. It extended the academic year to thirty-three weeks and initiated the process that would, over the next several years, add a number of integrated courses to the curriculum. It reduced considerably the time spent on anatomy and offered an applied anatomy course in the second year that involved co-operation with the radiology and surgery departments. An orientation to medical practice course, given in the first year, emphasized the interrelationship of the medical, behavioural and basic sciences through presentations by representatives of the various science and clinical departments. Later, this course was renamed "Man and His Environment" and was adapted to serve as an introductory course to clinical medicine. Given by the departments of community medicine, medicine, surgery and psychiatry, it emphasized the interaction of man and the environment in matters of health and disease.

For the second year, members of the clinical and medical science departments developed a major interdisciplinary course, entitled "Introduction to Medicine" that served as a bridge between the medical science and clinical years. Members of the various clinical departments also offered second-year courses in physical diagnosis and history-taking. In a survey of human disease course, offered in the third year, members of the departments of medicine, surgery and pediatrics presented individual cases. Preventive medicine continued to be offered in the last three years, but, in addition, certain aspects of the topic were treated from time to time in both clinical and preclinical courses. Both the third and fourth years were placed on a trimester system. Clinical clerkships were introduced into the third year, involving bedside clinics, mostly at the University of Alberta Hospital, small-group teaching and student assignments to individual patients. Fourth-year interns rotated through the various teaching hospitals of the city.[66] By the time the complete new curriculum was in place in 1959, it allowed one half day per week of free time in each year.[67]

Within three years of the accreditation team's visit, the dean was able to report that:

> Lecture hours have been sharply reduced, discussion groups are instituted and emphasized, students are given more responsibility for their own education, the curriculum is much less fragmented and large periods of uninterrupted time are available during clerkship periods which now extend over both third and fourth years. Students now have a continuing responsibility for patients and must keep their records on their cases up to date for discussion at any time.[68]

Some of the older professors, however, who had been at the school almost since its inception, were not enthusiastic about the new, experimental moves in medical education. Shaner, who had taught anatomy at the University of Alberta since 1921, remarked,

> It used to be assumed that a medical student had the imagination and the will power to learn something and to retain it, at least in outline, until he had use for it at some later time. The current trend among educators assumes just the reverse; that no one can learn anything except that for which he has immediate use. Hence the increasing practice of converting basic science teachers into casual pedlars of useful bits of information as required in clinical years.[69]

Dean Scott, well aware of some of these feelings, acknowledged that,

> some members of our basic science departments are not convinced that extreme integration of their subjects is valuable and they prefer to give a firm grounding in their subjects as separate disciplines and let the students integrate for themselves.[70]

Most faculty members felt that a good start had been made, but also understood the importance of a continuing review, both of changes taking place in medical education elsewhere and of the curriculum in their own school. In October 1961, Dean Mackenzie convened a study conference at Banff attended by all heads of departments and members of the Curriculum Committee at which Dr. George E. Miller, director of research in medical education at the University of Illinois and an outstanding authority on medical education, led the discussion periods. One outcome of this conference was the formation of a Committee for Research in Medical Education, with a mandate to study curricular changes, student selection procedures and evaluation methods. Dr. J.A.L. Gilbert, a full-time professor in the department of medicine, chaired this committee, that also included Dean Mackenzie, Assistant Dean D.F. Cameron, and a representative of the provincial Department of Education. It met on a regular basis for four years, organized several seminars, and invited authorities on the subject of medical education to visit the school.[71] The committee also examined the objectives of the school. Until the 1950s, the role of the medical school had been to produce knowledgeable and safe general practitioners. By the 1960s, however, the school offered graduate training programmes in the specialties and the medical sciences, and its graduates went into family practice, a specialty area, academic medicine or research. The faculty's new role, advised the committee, should be "to create an environment and provide educational opportunities to help the student in his individual development towards the medical profession."[72]

In 1966, at Dean Mackenzie's request, Gilbert studied curricular changes taking place elsewhere. He concluded that current changes in both the United States and Great Britain involved integration of courses, and reported that "all new educational systems in medicine have been developed along these lines." Such changes did require more staff, but they reduced didactic teaching time, and generated "a degree of enthusiasm amongst students and staff that is seldom, if ever, seen in the departmental based system."[73] He made four recommendations for the University of Alberta: a greater degree of integration at all stages; a reduction in didactic lectures; electives for those students who were in the upper two-thirds of their class; and improved methods of evaluation. As a result, electives in the medical sciences were offered in the first and second year in 1967 and were "received enthusiastically" by the students.[74] Second-year students circulated a questionnaire among themselves concerning electives, and the results supported this assessment and recommended that electives be extended over the entire four-year programme.[75] Total integration was impossible in a school with such a firmly established departmental system of teaching, but in 1968 the faculty introduced a trial integrated course in the neurological sciences, a course that included neuroanatomy, neurophysiology, neuropharmacology, neurology and neurosurgery.

Major Changes in the Curriculum Introduced in 1968
The Committee on Research in Medical Education dissolved in 1966, and a permanent Curriculum Advisory Committee assumed most of its functions. Simply stated, its purpose was to advise the dean and Faculty Council on matters relating to curriculum and to conduct studies in this area. Professor Gilbert remained as chairman.[76] An elected body, its members served for periods of three years, and a couple of years later it included student representatives.[77] After many meetings and consultations, and considerable discussion, the new committee proposed a radically different curriculum to go into operation in September 1968, dividing the four-year programme into three phases.

Phase I, given in the first year, constituted an introduction to medicine in which students received instruction in the basic sciences as they related to the practice of medicine, as well as a course in community medicine. The interdisciplinary course in neurological sciences continued in Phase II, the second year, but the biggest change in this phase was the introduction of a course entitled "Mechanism of Disease," taught by a multidisciplinary team on the "systems" method to small groups of students varying in number from fourteen to sixteen. Faculty members from various departments in both the medical and clinical sciences formed a multidisciplinary committee to co-ordinate the approach to each system The various teams taught the cardiovascular, endocrinological and metabolic, gastrointestinal, hematological, muscular, osteopathic, pulmonary and renal systems. Dividing the students into small groups meant individual instructors presented each system several times a year.[78] During this second phase, students received a certain amount of exposure to patients, and thus bridged the gap between the study of basic sciences and the student internship in the first year of Phase III.

The final phase, taught during the third and fourth years, was given on a continuous basis for eighty-six weeks, divided into fifty weeks of a rotating internship, thirty weeks of electives, and a six-week vacation period. Phases I and III effectively retained a departmental basis, although incorporating some team teaching, but Phase II made the leap to a fully integrated system. Unassigned time was also available in Phases I and II, and students could use this time either in electives or in taking extra time in areas of any weaknesses. Two half days a week were unassigned in Phase

I, but in Phase II the free time was so fragmented that it was not feasible to take an elective.[79]

The new curriculum ran into problems right from the start. Planned for introduction one year at a time from September 1968, it was delayed for a year because departments were not ready to present their new courses. The first-year students expecting to start on the brand new programme were sorely disappointed and decided to take matters into their own hands. Gilbert Dyck, the first-year student representative on the Curriculum Advisory Committee, organized a study group to ascertain whether the timetable could be rearranged to give his class all the necessary prerequisites for entry into the new curriculum in the second year. Despite the extra work commitment, his fellow students supported him wholeheartedly, as did the Curriculum Advisory Committee and Assistant Dean Cameron. So the Class of '72 became the first to graduate on the new curriculum.[80]

Both students and faculty, however, found fault with the new programme. The Medical Students' Association presented a "Student Opinion of the New Curriculum," which claimed that the curriculum was not radically changed and did not fulfil the objectives of the Committee on Research in Medical Education. While applauding the inclusion of electives in Phase III, it expressed concern about the lack of electives in Phases I and II, and a certain amount of rigidity in the first two years.[81] The students proposed some changes in the undergraduate internship programme, including a greater emphasis on the teaching of history-taking and physical examination, a one- or two-week orientation programme at the beginning of each rotation, and a clear definition of the responsibilities and duties of the student in the "clinical team approach."[82]

Some faculty members were equally unhappy, as the teaching load, particularly in Phase II, became very heavy. The team approach to teaching "systems" to small groups meant that faculty members taught the same material several times a year. The clinical faculty still included a large number of part-time teachers who found that the extra hours involved took much time away from their private practices. In addition to the extra work load—instruction periods increased from fifty to 560 hours a year—there was the added problem of maintaining enthusiasm with repetition every four weeks. While the new programme brought students onto the ward at an earlier point in their educational process, the staff of the medical school was not large enough to cope with the increased work load.

After three years, the groups gradually became larger and the programme moved away from integrated "system" teaching to block format instruction on pathological mechanisms of disease as they affected many organs.[83] Students later received some full class instruction in a more structured form in Phase III, and fewer elective hours. Electives were dropped from Phases I and II. A number of subjects that had not been included in the curriculum, such as geriatrics, allergy, nutrition and immunology, were incorporated in a Wednesday afternoon series of ninety-minute lectures.[84] In 1984-5 the faculty undertook another comprehensive review of the curriculum, once again seeking to reduce didactic teaching, to emphasize the acquisition of clinical skills, to provide the opportunity for more electives, and to stimulate independent learning.[85]

New Assessment and Evaluation Procedures Introduced

Changes in assessment and evaluation procedures accompanied changes in the curriculum. The Student Evaluation Board, established in 1970 with nine faculty and four student members, was the first in Canada. Under the guidance of this board, the faculty instituted multiple-choice comprehensive written examinations for the first time in 1971, although Faculty Council had accepted them in principle in 1963. To build up a "pool of questions," all departments submitted examination questions in their respective disciplines. They were stored in a computer, augmented and refined on a continuing basis, and weighted according to an accepted evaluation procedure.[86] The students then wrote only one comprehensive examination, developed from questions selected from this pool, after each of Phases I and II, rather than one for each subject as in previous years.

The final evaluation included assessments of personal attributes and abilities. Each department assessed students on an ongoing basis for 30% of their grade in Phase I, on in-class assessment and mid-term exams. At the end of the academic year, students wrote a multiple-choice, multidisciplinary examination, and the results of this examination represented the remaining 70% of their year-end grades. Phase II students also wrote a comprehensive examination at the conclusion of the academic year, that accounted for 70% of their year-end grades, but in addition they wrote a multidisciplinary examination at the conclusion of each "system," and this, together with a personal assessment, represented the other 30% of each student's grade. Phase III students received ongoing assessments and oral examination marks throughout their rotations for 30% of their final grade, while the final examination, made up of a series of multiple-choice, multidisciplinary written examinations, constituted 70% of their final grade.[87] In 1973, this ratio of written test to personal evaluation marks was changed to 60/40 in Phases I and II and 50/50 in Phase III.[88]

At the same time, students agitated for a pass/fail grading system. In 1971, the Medical Students' Association held its third annual pass/fail referundum, that once again showed that the majority of students favoured a change to this system.[89] It is of interest to note, however, that the percentage in favour decreased as the students advanced through the medical school. Ninety-one per cent of first year-students, as compared with 76% of fourth-year students favoured the change. Students in their final years were more aware of the importance of the traditional grading system, together with its accompanying class ranking, in the selection of students for awards and grants as well as opportunities for further postgraduate training. The faculty instituted a pass/fail/honours system in Phase II for a one-year trial period in 1972-3, but following this experiment another referendum showed that while 71% of students preferred some form of pass/fail grading, most of that group wanted the option of obtaining their marks or having them released to a third party. The school returned to the stanine 9-point grading system for all four years, but omitted the class ranking from the students' transcripts, although it was available upon request.[90] The same system prevailed through the 1980s, although students still discussed the advantages and disadvantages of a pass/fail alternative. The Canadian Federation of Medical Students launched a study of the pass/fail system, that has been adopted in a number of medical schools in the country.[91]

Prerequisites for admittance to medicine also came under review during this period of upheaval. For several years, prerequisites in only four subjects had been specified for entry into the medical faculty. With increasing competition for admission, academic standing played a large part in selection and some students took perceived "mickey mouse" courses to get a high overall standing. If they were not accepted into medical school, then their course content left little hope for acceptance into another discipline.[92] To improve the outlook for those students who did not get into medicine, and also to reduce the work load in Phase I, the faculty adopted a specific prerequisite programme for medicine. It included full courses in organic and inorganic chemistry, physics, biology, psychology, mathematics and statistics, genetics, microbiology, zoology and, in view of a perceived need for an improvement in written communication, English once again.[93] The faculty later readjusted the prerequisites, reducing the list to organic and inorganic chemistry, physics, biology, English and statistics. Students were encouraged to obtain a full baccalaureate degree, however, and to obtain more general arts and science courses. At the same time, nonacademic criteria for admission included an interview, letters of reference and an autobiography. The effect of these changes was to broaden the base of those eligible for admission.[94]

Graduate Training Programmes

Graduate training conducted by the Faculty of Medicine followed two routes—those proceeding to an M.Sc. or Ph.D. in one of the medical sciences or clinical departments under the aegis of the Faculty of Graduate Studies and Research, and those who, under the direction of the Division of Postgraduate Medical Education, were training in one of the various medical or surgical specialties. The latter sought certification or fellowship in the Royal College of Physicians and Surgeons of Canada, and the former worked towards a graduate degree of the University of Alberta, but both were taught by professors of the university's Faculty of Medicine.

The faculty made its first move to extend the medical course beyond a basic undergraduate programme in 1930 by offering a one-year programme of extra training in one of the basic medical sciences between the preclinical and clinical years. A student did research, submitted a thesis, and could earn a B.Sc.[95] Only one student, Stanley Hartroft, took advantage of this programme. In 1940, when the first two years of a B.Sc. programme became the prerequisite for medical school, students who wished to take advantage of the extra training programme worked under the aegis of the university's graduate school and received an M.Sc. Ten years later, when the B.Sc. prerequisite was dropped, the faculty revived the original programme,[96] but later the degree was changed to a B.Sc. (Med). Those who already had a baccalaureate could work toward an M.Sc. as before. In addition, graduate courses leading to masters or doctoral degrees in any of the basic medical sciences and some of the clinical sciences were offered through the Faculty of Graduate Studies and Research. In 1951, twenty-four students were registered in the graduate training programme, two of whom were graduates of other universities, and two years later the biochemistry department graduated its first Ph.D.[97] The graduate students were not usually M.D.s, but included those with science majors who wished to undertake graduate studies in medical sciences. In 1978, however, the faculty instituted an M.D. with honours in research that required a minimum of thirty-two weeks of work on an approved research project.[98]

In 1965, Dr. J.S. Colter, head of the department of biochemistry, was asked to chair a committee to investigate the development of a combined M.D. and Ph.D. programme. This committee proposed the establishment of such a programme for students interested in academic or research careers in one of the basic medical or clinical sciences. It required six or seven years of study, following the premedical training. Students could either break their medical programme after two years and take three years of Ph.D. training or complete the medical course without interruption but register in the appropriate medical science department during each intersessional break, and complete the Ph.D. programme following graduation as an M.D.[99]

As discussed in an earlier chapter, the Faculty of Medicine did not offer specialty training until after World War II,[100] but it did have some involvement with regulations concerning specialization. In fact, Alberta led the country in establishing regulations for the recognition of specialists when it amended the Medical Profession Act in 1926. This gave the Senate of the University of Alberta the power to assess the qualifications of those who wished to practise as specialists in the province. A committee, comprising Dean Rankin and other members of the faculty, the deputy minister of health and the registrar of the College of Physicians and Surgeons of Alberta, advised the Senate in their deliberations.[101] Minimum requirements at that time were a year as a graduate intern on a rotating service in a general hospital and "sufficient training for the chosen specialty" in a recognized teaching hospital.[102]

The growth of specialty training and practice escalated rapidly after the second world war. Residency training programmes in the specialties, and subspecialties, have developed under the auspices of the Royal College of Physicians and Surgeons of Canada (which was formed in 1929 by an act of Parliament primarily to improve standards of specialist practice in Canada). Changes in responsibility, standards and accreditation have taken place gradually over the years, until graduate training programmes became a joint responsibility of the Royal College, the teaching hospitals and the medical schools. The Royal College accredited such programmes and made an on-site review every five or six years. The provincial governments provided the major source of funding for the residency programmes in Canada and could thus control the numbers of postgraduate training positions in their provinces.[103] After 1973, the Alberta Hospital Services Commission, originally chaired by Dr. John Bradley, an alumnus of the University of Alberta, paid the residents. Annual negotiations established a quota of residents, set for 1973-4 at 176 positions.

The introduction of postgraduate training in Edmonton's hospitals added an additional impetus to the growth of the school. Residents provided stimulus for the instructors; took on some of the teaching of undergraduate interns; became involved in research activities; and provided increased patient care in the hospitals, as they assumed an integral role in the team approach.[104] Initially, most of the training took place at the University of Alberta Hospital, but shortly after the Royal Alexandra Hospital and then all Edmonton hospitals became involved in the programmes. In 1973, graduate medical education became a division of the Faculty of Medicine with responsibility for co-ordinating all residency training programmes. Each clinical specialty had a programme director and its own Residency Training Committee that planned and supervised the programme and the training of each candidate.[105] A Graduate Medical Society had been in existence for several years, and a committee of this society met on a quarterly basis with the Division of Postgraduate Medical Education to discuss mutual problems and concerns, including ongoing evaluation procedures. Postgraduate training in family practice began on a trial basis at Calgary's General Hospital in 1965-6 and family practice units were located later at the University of Alberta, Royal Alexandra and Misericordia hospitals in Edmonton.

Residency training followed the completion of two years of graduate internship and required a further three, four or five years, depending on the area of specialty. Each succeeding year of residency demanded increased responsibility in the team approach to patient care, and residents were encouraged to do research and prepare papers for publication or presentation to medical conferences. Over the years, a number of graduates of foreign medical schools have been accepted into the programme, but the majority have usually been Alberta graduates. Most of these remain in Alberta to practise, and a large number have taken positions in the Faculty of Medicine. By the late 1980s, the faculty had developed training programmes in some thirty-five specialties and subspecialties.

Continuing Medical Education

Continuing medical education programmes were first established to help practitioners overcome the deficiencies in their training. By 1930, however, with the rapidly expanding body of medical knowledge, the emphasis had changed and programmes were designed to enable practising physicians to keep up-to-date with current practices.[106] Alberta's Faculty of Medicine first became involved with continuing medical education in 1932 when it offered a five-day refresher course to local practitioners in co-operation with the Alberta Medical Association. Faculty members taught the courses, participants could live at the university residences at minimum cost, and the Alberta Medical Association covered the administrative expenses. Some sixty-six doctors attended the first course, and their evident satisfaction encouraged both the university and the association to offer a similar course the following year. The registration was a little less in 1933, but the interest in the programme was sufficient for it to become an annual event that grew in popularity over the years. Many doctors, particularly those from rural communities, availed themselves of the opportunity to up-date and refresh their medical knowledge and skills. Members of the medical faculty provided most of the instruction, but visiting guest lecturers also contributed their expertise. By 1940, more than one hundred doctors regularly attended the refresher course. When the programme first began, it cost the physician nothing, but later registrants paid a modest fee. Nevertheless, a "substantial financial surplus" accrued over the years and paid for the installation of a public address system in the large lecture room of the Medical Building in 1952.[107] Participants received a questionnaire to determine the areas of need of those attending, and the programme was based on the results of the replies. In 1941, voters identified the following priorities:[108]

49 for low back pain	29 for vaginal discharge
37 for skin lesions	28 for neurological examination
32 for sciatica	25 for injured corneas
31 for hypertension	24 for varicose ulcers
31 for infected hands	24 for wound treatment
29 for intravenouses	20 for injured shoulder

The refresher course continued during the war and in 1943 was tailored specifically for medical graduates in the armed forces then stationed in the area. There was a large attendance, and senior officers of the medical divisions of the Canadian armed forces, as well as representatives of the American College of Physicians, assisted with tuition.[109] Following the war, the faculty regularly brought in three or four guest speakers for each course from both Canadian and American medical colleges, and by 1951 attendance had surpassed two hundred. Many came from British Columbia and Saskatchewan, although 50% of the participants were alumni of the University of Alberta.[110] A full programme throughout the week included such topics as allergy in practice, modern treatment of syphilis, psychosomatic approach in practice, the Rh factor, and the interpretation of laboratory tests.

Special circumstances made for variations in course procedure, and in the 1950s, continuing medical education began to move outsideEdmonton. In 1956, the course was presented jointly with a sectional meeting of the American College of Surgeons—344 physicians attended. Four short courses of two or three days each in Edmonton or Calgary covered such topics as electrocardiography, orthopaedic surgery, and obstetrics and gynaecology.[111] Teams of speakers visited various districts. Instructors gave demonstrations in country hospitals and, in answer to requests, offered refresher courses in the basic sciences. They discussed topics ranging from arthritis to radioactive iodine and trained doctors in the latest diagnostic and therapeutic procedures.

The faculty established a department of continuing medical education in 1963, whose aim was to inform practising physicians about new medical knowledge and practices as they became available. In light of the number of drugs on the market—currently over 140,000 with an average of 237 new compound products appearing on the market each year—one of its first programmes was a three-day course presented in a different community each year entitled "New Drugs and Therapeutic Agents." "Trauma and Athletic Injuries," added a year or two later, was offered on a similar basis.[112]

The new teaching concepts invaded continuing medical education as well as undergraduate instruction: less emphasis on the acquisition of precise information and more on promoting attitudes and skills to select and evaluate information and to accept continuing education throughout a physician's professional life. Seventeen regional conference areas were established; each had a regional committee, and members of the university staff visited each area to lead wide-ranging discussions on specific cases selected previously by the committee. Other programmes included small-group teaching within a specific department in a hospital; a clinical traineeship for the physician who required detailed training in a specific field; and a visiting externship, an individually based programme enabling a physician to visit wards and attend rounds with members of the teaching staff.[113]

By the late 1970s, Wednesday evening seminars at the University of Alberta covering a variety of topics had been added to the established programmes. Telephone conferencing was introduced in 1979 to reach smaller communities. The major courses, however, were one-and-a-half to three-and-a-half day programmes held at Edmonton, Banff or Jasper.[114] Mainly for family practitioners, the curriculum was arranged in conjunction with the Canadian College of Family Physicians so that registrants could receive accreditation for continuing medical education as required by the college. Other courses were designed for paramedical professionals—physiotherapists and speech therapists, for instance. The American College of Physicians cosponsored a highly successful biennial course entitled "Advances in Internal Medicine."[115] In addition, the Division of Continuing Medical Education worked closely with both the College of Family Physicians and the Alberta Medical Association in research on the effects of continuing medical education.[116]

* * * * *

Many changes took place in all areas of teaching in the University of Alberta's Faculty of Medicine over its first seventy-five years: undergraduate, graduate and continuing medical education. They will continue to take place, here and elsewhere, as medical schools become more involved with community and public health concerns, and the team approach to professional health care. Changes in curriculum content will reflect these concerns as the school attempts to adopt the concepts of the GPEP Report.[117] The exponential growth of medical technology requires serious dialogue between medical educators, the profession as a whole and the general public. Medical educators, recognizing the dangers of slavish adherence to each advance, continue to seek ways of instilling an attitude of critical analysis in their students, and teach them to evaluate both the uses and the limitations of the new technology.[118] Changing a curriculum in a large medical school is a monumental task and, given the innate conservatism of the profession, takes a great deal of time and effort, not to mention the exercise of diplomatic skills on the part of curriculum committees. While changes in medical education for the twenty-first century continue to receive intense scrutiny, as pointed out in the introduction to this chapter, this has been going on since the time of Hippocrates.

* * * * *

CHAPTER 7

The Growth of Research in the Medical School

Research activities at the University of Alberta and the growth of support for medical research

"If I have one ambition greater than another it is that in the next ten years we will build up all the scientific departments into research departments and as far as my strength of mind and body will enable me to get the men and money I will do it. I will go farther in saying that every member of the staff who shows adaptability for research work will be given opportunity as far as possible to carry it on."

PRESIDENT HENRY Marshall Tory wrote these words to J. Bertram Collip in 1921,[1] and reiterated the sentiment when he spoke to the Congress on Medical Education held in Chicago in 1926. A university medical faculty, he felt, could only remain a vital teaching body if its members conducted their own research projects, and departments in which the teachers were content with a simple teaching schedule inevitably became sterile. The rewards of research activities were evident in three areas: first, an individual's personal satisfaction in being able to pursue his own interests; second, the stimulating effect upon co-workers; and, third, and most important, the exhilarating effect upon the students. "I have listened with a gratification I cannot describe to expressions of pleasure and pride among the students of my own university concerning the work of Dr. Collip."[2]

Even a man as forceful as President Tory, however, was not able to get blood out of a stone, and funding for research of any kind was sparse indeed in the lean years before the second world war. Tory himself was part-time president of the newly formed National Research Council (NRC), and for several years divided his time between that position and president of the university. Eventually, in 1928, he had to make a decision between the two, and he chose to become the first full-time president of the NRC. With this connection in research circles in eastern Canada, University of Alberta personnel felt that they were in an advantageous position to obtain funding. But medical research played a small part in the NRC's budget, despite the discovery of insulin in 1922 that had sparked a wide interest in medical research in Canada. The Connaught Laboratories were established in Toronto, and in 1928 Frederick Banting established the Banting Research Foundation, also in Toronto. It received no government funding, however, and had to raise money from public subscription.[3] Within a year, the foundation was in a position to give small grants for medical research, although its funds were extremely limited.

In 1936, Banting joined the National Research Council ''on condition that medical research would be supported on the same basis as the other sciences.''[4] Together with the Canadian Medical Association and the RCPSC the NRC proposed the formation of a medical research committee as an integral part of the council. Representatives of all medical schools and organizations in the country, together with federal and provincial departments of health, attended a conference in Ottawa in 1938 to discuss the aims and objectives of such a committee, and recommended the establishment of an Associate Committee on Medical Research.[5] The NRC agreed, appointed Banting as chairman, and the federal government began its support of medical research in Canada. The following year the departments of anatomy, biochemistry and physiology at the University of Alberta received research funds from the Associate Committee totalling $3,000.[6]

One of the Associate Committee's first projects was a fact-finding tour of all medical schools and teaching hospitals in Canada to establish the extent of current medical research in the country. Banting conducted this tour in 1938 and discovered that because of heavy teaching loads only a few instructors in each medical school were doing any research. Banting, Best, Collip and Hans Selye were conducting research projects at Toronto and McGill, and Wilder Penfield was working out of the Montreal Neurological Institute. Few staff appointments were made to medical faculties or teaching hospitals across the country during the depression, and most of them were part time, which precluded any available time for research. There were at least one or two researchers at each medical school, however, and most of these were in the preclinical sciences.[7]

Research in the Interwar Years

Two of the major research themes of the early days at the University of Alberta's Faculty of Medicine dealt with areas in which the school is at present a leading force: diabetes and cardiology. J. Bertram Collip, appointed to the medical faculty in 1915, was an avid researcher, and despite inadequate laboratory facilities, he managed to prepare several papers of publishable quality in the field of biochemistry. To obtain experience in laboratories with more modern equipment, he applied for, and received, a Rockefeller fellowship. He left Edmonton in 1921 to begin a year's sabbatical leave, a happenstance that led to his being at the right place at the right time to ensure his place in the annals of medical history. His important contribution to the isolation of insulin, an extract for the treatment of diabetes, has been discussed in an earlier chapter. Suffice it to say here that his role as a member of the "insulin team" benefited the University of Alberta in ways that would enhance its medical research facilities. According to the terms of the insulin patent, the university of each of the members of the team received a portion of the financial return from the sale of insulin, and in Collip's case this went towards the improvement of laboratory facilities in the biochemistry department. The Rockefeller Institute, the Carnegie Foundation and the College of Physicians and Surgeons of Alberta all contributed funding as well, which helped pay for laboratory assistants as well as more modern equipment.

Even though Collip was never recognized officially as a co-discoverer of insulin, he returned to Edmonton surrounded by the aura of one of the century's most important medical discoveries. In the university's biochemistry laboratories, he continued his investigations into the properties of the new extract to perfect the solution as it was applied to humans.[8] Furthermore, he worked with Heber Jamieson and the department of medicine on the clinical application of insulin to diabetic patients in the University of Alberta Hospital. By 1923, Collip was on to other research projects, as well as working toward his M.D. His investigations centred on the possibility of finding a substance similar to insulin in plant life as well as in animal life. He successfully isolated a similar substance, which he called "gluckonin," in yeast, as well as in other forms of plant life such as onions, beans and lettuce. Although it differed from insulin in some ways, he found it alleviated the symptoms of diabetes in dogs and rabbits, so his continued experiments attempted to establish its effectiveness in the treatment of diabetes in humans.[9] Collip was determined not to be denied credit for this discovery, as he had been in the case of insulin, and rather too hurriedly rushed his discoveries into print and presented a paper to the Society of Experimental Biology and Medicine in New York.[10] Unfortunately, he had not carried out sufficient testing and gluckonin proved to be ineffective and unstable, and Collip gradually lapsed into an embarrassed silence on the subject.[11]

He put this failure behind him quickly, however, and began work on another ductless gland, the parathyroid. Working on the theory that calcium metabolism in the blood was controlled by a secretion from the parathyroid glands, he spent long hours working diligently at the laboratory bench in his attempts to isolate and purify that substance. Eventually, he extracted the hormone that was responsible for regulating the concentration of calcium in the blood, and found it to be effective in helping those suffering from "parathyroid tetany."[12] Eli Lilly & Company produced and marketed the substance under the trade name "Para-Thor-Mone," and Collip gave the royalty rights to the university with the stipulation that the income was to be applied to furthering research in the department of biochemistry.[13] Collip left Alberta in 1928 to take up the chair of biochemistry at McGill, and was to become a major figure in the field of endocrinology. He became a member of the newly formed Associate Committee on Medical Research of the NRC in 1938 and assumed the chairmanship after Banting's death in 1941. Following the war, when this committee became the Medical Division of the NRC, Collip was appointed its first director. In this role,he visited the University of Alberta on several occasions and gave staunch support to assistance for medical research in the school where he began his career.

Collip received grants and awards for his work because of his association with the discovery of insulin, but for other departments in the medical school there was little funding from anyone. Ralph Shaner, in the department of anatomy, worked quietly and diligently for many, many years on cardiac embryology, investigating the development of the heart and the ways that defects developed. He began these investigations before he arrived at the medical school in 1921, when it was a "diverting and fascinating hobby" for him. "There will always be a need for the researcher who follows his own curiosity," he said, and he considered that imagination was the most important feature of a distinguished student.[14] In 1932, he received a grant of $150 from the Banting Research Foundation to study the development of the "tracts in the brain of the mammalian embryo."

In 1935, a Carnegie Corporation Research Grant of $75 enabled him to buy some photomicrographic equipment, and he was one of the first researchers at the University of Alberta to receive funding from the newly formed Associate Committee in 1939.[15] Fellow scientists and ex-students often sent him interesting specimens, and he sent his technician off regularly to Gainers Packing Plant to collect pig embryos that he used for his research. Despite little financial assistance, and inadequate equipment, Shaner published widely, achieved international status, and as a recognized world authority received invitations to speak and lecture. When the discovery of new surgical techniques made it possible to repair and restore hearts with congenital abnormalities, and the University of Alberta Hospital began its programme of open-heart surgery, the crucial importance of his work was suddenly recognized.[16] In 1961, Shaner was honoured by the Canadian Heart Association. He gave its first annual lecture, choosing the subject, "Congenital Anomalies of the Ventricle," which represented only a small part of his many years of meticulous research.[17]

Most of the research projects in the early years were carried out by basic medical scientists. For several years, the Provincial Laboratory, under the direction of Dean Rankin, a bacteriologist, and J.J. Ower, a pathologist, worked on the BCG vaccine to immunize cattle against bovine tuberculosis. This vaccine, which remained controversial, was developed and used successfully in Europe, but was not widely accepted on this continent.[18] In 1933, Harold Orr, developed a mycology unit in the Provincial Laboratory to investigate human fungus infections.[19] Two years later, a Carnegie Corporation Research Grant enabled Rankin to conduct research on fungi that were parasitic to man. The department of physiology, under A.W. Downs, conducted research on the effects of internal glandular secretions on the voluntary muscles.[20] In a clinical department, Irving Bell, of the department of anaesthesia, and Samuel Gelfan of the department of pharmacology, conducted experiments with the use of ethylene to improve anaesthesia, experiments that culminated in the first use of divinyl ether (Vinethene) as a general anaesthetic agent on a human subject in 1933.[21]

World War II created the second impetus to promote the need for medical research. Many research projects took place during the war, specifically for war-related medical problems such as wound healing, the effects of high-altitude flying on the lung, the treatment of burns, and the design and fitting of prostheses, to name but a few. These needs placed a heavy demand on the Associate Committee of Medical Research of the NRC, which set up a Committee on Aviation Medical Research and

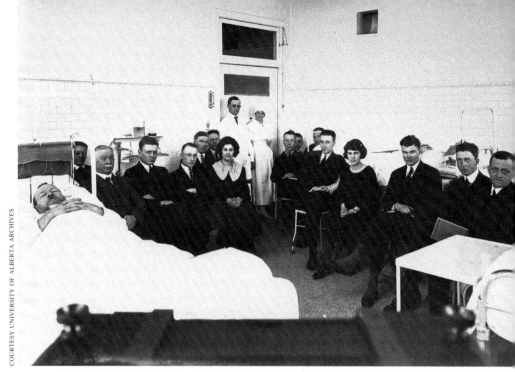

First graduating class at a bedside clinical class in 1923.

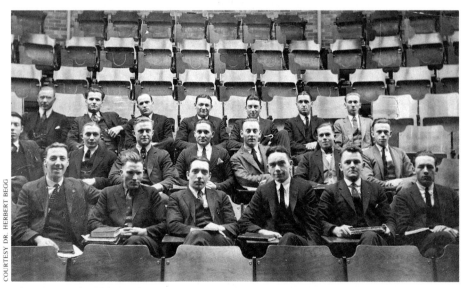

The class of 1928 in the large lecture room in the Medical Building.

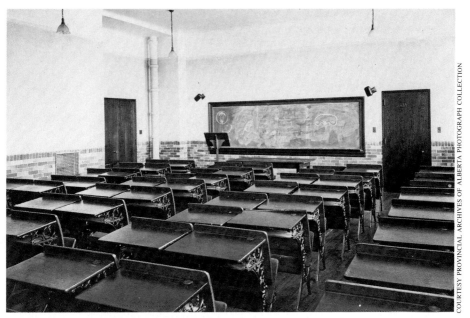

Classroom in the Medical Building c. 1925.

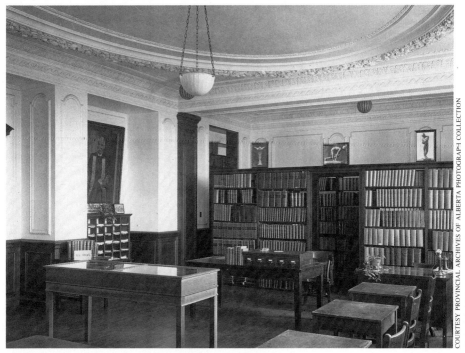

The Library in the Medical Building, c. 1925.

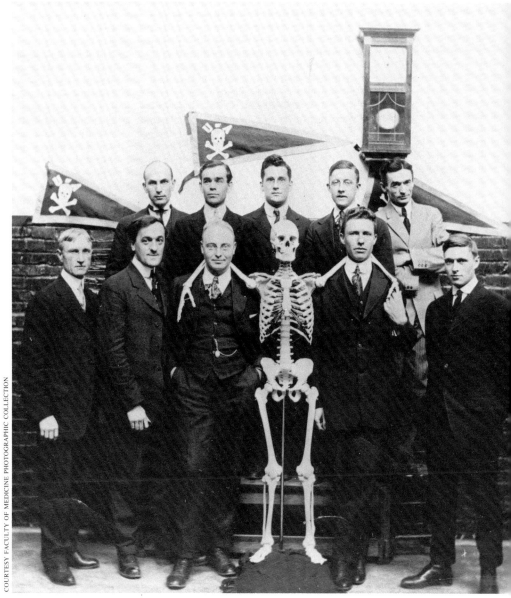

Anatomy Classes over the Years (*and next page*). Class in the old Anatomy Lab in the Power House in 1916. *Back row, left to right:* Gregory Novak, Joseph Riopel, Webster Bowles, Billy Hill, Nat Minish. *Front row:* Dr. D.G. Revell, H.S. Empey, Cecil Hankinson, ??, Percy Backus (who later practised in Harley Street in London, England) and J.B. Collip.

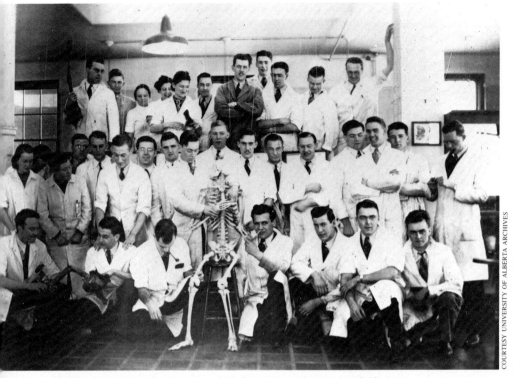

Medical class in the Anatomy Laboratory, January 1943.

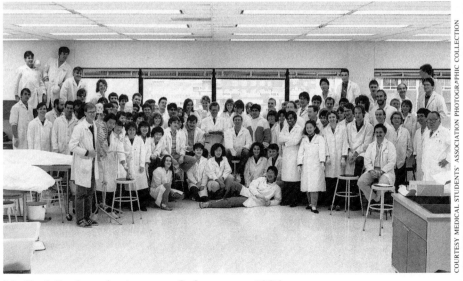

Medical Students in Anatomy Laboratory, 1986.

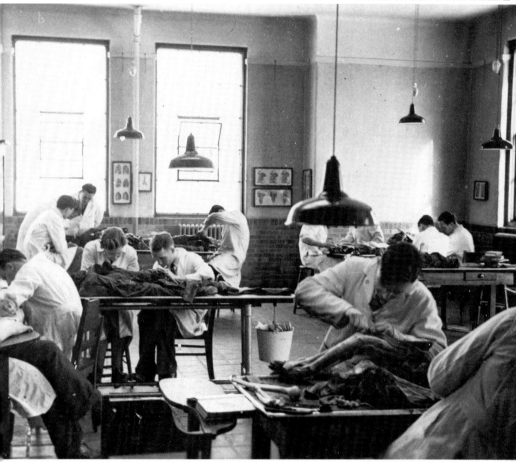

Anatomy dissection laboratory, 1941.

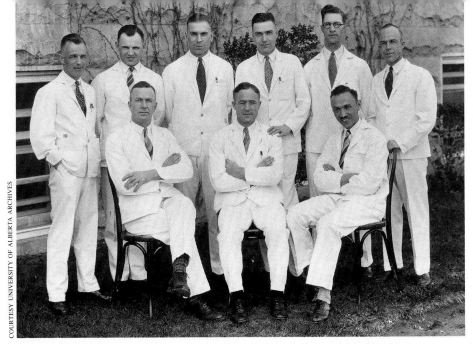

House physicians and surgeons, University Hospital, 1929-30. *Juniors, standing:* J. Calder, F.D. Johnston, F. Werthenbach, T.K. McLean, E.H. Watts, J.W. MacGregor. *Seniors, seated:* N.E. Alexander, J.R. Vant, Resident, M.M. Cantor.

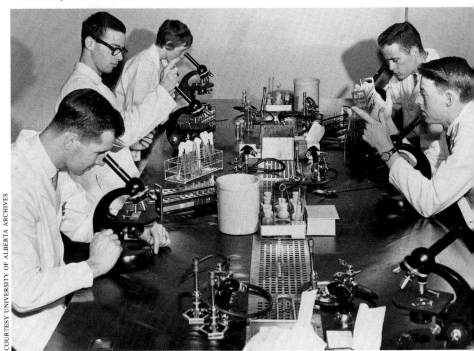

Bacteriology Department Laboratory, 1961.

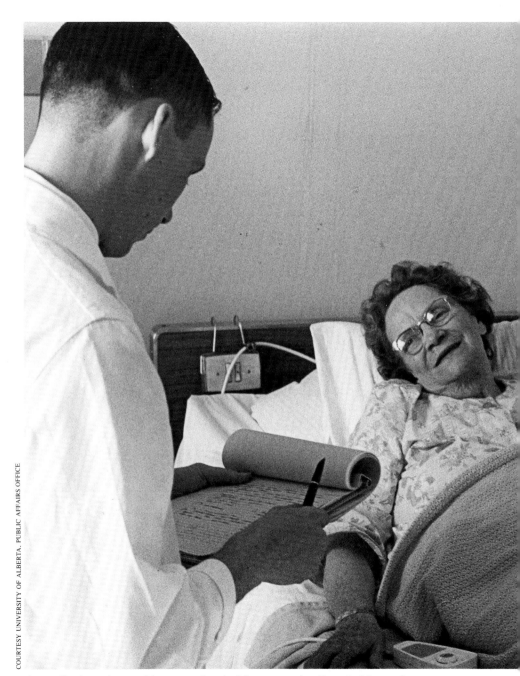

A medical student taking a patient's history at the Royal Alexandra
Hospital, 20 March 1969.

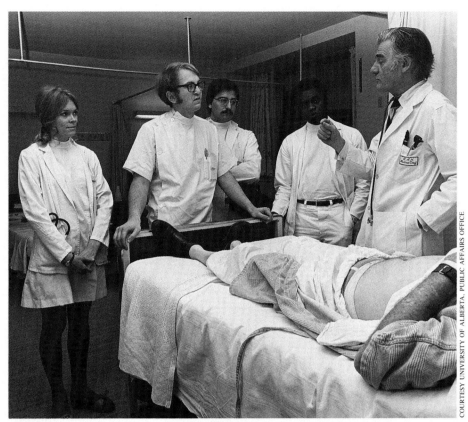

Bedside teaching at the
Royal Alexandra
Hospital, Dr. J.A.L.
Gilbert and interns,
c. 1969.

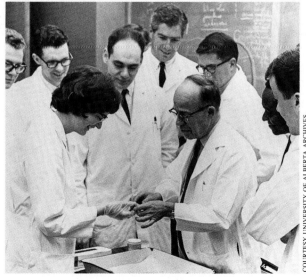

Dr. J.W. Macgregor,
Chairman, pathology
department, with a
group of students.

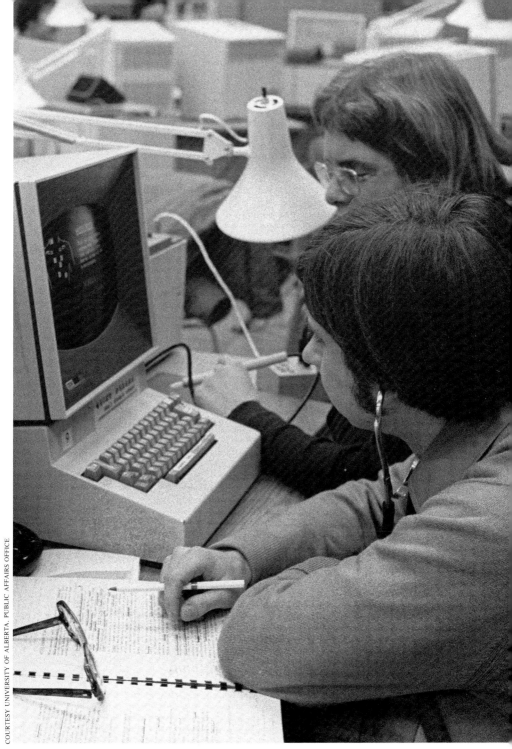

Computer learning.

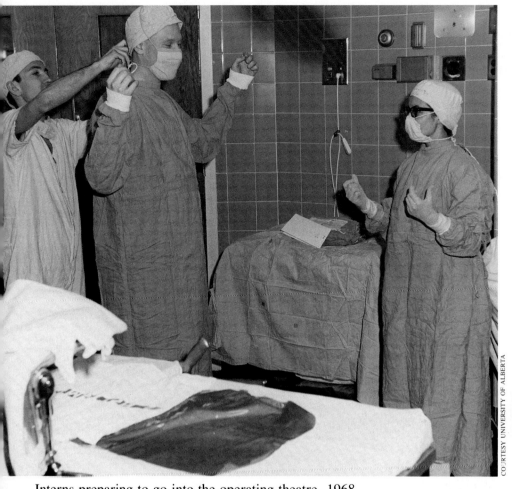

Interns preparing to go into the operating theatre, 1968.

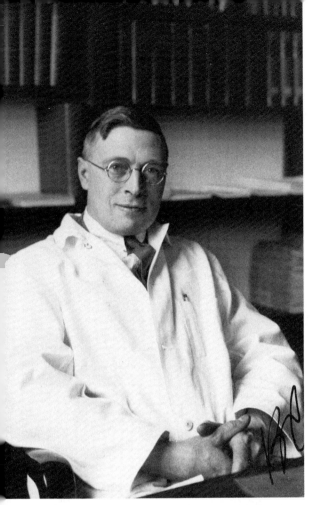

John Bertram Collip in his office, c. 1928.

Plaque commemorating Collip's discovery of the parathyroid hormone.

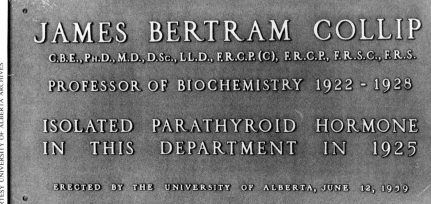

JAMES BERTRAM COLLIP

C.B.E., Ph.D., M.D., D.Sc., LL.D., F.R.C.P.(C), F.R.C.P., F.R.S.C., F.R.S.

PROFESSOR OF BIOCHEMISTRY 1922 - 1928

ISOLATED PARATHYROID HORMONE
IN THIS DEPARTMENT IN 1925

ERECTED BY THE UNIVERSITY OF ALBERTA, JUNE 12, 1959

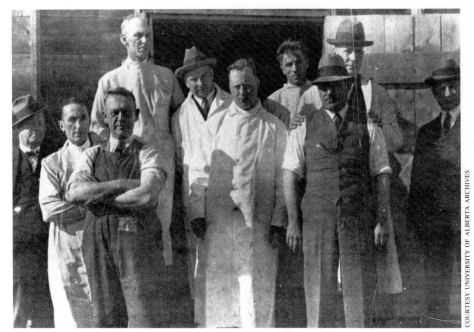

The BCG Research Committee, 1925. *Back row, left to right:* R.M. Shaw, bacteriologist; Professor J.J. Ower, pathologist; John Onyfrichuk, technician; P.R. Talbot, Provincial Veterinarian. *Front row:* W.C. Laidlaw, Deputy Minister of Health; L.L. McCullough, Provincial Mental Hospital; ? Haworth, veterinarian; H.M. Vango, pathologist; Dean Rankin, bacteriologist and chairman of the committee; A.H. Baker, Central Alberta Sanatarium.

Researcher working in the McEachern Laboratory in 1961. Here the combined effects of surgery and chemotherapy were studied in rats.

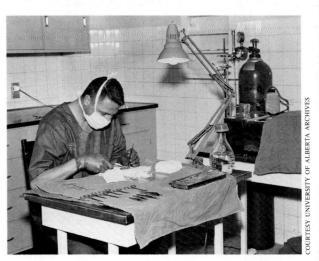

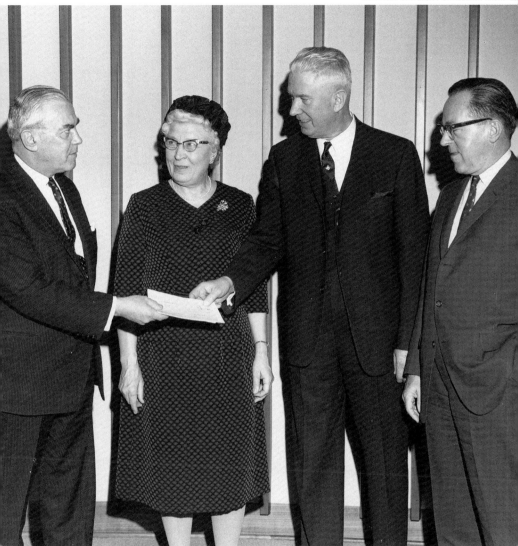

The M.D. Muttart Foundation has contributed sizeable amounts of money to the medical faculty over the years. Here Mr. and Mrs. M.D. Muttart present a cheque to President Walter Johns in 1966 to assist with diabetic research on the campus. Donald R. Wilson, head of the department of medicine, looks on.

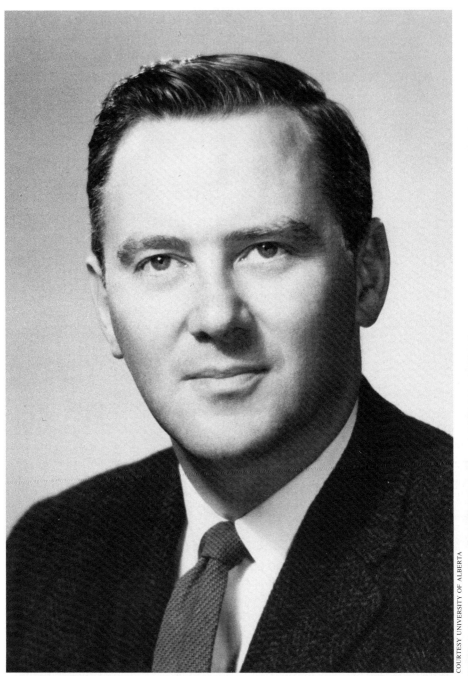

J.C. Callaghan, who developed the open-heart surgery programme at the University of Alberta.

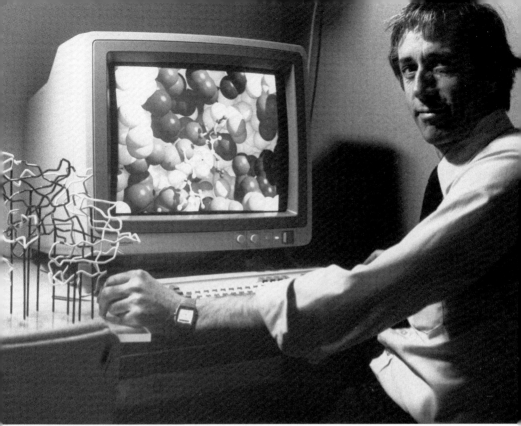

Michael James, a member of the MRC group in protein structure and function, is shown with a computer model generated by x-ray crystallography.

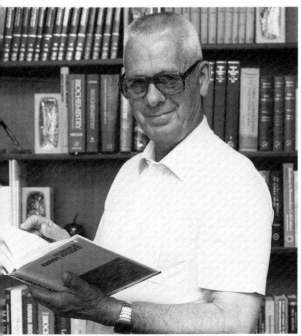

J.S. Colter, head of the department of bio-chemistry, 1961-87.

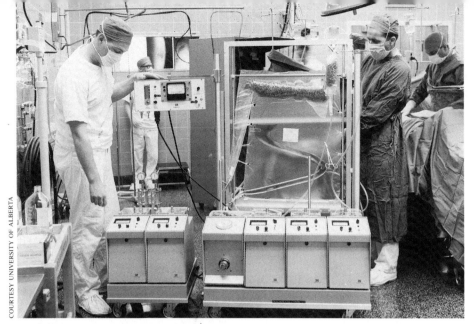

Operating room scene, showing the first type of disposable bubble oxygenator (Travenol), one of the early heart lung pumps used by Dr. J.C. Callaghan, this one in January 1967.

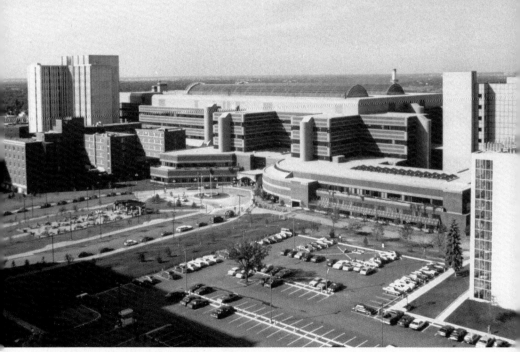

The Medical School/Hospital complex now. The new Heritage Research Centre is at bottom right.

subcommittees in naval medicine, wound infection, shock, blood substitutes, and many other areas of medicine and surgery.[22] Following the war, such intensive research projects, together with changes in the concepts of medical education made research activities more prominent. Medical schools were encouraged to promote research to stimulate both teacher and student. Financial support was still a problem, however, and those teachers who were interested in research needed facilities, technical assistance and a teaching load that left them enough time to pursue their research projects. None of these were available at Alberta's medical school, or at most other medical schools, as they struggled to cope with large numbers of veterans in prewar facilities.

Most of the wartime research activities were conducted in eastern institutions, particularly Toronto and the University of Western Ontario, where Collip was the dean. To stimulate an interest in medical research in the West the NRC initiated the establishment of a Western Regional Group of the Medical Division. From 1947 on, it held an annual meeting, hosted by the four western universities on a rotating basis, that was designed to help alleviate problems occasioned by the relative isolation of the West and the difficulties and expense of travel to the larger metropolitan centres in the East.[23] The University of Alberta hosted the second meeting in 1948, where Collip, now director of the Medical Division of the NRC, was a guest speaker. These meetings, usually well attended by both staff and residents, provided an opportunity for the participants to present the results of their investigations, share information on their research activities, and discuss, in an informal and friendly atmosphere, a variety of related problems. While most of the participants at the conferences were initially preclinical professors,[24] when Alberta hosted the 1958 conference at the Banff School of Fine Arts,[25] members of the departments of surgery and medicine, as well as biochemistry and physiology presented the results of various research projects.

Postwar Efforts to Promote Research Activities

The Faculty of Medicine at the University of Alberta also initiated some activities to promote an interest in medical research, particularly among the younger staff members and graduate students. One of these was the establishment of a Medical Science Research Club in 1946 for the purpose of "stimulating, reviewing and assuring cooperation in locally projected medical research problems." The preamble of the constitution read as follows:

Recognizing that the best interests of medical research are promoted by united interest and concerted effort, persons engaged in medical research and in affiliated fields of scientific and social endeavor, hereby organize themselves in conformity with the Constitution and By-Laws hereinafter stated.''

Open to both faculty members and students, the club planned to "study and correlate local research." Its monthly meetings were devoted to the presentation of "reports of current research by members or guest speakers, to assess feasible research projects for club members and assist them with their prosecution, and to give help in obtaining the necessary funding, facilities and assistance."[26] The following year, the name changed to the Collip Research Club, in honour of "one of our distinguished medical graduates who has been very sympathetic to our research problems."[27] The club remained active for nearly twenty years, and one of its major benefits was that it brought together both medical and clinical scientists. Later, fewer and fewer attended the meetings, however, and in 1964 the remaining members voted it out of existence. This was partly because of a growing lack of interest in widely disparate areas of research, but was unfortunate in that it constituted another break in the lines of communication between the basic and clinical sciences.[28]

Another faculty intiative was the organization of a Committee on Medical Research to "survey the field of research" and seek ways to promote an active interest on the part of both the university authorities and faculty personnel. This committee, together with Dean Ower and John Scott, met with the president of the university regarding the needs of the medical school in this area. President Newton received the proposal favourably and established two separate funds. The first one was a Medical Division of the University of Alberta Research Foundation, which could receive gifts and legacies from private sources in aid of medical research.[29] The second was a president's committee, approved by the Board of Governors in 1946, and known as the Committee on Allocation of Medical Research Grants.

This committee received money from two sources. First, it received interest on the original 1923 Rockefeller Institute endowment of $500,000 for the development of the medical faculty. By this time, it was invested in Province of Alberta debentures at a 3 1/2% interest rate. Second, the committee received interest on a capital sum of $201,350 given to the university under the province's debt reorganization programme, in lieu of bond interest that the provincial government had not paid during the years of depression.[30] Years later, in 1963, the Griesbach Cancer Research Fund, with a principal amount of $12,000, was also placed under the jurisdiction of this committee. Interest from these sources amounted to about $8,000 a year in 1946, increased to $11,000 by 1950, to $14,800 in 1960, and to $20,154 in 1966.[31] These sums appear small compared to today's dollars, but they provided a welcome source of funding for initial, or feasibility, studies on a variety of projects and promoted an interest in research within the faculty.

The fund was specifically for medical research, not for scholarships. Only faculty members who were fully qualified to undertake the research they proposed were eligible, although they were encouraged to employ graduate students as assistants on their projects. The policy of the Medical Reseach Fund changed little over the years. It gave modest support to research activities in both the medical and clinical sciences, essentially to pilot projects. It provided start-up funds for initial research, which, if viable, would then become eligible for funding from outside granting agencies. The fund did not cover the purchase of large items of equipment and did not supplement grants from outside agencies; it did supply salary support for summer students, but only when the assistance provided was an integral part of a project.[32] By the late 1960s a number of fellowships, and larger sums of money, were more readily available from outside funding agencies, and the eligibility rules changed somewhat. New staff members were given preference, and the committee attempted to use the funds on as broad a base as possible.

A committee, chaired by John Scott, and including Ralph Shaner, W.C. Mackenzie and J.W. Macgregor, assessed the applications and awarded grants. This was a president's committee, and President Newton took an active and knowledgeable interest in the decisions of the committee, which he had to approve. In 1949, the amounts awarded ranged from a minimum of $100 to a maximum of $1,200, for such proposed investigations as "oestrogenic potency of certain compounds related to carcinogens," "vaginal smears in cancer diagnosis," and "metabolic antagonisms in the frog heart."[33] By 1962, the amounts had increased only slightly, ranging from $200 to $1,500 and the topics included "tumor immunology," "dermatophytes in soil," and "a preliminary study of electronarcosis."[34]

Other avenues of research funding opened up after the war. In 1946, the Associate Committee of the NRC became the Medical Division of the Council, and by 1955 it had a budget of $725,000. Unlike most other countries it decided to expand its support of medical research in Canadian medical schools and hospitals, rather than establish its own laboratories.[35] Another survey of medical research in Canadian medical schools in 1948 showed a much increased interest in research by both faculty and the student body; but heavy teaching loads and increased student enrolment left little time for any investigations. Many of the younger faculty members who had served in the war and been exposed to research activities were enthusiatic, but adequate funding was still unavailable. In response to a proposal from the Association of Canadian Medical Colleges that the Medical Division be separated from the NRC, a Medical Research Council (MRC) was established in 1960. Initially, MRC was not in control of its own budget, and its independence from NRC was not complete until 1968, and the passage of the MRC Act. Since that time it grew rapidly.[36]

National organizations, such as the National Cancer Institute, the Canadian Heart Foundation, the Canadian Tuberculosis Association, and other "disease oriented" associations, as well as their provincial branches, provided grants, research associateships and fellowships and funded "research beds." In 1949, both the Kinsmen Club and the Alberta Cancer Society endowed a research bed in the University of Alberta Hospital.[37] The Muttart Foundation donated $18,000 to establish a chair in medical research in 1954, and the following year Robert Fraser was appointed the Muttart Research Associate Professor.[38] The family of Dorothy Jean Usher provided a memorial scholarship fund of $10,000 to support a yearly research scholarship of $275 in a field of medicine relating preferably to leukemia,[39] and the College of Physicians of Surgeons of Alberta showed its support by establishing a fellowship in research in the basic medical sciences for undergraduates.[40]

Among the major fellowships to support research in the medical school were those offered by the John and Mary Markle Foundation. Established in 1927, this foundation supported medical scholars in the United States and Canada. A $30,000 scholarship for the support of academic physicians and their research was granted to the university at a rate of $6,000 a year over a five-year period. The university made the application for a Markle scholarship, and the grant supplemented the rate paid to the recipient by the university, and also supported the recipient's research activity. This enabled medical faculties to acquire the full-time services of a physician who would then have time for research and teaching.[41] Donald R. Wilson received the first one in 1949. Five years later, in 1953, Robert S. Fraser received another, and a third was awarded to Lionel E. McLeod, another Alberta graduate, in 1958.

All three Markle scholars contributed to research in their own fields. Wilson began to develop an endocrine laboratory, and the University of Alberta Hospital provided him with a small laboratory, ''a little room behind the elevator shaft in the old 1912 wing,''[42] where he began research in the field of steroids and steroid metabolism.[43] Fraser established a cardiovascular unit, the second subspecialty unit in the department of medicine, which ''provided special facilities for the investigation of all types of heart diseases'' and would become closely connected with open-heart surgery at the University of Alberta Hospital. When McLeod received his Markle scholarship, Donald Wilson, now head of the department of medicine, obtained a grant from the NRC to set up a metabolic unit in the University of Alberta Hospital. McLeod became its director and developed a programme of clinical investigation in endocrinology and metabolism. The activities of this unit became closely integrated with the artificial kidney programme because of his specific interests, and McLeod also developed one of the early programmes for treating renal failure.[44]

The McEachern Laboratory
Meanwhile, the faculty's Committee on Medical Research continued to solicit funding for research and approached the Alberta Division of the Canadian Cancer Society for assistance. Initially, the society endowed a bed at the University of Alberta Hospital for clinical research in cancer and made a grant of $2,500 to purchase equipment;[45] but its major contribution was a joint venture to develop a laboratory to be used for basic research in cancer. The society contributed $150,000 for the construction, and the university was responsible for the administration of the building and equipment and had sole control and direction of research activities. The laboratory, a two-storey structure built at the rear of the Medical Building, between the east and west wings, was named for John Sinclair McEachern, OBE, a physician who practised in Calgary for more than forty years and was responsible for the formation of the Canadian Cancer Society.[46] It was constructed in such a way that it could be incorporated into the centre wing of the Medical Building, should one be built in the future. The sod-turning ceremony took place in 1951, and Mrs. McEachern presided at the formal opening on 1 November 1952. Many people attended as the opening coincided with the installation of the new Chancellor, Dr. E. P. Scarlett, another noted Calgary physician.[47] The provincial government did send a representative to the opening, but its attitude toward funding medical research at that time was indicated in a letter from Premier Manning:

> ...it should not be assumed that the government will assist in the costs of continuing the work [at the McEachern Laboratory] should there be any change in the anticipated grants. The government is not prepared to make any future commitments regarding financial assistance for the project.[48]

The McEachern Laboratory was equipped with biochemical and radio-isotope equipment, and two surgical research teams were already at work in the building before the official opening took place.[49] A university committee, chaired by Ralph Shaner, administered the building, approved expenses for equipment, and arranged for the use of facilities by the various departments. It was "open to any qualified investigator... whose project came within the intent of the founders." Research in the building was financed by granting agencies, such as the NRC, the Defence Research Board and the Canadian Cancer Institute, and individual researchers themselves had to obtain funding to cover the necessary expenses of their projects.[50]

When K.P. Kowalewski, an assistant professor in experimental surgery, received a Canadian Cancer Society Research Fellowship in 1953, he began to work in the McEachern Laboratory and later became its director. He not only engaged in his own research but also was responsible for assisting and supervising the work of others in the laboratory.[51] In his first full-time year, laboratory staff prepared seven papers for publication, and he was involved in five of them. The following year, 1954, Kowalewski began a study of "the reaction of radioactive iodine in thyroid tumours," and the first intimation of a correlation between smoking and lung cancer was recorded in the annual report:

> ...the hitherto unsuspected prevalence of cancer in the lung and its possible connection with smoking has stimulated a widespread investigation of the lung.[52]

Cancer research was in its early stages and, as the laboratory was always short of funds, personnel qualified to conduct cancer research were not readily available. Almost from the beginning, the Board of Directors of the McEachern Laboratory stipulated that any "worthwhile basic research project" would be sanctioned "until such time as it could become a pure cancer research institute." Over the years, gradually less and less cancer research was carried on, and the laboratory began to be used mostly by members of the department of surgery. During this period, in fact, three members of the surgical department who conducted research in this institution—R.C. Harrison in 1953, William Lakey in 1956 and Peter Allen in 1959—won the Gold Medal of the Royal College of Physicians and Surgeons of Canada for "outstanding basic surgical research done in Canada."

The Surgical Medical Research Institute

In 1955, lack of funds for day-to-day "housekeeping" expenses, together with administrative problems, led to a reorganization of the running of the McEachern Laboratory. The university agreed to contribute $10,000 annually to the general budget, and asked the department of surgery to assume responsibility for the day-to-day operations. It still ran on a shoestring; there was no office space, although Kowalewski did have a secretary, and the only technician looked after the animals. Through his connections with the City of Edmonton, Walter Anderson, a surgeon at the Royal Alexandra Hospital, approached the Edmonton Civic Employees Welfare Chest Fund for financial support for the laboratory. Since that time, this organization consistently supported surgical research fellowships as well as specific projects, initially in the McEachern Laboratory and since1961 in the Surgical Medical Research Institute.[53]

Walter Mackenzie, then head of the department of surgery, began a campaign to obtain more space and money for research in experimental surgery. His efforts were rewarded with the construction of the central wing of the Medical Building in 1960. The original McEachern Laboratory building was renovated and included in it, and at the same time surgical research activities moved into an additional 22,000 sq. ft. of space in the new wing. Called the Surgical Medical Research Institute (SMRI), it was a division of experimental surgery, under the direction of Kowalewski. Here, surgical residents were required to spend one year of their training, and they were encouraged to bring problems from the bedside and try to work them out at the laboratory bench.[54] Mackenzie arranged for Kowalewski to travel to Europe and the United States to study other surgical institutes. More money became available for technicians, and over the years SMRI attracted a number of scholars from other provinces and from other countries. When Kowalewski retired from the SMRI in 1977, more than five hundred papers had been prepared for publication from the McEachern Laboratory and the SMRI.[55] After the Faculty of Medicine moved into new buildings, the SMRI remained in the Medical Building (renamed the Dental/Pharmacy Building) and offered research facilities for clinical faculty in the fields of experimental surgery or medicine, offered a postgraduate Ph.D. course in experimental surgery, and housed a histology and biochemistry laboratory.

The development of the SMRI freed up the McEachern Laboratory for research directly related to cancer. The building was renovated extensively to bring it up to the standard consistent with current cancer research, and Alan R.P. Paterson was appointed director. The Canadian Cancer Society (Alberta Division) and the University of Alberta paid for the renovations, and the provincial government, now willing to assist with research funding, contributed $20,000.[56] Complementing work being done in the department of biochemistry, research in the McEachern Laboratory placed particular emphasis on the structure and physiology of the cell, and biochemical aspects of cell growth.[57] Investigations ranged from biochemical changes in body cells to the development of surgical techniques, from purely basic research to the applied, and from the individual efforts of one researcher to the combined efforts of several members of a team.[58] Subsequently, the McEachern Laboratory moved to the Medical Sciences Building and housed the University of Alberta's Cancer Research Unit.

Extramural Support for Medical Research
During the late 1940s and early 1950s, the lack of facilities, money and staff contributed to the paucity of major research projects in the medical school.[59] Heavy teaching and administrative loads left little time for faculty members to plan and carry out co-ordinated and continuous research projects that would lead to improved patient care. The medical science departments continued to be more active in this area, and twenty three separate research projects were underway in 1950, with financial support from the Medical Division of the NRC, the National Cancer Institute, the Cancer Society of Alberta, the Alberta Tuberculosis Association, and the university's Medical Research Fund.[60] The accreditation report of 1956, which identified a lack of research activity at the school, resulted in an increased budget and the sudden infusion of more full-time staff as well as improved facilities. Research activities began to increase in the late 1950s and by the end of the decade funds totalling more than $240,000 were allocated to the school for a variety of research projects. In 1960, the addition of the central wing to the Medical Building provided space for more investigators, and the increase in research activities in the faculty was reflected in a sharp increase in grants-in-aid of research during the 1960s. J.W. Pearce was appointed chairman of the Research Committee in 1961, and that year faculty members published 140 papers and gave 273 presentations to various

local, national and international bodies.[61] The school had few pieces of expensive equipment until the 1960s when, thanks to the MRC, it acquired an electron microscope, which was managed by Theodor Shnitka, and a Kiil Artificial Kidney, which enabled long-term studies in the field of chronic kidney disease.[62]

Throughout the 1960s extramural support for medical research in the University of Alberta rose steadily. Research grants from outside agencies increased from $22,365 in 1948-9 to $1,393,470 in 1966, and to $5,710,836 in 1980-81. (Table 11 shows the extramural research grants to the various departments from 1949 to 1961.[63]) By the 1970s, research projects and funding from outside sources had reached a stage where some of the larger departments appointed their own research co-ordinators or research committees.[64]

TABLE 11: RESEARCH FUNDS OBTAINED FROM EXTRAMURAL SOURCES BY DEPARTMENT 1949-1961

Department	1949	1952	1955	1958	1961
Anatomy	3,380	3,300	700	975	10,300
Bacteriology	0	500	2,700	5,800	29,200
Biochemistry	12,335	16,950	19,550	54,650	215,000
Medicine	3,000	15,450	29,600	49,095	142,000
Pathology	0	1,100	1,000	0	19,000
Pediatrics	0	0	0	6,338	40,500
Physiology	3,650	8,700	7,600	45,375	50,500
Radiology	0	0	1,000	0	21,000
Surgery	0	2,900	29,825	78,587	168,000
Total	**$22,365**	**$48,900**	**$91,975**	**$240,820**	**$695,500**

Student Research

Research among the student body also began to increase in the 1960s. Michael Emery promoted the concept of an annual Student Research Day in 1968 in an effort to engage student interest in research and to develop a knowledge of investigative techniques. While only a small percentage of students went on to a career in research, involvement in research activities provided an awareness of experimental techniques and approaches in the practice of medicine. On Student Research Day, students presented their research projects and findings, and a panel of judges assessed them and awarded prizes. Since the advent of the Alberta Heritage Foundation for Medical Research, this programme benefited from the impetus of summer studentship awards. Many took the opportunity to participate in research during the summer months. By the late 1980s, prizewinners were receiving $300, courtesy of the Medical Alumni Association, and the three top winners went on to present their work at a national forum for student research.[65]

Major Research Projects
Major new research projects were initiated in the early 1970s. One of the first was the development of a transplantation immunology laboratory, a project supported by an MRC grant of $1,250,000. John B. Dossetor, an active researcher in rejection of organ transplants in Montreal, joined the medical faculty in Edmonton in 1969. Together with Erwin Diener, they set up the Immunology Laboratory to conduct research on the body's immunity to transplanted tissue, and to find a method of preventing or reducing the body's reaction to another's organ. Dossetor and Diener put together a broadly based interdisciplinary team of scientists, which has achieved an international reputation, and investigation involved both the immunobiology of transplanted tissue at an experimental level, as well as clinical studies focused, initially, on kidney transplants.[66]

Research activities in neurosurgery began about the same time. Thomas Speakman and William O'Callaghan studied the complexities of spinal cord regeneration and, later, George Monckton, generously supported by the Muttart Foundation, established a neuromuscular disease laboratory. B.K.A. Weir's research contributed to a better understanding of bleeding around the brain, and resulted in improved clinical treatment. The growth of neurosciences research has featured both diversification and technical innovation. Recent research activities have used computer technology, advanced engineering techniques, and laser phototherapy to address a number of neurological problems, including those suffered by people who were paraplegic or quadriplegic, have brain tumours, or fall victim to multiple sclerosis.[67]

Many other important research projects have been developed, and since the beginning of the 1980s and the inception of the Alberta Heritage Foundation for Medical Research (AHFMR), the expansion of medical research has been phenomenal. A number of the research projects have received national and international recognition and have been instrumental in advancing improved patient care. There are far too many to be enumerated here, thus the remainder of this chapter will describe the establishment of the AHFMR and outline three specific research projects.

Alberta Heritage Foundation for Medical Research

Since the beginning of the 1980s, undoubtedly the major influence on medical research at the University of Alberta was the establishment of the AHFMR. When Science Minister Judd Buchanan was in Edmonton in 1978, Walter Mackenzie told him that "inadequate federal funding of medical research is preventing young scientists from breaking into the field."[68] Research grants that were available usually went to established researchers, and competition for funding was fierce, both for federal funds and for grants from national and provincial agencies and institutions. While Alberta received an equitable proportion of the grant monies available, an application for funding became both a time-consuming procedure and an art form in itself. The department of medicine employed a part-time editor to assist applicants in their applications.[69]

At this time, the province was approaching the height of its oil boom, and the government had set aside vast sums of money as a Heritage Savings Trust Fund "for future generations." The two Alberta medical schools felt that the time was ripe to appeal to the province for an endowment fund for medical research. Lionel McLeod, then dean of medicine at the University of Calgary, and Dean Cameron met with Premier Lougheed to discuss the proposal.[70] The premier appointed John E. Bradley, an Alberta medical school graduate, to investigate the concept and to develop a proposal to establish such a fund. After spending two years in consultation with authorities in Canada and elsewhere, Bradley proposed the establishment of a foundation that would operate at arm's length from the government, and would be financed by an endowment from the Heritage Savings Trust Fund. Lougheed approved the proposal and guided it through the Legislature, and it was he who suggested an amount for the endowment. According to Dean Cameron, "We were hoping for $30 million, we got $300 million." The proposal was approved by the legislature in 1979 and enacted that same year.

> The revenue was to be made available to support basic and clinical medical research and the government hoped that this thrust would attract outstanding scientists to carry out research in Alberta and to participate in this exciting program and encourage young people to entertain careers in research.[71]

The foundation operated at arm's length from the government so that it would be unaffected by political pressures and economic fluctuation. Bradley was the executive director during the initial organizational stages and while a board of trustees was appointed. Lionel McLeod, dean of medicine at the University of Calgary and a graduate of the University of Alberta, was appointed its president in 1981. A Scientific Advisory Council advised the trustees on policies and programmes and also acted as "a peer review system" to maintain a high standard of quality in the allocation of grants. A board of review, composed of international scientists, assessed the work of the foundation on a regular basis.

Grants from the AHFMR were designed to complement other sources of funding. The foundation supported the salaries of trainees and independent researchers, gave awards and scholarships, fellowships, studentships, supported visiting scientists, professors, lecturers and conferences, and made major equipment awards. The AHFMR became a major contributor to research funding and was responsible for the tremendous expansion of medical research in Alberta in the 1980s. As well as promoting scientific discovery within the medical school, the foundation attracted world-class scholars. It encouraged the formation of interdisciplinary groups, comprising basic, medical and clinical scientists, which were able to take research from the bench through to the bedside. Some research projects were delayed only because of a lack of laboratory space, but this was overcome by the construction of the Heritage Medical Research Centre, which was partly funded by the AHFMR. When the first section of this building opened in November 1988, three research teams were ready to move in immediately. The buildings were heated by a passive solar system and constructed in such a way that they could be readily "modified as technology and research personnel change."[72]

Shortly after his appointment in 1984, Dean Douglas Wilson, with the assistance of the new Associate Dean (Research) Mark Poznansky, established planning groups to recommend new interdisciplinary research that could integrate individual research strengths and work at the leading edge of biomedical science. Within five years, seven research groups had been approved for development in association with the Heritage Medical Research Centre. These were in the areas of lipid and lipoprotein metabolism, cardiovascular diseases, rehabilitation neuroscience, microbial pathogenesis, human molecular genetics, clinical and molecular immunology, and protein engineering and drug design. By the late 1980s, members of the first three groups had already been recruited from points in Canada, the United Kingdom, the United States and Japan and were actively pursuing their research goals.[73]

The International Board of Review for the AHFMR issued this comment in its 1987 report to the Government of Alberta:

> There is no doubt whatsoever that the Foundation has had a profound effect on medical research and education and a beginning and expanding influence on patient care in the Province of Alberta.... The programs of the Foundation have produced a unique medical research milieu that is likely not matched elsewhere in the world.[74]

Muttart Diabetes Research and Training Centre

In 1980, G.D. Molnar, chairman of the department of medicine, submitted a proposal to the Gladys and Merrill Muttart Foundation seeking financial support for a diabetes research and training centre at the University of Alberta. Mrs. Muttart, who was a diabetic, was instrumental in the formation of the Canadian Diabetic Association, and the foundation had always been a great supporter of medical research.[75] Molnar requested a donation of $1.2 million for a centre that would establish research into the cause, treatment, cure and prevention of diabetes mellitus. At the time there were about ten individual research projects being carried out in different departments of the university which dealt with some aspect of the disease. The proposed centre would provide laboratory facilities for all those investigators who shared this common interest and give the opportunity for "interdisplinary interaction" and an "interchange of ideas and information" throughout the university. As the university already had research groups with "international reputations in the areas of biochemistry, immunology and glucose regulation" Molnar felt that such a centre would attract additional scientists who were active in the field. The main objectives of the proposed centre were: to provide laboratory and animal facilities for researchers; to provide start-up funding for pilot projects; to train investigators; and to encourage interaction between investigators in various disciplines.[76]

The Muttart Foundation approved the proposal to establish a centre, and a diabetes research team consisting of Ray Rajotte, Garth Warnock and Norman Kneteman also received support from the AHFMR. They formed a truly multi-disciplinary team: Rajotte was a basic scientist with an engineering degree, while Warnock and Kneteman were University of Alberta medical graduates with science degrees, surgical specialty training, and research training in the United States and England. Rajotte's original research dealt with freezing kidney tissue to ultra low temperatures, but he branched off into work on the Islets of Langerhans. These islets, very small structures located in the pancreas, are composed of several types of cells, one of which produces insulin. In diabetics these islets are deficient. In 1972 replacement therapy treatment was successfully applied to rodents in St. Louis, where it was shown that replacement of islets could reverse the diabetes. Since then, research has investigated how this procedure can successfully be applied to humans.[77]

The whole pancreas was transplanted in selected patients, but it was a major operation with a number of healing problems. The success rate improved during the late eighties and there was some reversal of the diabetic condition. The main objectives of the Alberta team were to acquire, bank and preserve insulin producing cells, continue the study on tissue banking and its preservation, and prevent rejection of the transplanted cells using "sensible, safe, anti-rejection treatment." The next step was to transplant just the islets which were placed in the diabetic's liver or spleen. Some patients received this treatment, with some degree of success, but not enough to reverse the need for insulin. There were still many technical difficulties which needed considerably more research. The centre was the only programme for islet transplantation in Canada, and was also working on islet isolation, preservation of islets, prevention of rejection, and human trials. It was well known internationally for its islet preservation technology, and was an important source for the Islets of Langerhans. More than 160,000 are necessary for each transplant and the team was stockpiling donated healthy tissue for their clinical experiments.[78]

The Diabetic Research team of nine people included one basic scientist, two surgeons, two endocrinologists and two diabetologists. Other research activities dealt with investigations to discover the causes of diabetes, the reasons for the attack on cells that makes them deficient; molecular studies to prevent immune attacks on cells; and metabolic studies on islet transplants in animals. The Transplant Immunology Group, mentioned above, was also working on the immunologic aspects of diabetes.

The Department of Biochemistry and the MRC Group in Protein Structure and Function

The Faculty of Medicine's department of biochemistry seems always to have been more active in research activities than any of the other departments, from the time of its first head, J. B. Collip. It consistently attracted financial support from outside funding agencies, and over several years in the 1980s attracted more extra-mural research funds than any other department in the entire university: more than $5 million each year.[79] The department moved into the area of molecular biology and achieved and maintained an international standing of high repute for many years.[80] Since 1953 it has offered a Ph.D. programme, and developed an active graduate student programme which resulted in high quality research. Both the masters and doctoral programmes were based on primary research, and this was reflected in the number of graduate student publications in scholarly scientific journals, both in Canada and abroad.[81]

J.S. Colter, who took his honours baccaleurate in chemistry at the University of Alberta, returned to his *alma mater* as head of the department of biochemistry in 1961, and remained in that position for 26 years.[82] He came from the Wistar Research Institute in Philadelphia and brought with him an "extensive experience of virology and nucleic acid chemistry."[83] Over the years the department expanded and careful selection of new staff members created a department that achieved a high standing in both research and teaching, as well as one in which all members interacted congenially. The recruiting programme resulted in research groups that worked well together, discussed common problems, collaborated on both a formal and informal level, and reinforced each others' expertise.[84] The department was equally successful in obtaining research funds, demonstrated by the fact that eight of the twenty staff members were in research positions funded by external granting agencies. As would be expected with its success in attracting research funding, the department was extremely well equipped and had many "state-of-the-art" pieces of equipment.[85]

All members of the academic staff were involved in research programmes. These included studies of infectious viral and bacterial agents; membrane biochemistry; DNA replication, repair and recombinations; and a group working in the McEachern Cancer Research unit on biochemical pharmacology of drugs used in chemotherapy. However, the Protein Structure and Function Group, funded by the MRC, developed the highest profile. The members of this group, which originated in 1974, have included Larry Smillie, Cyril Kay, Wayne Anderson, Michael James, Brian Sykes, Robert Hodges and R.J. Fletterick, and they comprised one of the most prominent research teams in Canada. A major MRC group, it received funding of more than two million dollars a year for five-year periods, which were renewed continuously. Each member of the group brought strengths in particular areas and it offered a multi-faceted approach to problems in protein structure and function. When the department of biochemistry was reviewed in the early 1980s, this group was termed "a national resource," which was a great source of pride to all members of the department.

One of the group, Michael James, established the first protein crystallography laboratory in the country in 1968, and became "one of the world's leading x-ray crystallographers." This is a process which determines very precisely the three dimensional structure of a protein molecule, positions every atom in relationship to every other, and can reproduce what is likely happening to atoms in the molecule when any movement takes place. X-ray crystallography is an essential part of drug development. James worked on studies of proteins which would block enzymes, proteases, some related to emphysema, and in 1988 he and his colleagues solved the structure of renin, a key enzyme in the kidney that plays a role in the early development of high blood pressure.[86]

The Cardiovascular Unit and Open-Heart Surgery

A Cardiovascular Unit established in 1953, with funds provided by the Muttart and the Markle Foundations as well as the University of Alberta Hospital, provided facilities for the investigation of all types of heart ailments, with particular emphasis on the diagnosis and treatment of the more difficult and serious types of heart disease. The first cardiac catheterizations in Alberta took place here, and heralded a "new era of cardiologic diagnosis," as prior to World War II, physicians had been able to offer little more than palliative care to those suffering from heart disease.[87] This new procedure facilitated the diagnosis of abnormalities of the heart by inserting a catheter into a vein in the groin or the arm and passing it along until it reached the chambers of the heart. Robert S. Fraser was its director. Together with Joseph Dvorkin, another Alberta graduate, and two assistant research fellows, they conducted an active programme of clinical research and experimental cardiology with the use of animals.[88] In its first two years over 500 patients were referred to the unit from all parts of the province for investigation and diagnosis, and ninety catheterizations were performed in 1956.

As a result of its success, the unit was considerably expanded and acquired extra equipment and maintenance.[89] One of the research fellows, Brian Sproule, developed an interest in the pulmonary aspects of cardiovascular disease and received a fellowship from the Canadian Life Underwriters Association to carry out further study in this area in the United States. He later returned and rejoined the team.[90] In 1957, Richard E. Rossall, from the University of Leeds, became the second geographic full-time professor in cardiology, and activity in the Cardiovascular Unit increased enormously. However, as Fraser has since remarked; ''We could prove a patient had a hole between connecting chambers of the heart but nobody could do anything with the information. Then John Callaghan arrived on the scene with cardiovascular surgery.''[91]

John C. Callaghan joined the surgical department in 1955. He was a young and highly respected surgical trainee in eastern Canada, and had a long and specialized training in the cardiovascular field. Walter Mackenzie, then the head of the surgical department and determined to have an open-heart surgery programme at the University of Alberta, recruited Callaghan to come to Edmonton and initiate the procedures. Research in heart surgery began in the SMRI, and Callaghan worked in close co-operation with Fraser and Dvorkin and the Cardiovascular Unit, as well as those in other departments who were involved in congenital heart disease.

The equipment necessary for open-heart surgery had first to be developed and tested under experimental conditions. The first heart lung pump to be used ''was strictly homemade, with large plastic tubes through which the oxygen bubbled into the blood and escaped into the room air.''[92] By 1956, the experimental and investigative research on open-heart surgery had reached a stage when it could move into the University of Alberta Hospital, and the team conducted its first open-heart operation in the fall of that year. A few months later, and after the first successful ''blue baby'' operation, the cardiac surgical/medical team was well on its way to a highly successful programme. Joint open-heart rounds in the hospital provided a common meeting ground for staff of all the disciplines involved — surgeons, cardiologists, radiologists, pediatricians, anaesthetists, senior nurses and pump technicians.[93]

As the years went by, more and more complicated procedures took place, requiring more sophisticated equipment, and all were based upon experimental and investigative work in both surgical and medical fields. Thirty-five operations were performed in the first year, on patients ranging in age from newborn to thirty-eight years, all of whom were suffering from heart defects for which there had been no satisfactory treatment prior to the development of intracardiac surgery. The 1,000th took place in 1967, and by 1985, when Callaghan received the Order of Canada, the team had performed over 7,000 open-heart operations.[94] The programme achieved a high public profile and patients were referred from all parts of the province.[95] As well as being an excellent surgeon, John Callaghan was also a good ''public relations'' man. His successes at the operating table made headlines in both the local and national press, and he also arranged for the CBC to film an operation to replace an aortic valve. Callaghan supplied the narration, and it was shown in both North America and Europe. On another occasion, Premier Manning and his cabinet watched an operation from the dome over the operating room.[96]

Ongoing research for this programme, together with the study of immunology and the pharmacology to control immune activity, led inevitably to the next step in the process. In 1984, Dennis Modry, another University of Alberta graduate, returned to Edmonton from Stanford University, "the mecca of cardiac transplantation," charged with the responsibility of setting up a human heart transplantation programme at the University of Alberta Hospital. In 1986, Modry and his team conducted western Canada's first heart transplant.[97] The University of Alberta Hospital later developed a heart and lung transplant programme, and became a major centre for pediatric heart disease. A newly established Heritage Research Group on Cardiovascular Diseases began working on new research in the understanding of heart function.[98]

* * * * *

Since the University of Alberta's first president, Henry Marshall Tory, expressed his decided views on the importance of research to a medical faculty in the 1920s, several others have reiterated them. In 1948 Dean Ower said that "in order to establish and maintain its reputation in the community of medicine [the medical school] must make an attempt to contribute new knowledge. Research . . . stimulates the individual to be more critical and dynamic in his thinking and teaching."[99] Dean Scott, in 1955, concurred: "If members of the teaching staff were satisfied merely with the handing on of knowledge they would soon become disinterested and ineffective teachers. . . ."[100] Furthermore the school had the stimulus of a world-class researcher in its midst: while J.B. Collip did not receive a Nobel Prize, one of his co-researchers, J.J.R. Macleod, shared his award with him.

It is perhaps too easy to say that there was no money available for research and facilities were inadequate. Some people, a very few, did seek answers to their questions. Nevertheless, it was difficult if not impossible to carry out research activities in overcrowded laboratories, while carrying a heavy teaching load and conducting a private medical practice. And despite the fact that medical research in Canada received a tremendous boost by the discovery of insulin, governments and national agencies were slow to support, let alone encourage, research activity.

Ironically, some of the results of war are beneficial, and the change in attitude towards research seems to have started in the early forties, with the many research activities dealing with war-related problems. After the war, many young physicians joined medical faculties after their release from the services: they had been exposed to medical research during their war service and became increasingly aware of its importance and potential for improvements in patient care. Money was still scarce, and the teaching load heavy, but they created a growing demand for increased opportunities for medical research. Governments began to realize the potential and, following the Hall Commission and the establishment of the Medical Research Council, federal funding became increasingly available. In Alberta this was considerably augmented by the establishment of the AHFMR in 1979.

Research at the University of Alberta followed the national trend, although it lagged behind. Until 1945, it was the youngest medical school in the country (and probably the poorest), suffered severe financial restraints during the depression, and was slow to adopt the geographic full-time concept.(Part-time professors have little available time for research projects.) After a cautionary accreditation report in 1956, budgets, buildings, and full-time staff increased, and since that time the school has fitted into the mainstream of medical research in Canadian medical schools.

* * * * *

Conclusion

IN ITS first seventy-five years, Alberta's Faculty of Medicine has faced, and overcome, many challenges. It began as a two-year preclinical school in 1913, the fifth academic department in a university that was only five years old. Located in a frontier community, it was completely dependent on fees and government funding. A faculty of six professors met a class of twenty-seven students in the first premedical year. In 1988, 118 students entered the first year of the professional programme[1] and the faculty comprised over one thousand full and part-time academic staff.[2] In addition, about four hundred interns and residents participated in postgraduate education in more than thirty specialties, the medical science departments offered masters and doctoral programmes, and the faculty also provided health-service administration courses. To help the medical practitioner in the field keep up with the fast-moving pace of advances in all fields of medicine, an active Division of Continuing Medical Education provided a variety of programmes for those practising in and around Edmonton and in northern Alberta.

From working with one teaching hospital in 1922, when the school began its expansion to a full degree-granting programme, by 1988 the faculty had developed affiliations with six other local institutions. In addition to the University of Alberta Hospital, the Royal Alexandra, Edmonton General, Misericordia, Charles Camsell, Cross Cancer Institute and the Glenrose Provincial hospitals all provided teaching facilities for students, interns and residents of the medical school. The change in the basic philosophy of the school and its major teaching hospital was exemplified by the University of Alberta Hospital voluntarily giving up its internship programme in the early 1980s: it had become so specialized that it was not considered a good training ground for first-year graduate interns.

Six people attended the first Faculty Council meeting in April 1914—and one of those was late. In 1988, Faculty Council had over four hundred members. In comparison, it seems that life was simpler in those early days. But those six members of the first Faculty Council confronted a large task—the development of a medical school in a newly settled and isolated part of the country, with few facilities and little support from the medical fraternity. It was an ambitious undertaking, even under ordinary circumstances, but within a few months it faced a string of extraordinary crises: a world war, followed by a recession, a major depression, and a second world war.

Throughout its history, the Faculty of Medicine suffered from a shortage of both qualified staff and adequate physical facilities. Its growth was sporadic; only overcrowded conditions eventually resulted in new buildings or additions, which quickly became overcrowded again. Yet, its first home, the Medical Building, was often regarded as the most handsome on the university campus, and was certainly the most photographed. The faculty celebrated its seventy-fifth anniversary in its new home, the Walter C. Mackenzie Health Sciences Centre, which also attracted a great deal of interest, from both an architectural and a medical standpoint. Designed by a consortium of architects, including the Toronto firm that built that city's Eaton's Centre, it was open, airy and attractive; yet, it incorporated classrooms, laboratories, office space and examining rooms, a fine library, 834 hospital beds and easy indoor access to the medical and clinical science buildings.

In its formative years, the school's main objective was to produce "safe and capable" general practitioners for service in small towns and rural communities in the province, as well as the larger centres. Its basic mission remained to train physicians for primary medical care, but in the modern context. As medical science advanced technologically, both the profession and society demanded more specialized training, and graduates of Alberta's medical school divided more or less equally between family medicine and a specialty practice. In a survey conducted jointly by the medical schools of the Universities of Alberta and Calgary in 1988, the results showed that 49% of the University of Alberta's graduates between 1973 and 1985 entered family practice, and 51% were involved in one of thirty-five specialties. That same survey revealed that about 10% practised in villages and rural communities, even though 20% of Alberta's population lived in those areas.[3] After seventy-five years, the school still saw a need to encourage students to consider practice in rural settlements. By electives and a programme of education and service in northern communities, the faculty hoped to promote this objective in the future.

The medical faculty, unlike other schools and faculties in a university, is intimately involved with the standards and provision of service of its discipline throughout the province, and most innovative medical methods originate in a medical school. Furthermore, unlike medical research in a number of other western countries, most medical research in Canada is conducted in its medical schools and teaching hospitals. The traditional roles of medical schools are three-fold: the training of medical practitioners; research activities; and service to the community. These three should be inextricably entwined. At the University of Alberta's medical school, changes have taken place in each area.

To meet the need for change in medical education, a Division of Studies in Medical Education was established in 1986, with the initial aims of establishing an examination centre; furthering computer assisted and independent self-learning techniques; developing workshops designed to improve teaching techniques of residents and faculty members; and conducting research into medical education with a view to changing the curriculum. Other studies examined the future direction of health-care needs in Alberta so as to adapt the educational programme to meet demands for involvement in community medicine, disease prevention, geriatric care, health promotion, and the team approach in which physicians work more closely with other health-care professionals.

The biggest change came in the area of research, not only at the University of Alberta but also at all Canadian medical schools. Research activity increased rapidly during the 1970s and 1980s, mainly in response to improved funding from the Medical Research Council of Canada (MRC) and, during the 1980s in Alberta, the Alberta Heritage Foundation for Medical Research (AHFMR). To the public, these became the most visible activities of the medical school. Just as J.B. Collip's association with the discovery of insulin and his biochemical research activities in the 1920s focused public attention on Alberta's fledgling medical school, since 1974 the highly successful MRC group of protein structure and function, within the same department, achieved an international standing. Other high-profile research projects, such as the transplant immunology group and the diabetes research team, gave the university prestige and international recognition. The AHFMR supplied funding for state-of-the-art laboratory equipment as well as start-up costs, funds that were never included in the university budget but are a basic requirement to attract highly qualified international scholars. The AHFMR enabled the school to recruit scientists from all over the world, and the required qualifications for teachers have since included a significant level of training in research.

An essential role and responsibility of the medical school has always been to research and investigate methods that will improve the delivery of health-care. For many years, there was comparatively little interest in research by clinicians in most medical schools. Much of the research was conducted by medical scientists, but they needed to work with people who could provide a practical application so as to pass on the results to a patient-care setting. In the early 1980s, attitudes began to change as some clinicians and medical scientists collaborated on their research activities. Successful research projects gave the university prestige and international recognition, which in turn attracted high-calibre scholars from all parts of the world who would not previously have been available to the school. Success in research also enabled departments to recruit young research fellows and graduate students, both for their research and teaching ability. Research fellowships in turn provided more teaching positions and so enhanced the quality of tuition, and relieved some financial problems for university budgets that were never sufficient to provide an adequate number of instructors. Furthermore, with the advent of the AHFMR, students gained access to funding for summer research projects. While few planned academic careers, research offered a good training and taught them to evaluate problems scientifically.

As the Faculty of Medicine entered the last quarter of its first century, it faced many challenges. Burgeoning technology in the field of medicine imposed both technical and ethical questions to be resolved by both the medical fraternity and society as a whole. One of the major problems faced by medical educators was to find a way of training doctors to assess technological advances critically; to appreciate both the values and the limitations of such developments and still treat the patient as an individual.[4] One of the disadvantages of such developments is that they have tended to reduce the human factor in the doctor/patient relationship—the treatment can become more important than the patient. An aspect of this problem is the selection of effective medical students. Selection procedures have raised questions for many years, but scientific and technological advances placed more emphasis on personal qualities, an ability "to learn independently" and "to acquire critical analytical skills." These attributes are, however, much more difficult to assess than scientific ability and cannot be judged by examination or grade point averages.

Increased funding from federal sources and agencies, such as the MRC, national associations and corporations, and, in particular the AHFMR have made significant changes in the medical school. Extramural support expanded both the role and the concept of research activities. As attitudes on the part of clinicians changed, teams rather than individuals conducted most investigative procedures, teams sometimes composed of people from a variety of disciplines. The bridge between the laboratory bench and the bedside was more readily accessible, and the next step was to take the beneficial results of that research into the commercial field. Such rapid development, however, created new problems. Researchers who were funded by outside agencies were sometimes limited, by the terms of their agreement, to the time they were able to give to teaching. This raised questions concerning an equitable distribution of the medical educator's time between teaching and research and concerning the protection of academic freedom. Those research positions financially dependent upon outside agencies, rather than the school, can create conflicts of interest for the researcher, who might develop a greater loyalty to the agency than to the school. Corporate sponsorship of academic medical research had already raised these questions in United States medical schools, and they were being actively addressed at the University of Alberta.[5]

These are, however, the dilemmas of incredible growth and complex problems, rather than the original challenges of establishment and survival. Henry Marshall Tory sought to bring the University of Alberta into the mainstream of medical education and research. The Faculty of Medicine's involvement at the heart of modern health-service technology demonstrates the success of that enterprise seventy-five years later.

* * * * *

Appendix

(in chronological order from year of establishment)

Canadian Medical Schools*

1829   McGill University, Montréal, P.Q.
1843   University of Toronto, Toronto, Ont.
1843   Université de Montréal, Montréal, P.Q.
1852   Université Laval, Québec City, P.Q.
1854   Queen's University, Kingston, Ont.
1867   Dalhousie University, Halifax, NS.
1881   University of Western Ontario, London, Ont.
1883   University of Manitoba, Winnipeg, Man.
1913   University of Alberta, Edmonton, AB.
1926   University of Saskatchewan, Saskatoon, Sask.
1945   University of Ottawa, Ottawa, Ont.
1949   University of British Columbia, Vancouver, B.C.
1967   University of Sherbrooke, Sherbrooke, P.Q.
1969   McMaster University, Hamilton, Ont.
1969   Memorial University, St. John's, NFLD.
1970   University of Calgary, Calgary, AB.

---

* From J.A. MacFarlane, et. al., *Medical Education in Canada* (Canada: Royal Commission on Health Services, 1965), p. 16.

Presidents of the University of Alberta

1908-1928	Henry Marshall Tory
1928-1936	Robert C. Wallace
1936-1941	W.A.R. Kerr
1941-1950	Robert Newton
1950-1959	Andrew Stewart
1959-1969	Walter H. Johns
1969-1974	Max Wyman
1974-1979	Harry Emmett Gunning
1979-1989	Myer Horowitz
1989-	Paul Davenport

Deans of the Faculty of Medicine

1920-1945	Allan Coates Rankin
1939-1943	John J. Ower (Acting)
1945-1948	John J. Ower
1948-1959	John W. Scott
1959-1974	Walter C. Mackenzie
1974-1983	D.F. (Tim) Cameron
1983-1984	Robert S. Fraser (Acting)
1984-	Douglas R. Wilson

Executive Secretaries, Assistant and Associate Deans

1938-1950	H.E. Rawlinson
1950-1953	W.R. Salt
1953-1962	J.S. Thompson
1962-1974	D.F. Cameron
1968-1979	L.C. Grisdale
1970-1977	R.E. Rossall
1975-1986	F.B. Cookson
1977-1978	D.M. Paton
1977-1979	S. Kling
1978-1985	T.A. McPherson
1979-1984	R.S. Fraser
1979-1986	L.M. Anholt
1983-	D. Fenna
1983-	A.B. Jones
1985-	M.J. Poznansky
1986-	G. Goldsand
1986-	C.H. Harley
1988-	C.I. Cheeseman

Department Heads/Chairmen

Anaesthesia

1956-1975	E.A. Gain	1984-1988	W.B. MacDonald
1975-1984	G. Moonie	1988-1989	D.B. Duval (Acting)
		1989-	B.T. Finucane

*Anatomy and Cell Biology**

1913-1937	D.G. Revell	1963-1983	T.S. Leeson
1937-1960	R.F. Shaner	1984-1987	K.D. McFadden (Acting)
1960-1962	H.E. Rawlinson	1987-	R.A. Murphy
1962-1963	W.R. Salt (Acting)		

Applied Sciences in Medicine

1982-	D. Fenna

Bacteriology and Hygiene, Provincial Laboratory of Public Health

1907-1913	D.G. Revell	1919-1945	A.C. Rankin
1914	A.C. Rankin	1945-1949	R.M. Shaw
1914-1919	H.C. Jamieson (Acting)	1950-1959	R.D. Stuart

Directors of Provincial Laboratory

1959-1967	R.D. Stuart	1988-1989	D.L.J. Tyrrell (Acting)
1967-1988	J.M.S. Dixon	1989-	W.L. Albritton

Biochemistry

1920-1921	A.W. Downs	1929-1949	George Hunter
1921-1928	J.B. Collip	1949-1961	H.B. Collier
1928-1929	J.W. Scott (Acting)	1961-1987	J.S. Colter
		1987-	W.A. Bridger

Community Medicine (Preventive Medicine)

1927-1956	M.R. Bow	1959-1981	S.E. Greenhill
1956-1959	C.R. Amies		

Geriatrics

1980-1986	D. Skelton
1986-1987	J.A.L. Gilbert/G.R. Zetter (Acting)
1988-	P. McCracken

Health Services Administration and Community Medicine

1967-1981	C.A. Meilicke	1981-	C.B. Hazlett

Immunology

1971-1974	T.A. McPherson (Acting)	1988-1989	B. Singh (Acting)
1974-1988	E. Diener	1989-	T. Mossman

---

* Cell biology was added in the 1980s.

Medicine and Clinical Medicine

1923-1944	E.L. Pope	1974-1975	B.J. Sproule (Acting)
1944-1954	J.W. Scott	1975-1986	G.D. Molnar
1954-1969	Donald R. Wilson	1986-	E.G. King
1969-1974	R.S. Fraser		

Medical Microbiology

1959-1966	G. Myers	1967-1986	F.L. Jackson

Medical Microbiology and Infectious Diseases

1986-   D.L.J. Tyrrell   —————

Obstetrics and Gynaecology

1923-1941	L.C. Conn	1981-1983	T.R. Nelson (Acting)
1941-1962	J.R. Vant	1983-1986	D.L. Dunlop (Acting)
1962-1965	W.M. Paul	1986-	B.F. Mitchell
1965-1981	R.P. Beck		

Ophthalmology and Otolaryngology   *Ophthalmology*

1923-1940	R.B. Wells with	1969-1980	T.A.S. Boyd
	C.V. Jamieson	1980-	H.T. Wyatt
1940-1954	M.R. Marshall		

Pathology

1920-1951	J.J. Ower	1980-1987	T.K. Shnitka
1951-1970	J.W. Macgregor	1987-	K. Solez
1970-1980	G.O. Bain		

Pediatrics

1957-1971	J.K. Martin	1984-1986	F.L. Harley (Acting)
1972-1984	E.E. McCoy	1986-	P.M. Olley

Physiology and Pharmacology

1914-1916	H.H. Moshier	1949-1955	H.V. Rice
1916-1920	J.B. Collip (Acting)	1955-1961	J.W. Pearce
1920-1948	A.W. Downs		

Pharmacology   *Physiology*

1961-1972	E.E. Daniel	1961-1965	J.W. Pearce
1972-1980	J.S. Charnock	1965-1986	M. Schachter
1980-	D.A. Cook	1986-	P.K.T. Pang

Psychiatry

1954-1955	R.R. MacLean	1957-1975	K.A. Yonge
1955-1956	S.S. Spaner	1975-1990	W.G. Dewhurst
1956-1957	Stanley Smith	1990-	R.C. Bland

Radiology
1954-1965 H.E. Duggan
1965-1971 F. McConnell

1972-1984 J.D.R. Miller
1984-   D.B. Russell

Surgery and Clinical Surgery
1922-1929 F.H. Mewburn
1929-1938 A.R. Munro
1938-1949 W.F. Gillespie
1949-1950 H.H. Hepburn

1950-1960 W.C. Mackenzie
1960-1975 R.A.L. Macbeth
1975-1986 H.T.G. Williams
1987-   B.K.A. Weir

Directors — Divisions of the Department of Medicine

Anaesthesia
1936-1955 E.H. Watts

1955-   Departmentalized

Cardiology
1922-1944 C. Hurlburt
1955-1969 R.S. Fraser

1969-1988 R.E. Rossall
1988-   T.J. Montague

Dermatology
1930-1952 H. Orr
1952-1977 P. Rentiers
1977-1986 J. Brown

1986-1989 E.H. Schloss
1989-   K. Jimbow

Endocrinology and Metabolism
1947-1964 D.R. Wilson
1964-1968 L.E. McLeod
1968-1973 M. Watanabe

1973-1988 P. Crockford
1988-   J. Ginsberg

Family Medicine
1978-1979 L.C. Grisdale
1979-1983 G.L. Higgins

1983-   Departmentalized

Gastroenterology
1965-1968 R.W. Sherbaniuk
1968-1980 R.H. Wensel

1980-1987 R.W. Sherbaniuk
1987-   A.B.R. Thomson

General Internal Medicine
1970-   A.G. Richards
1970-1972 J. Sprague
1972-1979 L.M. Anholt

1979-1987 J.A.L. Gilbert
1987-   J.A.L. Gilbert and
           A.M. Edwards

Hematology
1969-1974 A.S. Little
1974-1979 M. Mant (Acting)
1979-1983 J.R. Hill

1983-1985 R.N. MacDonald (Acting)
1985-   A.R. Turner

Immunology and Nephrology
1969-1985   J.B. Dosseter   1986-   P. Halloran
1985-1986   R. Ulan (Acting)

Infectious Diseases
1969-1985   G. Goldsand   1987-1988   E.A. Fanning (Acting)
1985-1987   D.L.J. Tyrrell   1988-   L.J. Miedzinski

Medical Oncology
1977-1981   R.N. MacDonald   1987-1989   A.L.A. Fields
1981-1982   J.G. Pearson (Acting)   1989-   A.R. Blench
1982-1987   R.N. MacDonald

Nephrology
1962-1968   L.E. McLeod   1969-   Combined with
1968-1969   R. Ulan   Immunology

Neurology
1957-1978   G. Monckton   1988-   M.H. Brooke
1978-1988   D.R. McLean

Pediatrics
1923-1956   D.B. Leitch   1957-   Departmentalized

Psychiatry
1954-1955   R.R. MacLean   1956-1957   S. Smith
1955-1956   S.S. Spaner   1957-   Departmentalized

Pulmonary Diseases
1960-1988   B.J. Sproule   1988-   S.F.P. Mann

Rheumatology
1956-1966   E.G. Kidd   1987-1988   A.S. Russell (Acting)
1966-1987   J.S. Percy   1988-   A.S. Russell

Directors — Divisions of the Department of Surgery

Biochemistry
1968-   J.C. Russell

Experimental Surgery (SMRI)
1954-1960   R.C. Harrison   1978-1987   G.W. Scott
1960-1978   K. Kowalewski   1988-   R.V. Rajotte

General Surgery
1985-1987   H.T.G. Williams   1987-   W.W. Yakimets

Neurosurgery

1932-1951	H.H. Hepburn	1970-1982	P.B.R. Allen
1951-1965	G.K. Morton	1982-1987	B.K.A. Weir
1965-1969	T.J. Speakman	1987-	K.C. Petruk

Opthalmology

1954-1960	M.R. Marshall	1964-1969	T.A.S. Boyd
1960-1964	J.W. Duggan	1969-	Departmentalized

Orthopedic Surgery

1924-1944	Hastings Mewburn	1976-1978	L.A. Davis
1944-1958	R.G. Huckell	1978-1987	J.R. Huckell
1958-1976	Olav Rostrup	1987-	M.J. Moreau

Otolaryngology

1960-1973	K.A.C. Clarke	1978-1979	R.W. Mallen
1973-1977	R.W. Mallen	1979-	D.J. Oldring
1977-1978	K.A.C. Clarke		

Plastic Surgery

1965-1987	J.D.M. Alton	1987-	G.W. Lobay

Thoracic/Cardiovascular Surgery

1960-1987	J.C. Callaghan	1988-	D.L. Modry
1987-1988	E.T. Gelfand		

Urologic Surgery

1923-1935	E.C. Smith	1975-1987	W.H. Lakey
1935-1959	G.N. Ellis	1987-	M.S. McPhee
1959-1975	J.O. Metcalfe		

Presidents of the Medical Undergraduate Society

Medical Students Club

1917-1918	Ann A. Curtin
1918-1919	W.J. Dorrance
1919-1920	J.L. Jackson
1920-1921	A.H. Meneely
1921-1922	Wm. A. Henry
1922-1923	Julius C. Grimson
1923-1924	Eldon J. Liesemer
1924-1925	George M. Lewis
1925-1926	Thomas C. Michie
1926-1927	George C. Haworth
1927-1928	William H. Cassels
1928-1929	Nesbitt E. Alexander
1929-1930	Almer M. Borrowman
1930-1931	R. Julian Brown
1931-1932	Herbert L. Newcombe
1932-1933	William N. Gourlay
1933-1934	John Smith Gardner
1934-1935	Harry E. Gibson
1935-1936	Albert W. Hardy
1936-1937	John B. Wood
1937-1938	John P. Wellwood
1938-1939	Rickard Younge
1939-1940	J. Douglas D. Wallace

Medical Undergraduate Society

1940-1941	William R. Bell
1941-1942	Alfred K. Gibbons
1942	John W. Duggan
1943	James B. Wallace
1943-1944	Reginald G. Christie
1944	Richard C.B. Corbet
1945	Patrick J.E. Kimmitt
1945-1946	Donald B. Wray
1946-1947	Gordon M. Fierheller
1947-1948	Allan L. Hepburn
1948-1949	Erenest C. Shortliffe
1949-1950	Donald B. Baker
1950-1951	George D. Molnar

1951-1952	Richard MacDonald Jr.
1952-1953	Ralph L. Hay
1953-1954	Frederick C. Marshall
1954-1955	David R. Shea
1955-1956	Mario I. Tedeschini
1956-1957	Robert F. Clark
1957-1958	David M. Gilmour
1958-1959	John A. Cairns
1959-1960	John N. Chappel
1960-1961	Roderick A. Morgan
1961-1962	Robert J. Raine
1962-1963	Roger A. Cumming
1963-1964	Alan L. Maberley
1964-1965	Douglas F. Waller
1965-1966	William M. Sereda
1966-1967	Dennis Jirsch
1967-1968	Derek A. Younge
1968-1969	Blayne C. Hirsche

Medical Students' Association

1969-1970	Clark B. Jamieson
1970-1971	Robert B. Haynes
1971-1972	Harv H. Haakanson
1972-1973	David L. Shragge
1974-	Judy Cooney
1974-1975	Frank J. Moffet
1975-1976	Michael S. Wilson
1976-1977	Gregory Baker
1977-1978	David Bond
1978-1979	Tom Davies
1979-1980	Andrew Wilkinson
1980-1981	John D. Epps
1981-1983	Ian Cowan
1983-1984	Gary May
1984-1985	Tim Dewhurst
1985-1987	Louis H. Francescutti
1987-1988	Marion Doberthein
1988-1989	Kenneth Brown

Presidents of the Medical Alumni Association

1947-1948	Percy H. Sprague	1967-1968	William T. Boyar
1948-1949	William W. Eadie	1968-1969	Bohdan Michalyshyn
1949-1950	John Smith Gardner	1969-1970	G. Sigurd Balfour
1950-1951	Herbert E. Rawlinson	1970-1971	Robert E. Hatfield
1951-1952	C. Angus McGugan	1971-1972	Edward G. Kidd
1952-1953	Nesbitt E. Alexander	1972-1973	Joseph Dvorkin
1953-1954	Edward Hitchin	1973-1974	Calvin J. Fairbanks
1954-1955	M. Olav Rostrup	1974-1975	Neil F. Duncan
1955-1956	Reuben E. Jespersen	1975-1976	J. Murray Cowan
1955-1956	Leonard O. Bradley	1976-1977	John R. Settle
1956-1957	Samuel Hanson	1977-1978	John D.M. Alton
1957-1958	Hugh A. Arnold	1978-1979	F. Gordon Gore-Hickman
1958-1959	Arthur V. Follett	1979-1980	James H. Hook
1959-1960	Joseph A. O'Brien	1980-1981	Donald S. Wallace
1960-1961	Jack L. Edwards	1981-1982	William H. Lakey
1961-1962	Nelson W. Nix	1982-1983	Margaret G. Pearson
1962-1963	Allan L. Hepburn	1983-1984	John Higgin
1963-1964	John E. Bradley	1984-1985	Robert J. Sommerville
1964-1965	Lloyd W. Johnston	1985-1986	Frank C.Haley
1965-1966	Norris R. Bertrand	1986-1987	Robert E. Pow
1966-1967	Douglas C. Ritchie	1987-1988	Alvin R. Backstrom
		1988-1989	Gerald M. McDougall

Outstanding Achievement Award Winners
Medical Alumni Association

1963	T. Blair McLean	1974	H. MacKenzie Freeman
1964	George Morris Lewis	1975	William Stewart Simpson
1965	Edward F. Donald	1976	Lionel E. McLeod
1966	Eliot Corday	1977	Helen E. Reid
1967	Lloyd Douglas Maclean	1978	Helen I. Huston
1968	Gordon Barry Pierce	1979	John E. Bradley
1969	J. Douglas Wallace	1980	A. Earl Walker
1970	David Landner	1981	Frank M. Christie
1971	J. Frank Elliott	1982	Rupert Clare
	H. Lionel Dobson	1983	Theodor K. Shnitka
	John W. MacGregor	1984	Leonard O. Bradley
1972	R. Kenneth C. Thomson	1985	Robert A. Macbeth
	Hugh J. Arnold	1986	Hector E. Duggan
	Matthew Matas	1987	Lloyd C. Grisdale
1973	John Smith Gardner	1988	John S. Lewis
		1989	Gordon Brown

* * * * *

Notes

Introduction

[1] J.M. Large was a medical student, class of 1930; D.G. Revell was the head of the Anatomy Department; and E.F. Cain was a medical student, class of 1929.

[2] William Hardy Alexander. "In the Beginning," *Alberta Historical Review*, (Spring 1960), p. 15.

[3] E.A. Corbett, *Henry Marshall Tory, Beloved Canadian.* (Toronto: Ryerson Press, 1954), p. v.

[4] Hilda Neatby, "The Medical Profession in the North-West Territories," *Saskatchewan History*, Volume II, Number 2, (May 1949), pp. 2-3.

[5] Minutes of the CPSA, 18 October 1906.

[6] Dean J.J. Ower Diaries, 15 November 1934.

[7] Minutes, CPSA, 20 November 1916.

[8] For these and following cases see Attorney Generals' Files. f.75.126/760a-d.

[9] CPSA minutes, 8 November 1921.

Part I
Chapter 1
The Early Years 1913-1921

[1] Letter, Tory to Rutherford, 6 March 1906. Chancellors' Papers, UAA.

[2] W.H. Alexander, E.K. Broadus, F.J. Lewis and J.M. MacEachran. *These Twenty-Five Years. A Symposium.* (Toronto: Macmillan Company of Canada Limited, 1933), p. 6.

³ *Statutes of Alberta*, 1907. This amendment was passed 15 March 1907, and was subsequently repealed in 1910.
⁴ Letter, Low to Rutherford, 2 November 1906. Chancellors' Papers. UAA.
⁵ Robert Newton, *I Passed This Way, 1889-1964*, unpublished memoirs, UAA., p. 284.
⁶ *Journals of the Legislative Assembly of Alberta, 1906-1910.* 17 February 1910.
⁷ D.G. Revell, "The Medical Faculty - University of Alberta," *Historical Bulletin*, Calgary Associate Clinic, Vol. 13, No.4 (February 1949). p. 70.
⁸ G.D Stanley, "Dr. Daniel Graisberry Revell," *Historical Bulletin*, Calgary Associate Clinic. Vol. 14 (1949), p. 52.
⁹ Letter, Revell to W.A.R.Kerr, Acting President, 2 August 1918, Presidents' Papers (hereinafter referred to as P.P.), f.150. UAA.
¹⁰ Corbett. *op.cit.* p. 94.
¹¹ Minutes of the University of Alberta Senate, 10 June 1909.
¹² Heber C. Jamieson, *Early Medicine in Alberta, the First Seventy-Five Years*, (Edmonton: Canadian Medical Association, Alberta Division, 1947), p. 65.
¹³ Letter, Tory to Rev. C. Carruthers, 1 April 1922, P.P. f.161. UAA.
¹⁴ *Journals, 1906-1910, op.cit.*
¹⁵ *Alberta Revised Statutes*, 1922, Vol. I, "The University Act," Section 25.
¹⁶ *ibid.*, Section 39.
¹⁷ Minute Book, College of Physicians and Surgeons, 18 October 1906.
¹⁸ By 1913, qualifying examinations for all organizations in the province requiring higher educational qualifications were held through the university, including the Law Society, Land Surveyors Association, Association of Architects, Dental Association, Chartered Accountants and Pharmacists associations. (Sessional Paper, No. 88, 1914, PAA). The composition of the Senate included representatives from all societies whose examinations for status were conducted by the university.
¹⁹ Alexander McPhedran, professor of medicine, University of Toronto, "Undergraduate Training and Requirements for License to Practise," *The Western Medical News*, Vol. 4, No. 4 (April, 1912), pp. 80-81.
²⁰ Minutes, CPSA, 8 November 1917.
²¹ Dr. Walter Anderson, interview.
²² *The Gateway*, 15 May 1925, p. 1.
²³ H.M. Tory. Untitled article in *Medical Alumni Bulletin*, Vol,1., No.1., 8 May 1942.
²⁴ Lease Agreement, in P.P., f.155., UAA.
²⁵ Angus C. McGugan. *The First Fifty Years. The University of Alberta Hospital, 1914-1964.* (Edmonton: 1964). p. 6.
²⁶ Letter, Revell to Kerr. 2 August 1918, P.P., f.150., UAA.
²⁷ Revell, "The Medical Faculty," *op.cit.* p. 66.
²⁸ Interview with Dr. W.H. Mulloy whose father was one of the students in the first medical class and who signed the petition.

29 Kenneth M. Ludmerer, *Learning to Heal. The Development of American Medical Education*, (New York: Basic Books, Inc., Publishers, 1985), pp. 92-96.

30 N. Tait McPhedran, "The Evolution of Medical Education in Canada." Unpublished manuscript, 1988, p. 5.

31 H.M. Tory, "The University's Function in Medicine," *The Canadian Medical Association Journal*, Vol. XVI, No. 11 (November, 1926), pp. 1301-06.

32 *ibid.*

33 E.P. Scarlett, "A Doctor's Notebook," *Alberta Medical Bulletin*, Volume 28, No.4 (November 1963), p. 164.

34 Ludmerer, *op.cit.*, pp. 92-96.

35 Sessional Paper (hereinafter referred to as S.P.), No. 77, 1913. PAA.

36 Letter, Tory to Adami, December 1914, P.P., f.141, UAA.

37 Senate Minutes, 28 April 1915. UAA.

38 S.P. No 77, 1913. PAA.

39 John W. Scott, *The History of the Faculty of Medicine of the University of Alberta, 1913-1963*, (Edmonton: The University of Alberta, 1963), p. 6.

40 Ralph Shaner. "Dr. Daniel Graisberry Revell," Obituary notice, *Proceedings of American Association of Anatomists*, Vol. 122. No.4 (1955), p. 640.

41 Miss G.A. Revell, interview.

42 Donald R. Wilson, "James Bertram Collip," *Annual Report of the Alberta Medical Association* (1982), p. 21.; and Stanley, *op.cit.*, p. 54.

43 Taped interview of J.S. Gardner and James Nixon by Allan Hepburn, 1973. UAA.

44 Minutes of City of Edmonton Names Advisory Committee, 19 March 1986, when Revell's name was being considered for a street in a new subdivision. (Biography file, UAA.)

45 Minutes, Council of the Faculty of Medicine (hereinafter referred to as FCM.), 22 March 1922.

46 J.J. Ower, "Citation," *Medical Alumni Bulletin*, 20 April 1946, p. 11.

47 Mrs. Mary (Jamieson) Petley-Jones, interview.

48 S.P. No. 88. 1914. PAA.

49 Revell, "The Medical Faculty," *op.cit.*

50 University of Alberta Calendar, 1915-16, pp.15-16.

51 Walter Morrish, "Memoirs re Medical and Political Experiences," unpublished manuscript, c. 1963. GAI.

52 *The Gateway*, Special Number, April 1914.

53 University of Alberta Calendar, 1914-1915.

54 *ibid.*, several issues.

55 John W. Scott, "Early Medical Education and Practice in the Province of Alberta," Unpublished manuscriopt, (November, 1975).

56 University of Alberta Calendars, 1913 to 1920.

57 FCM. 26 April 1915.

58 *The Gateway*, Special Number, April 1915.

59 Morrish, *op.cit.*
60 Revell, "The Medical Faculty," *op.cit.*
61 Letter, Revell to Kerr, Acting President, 31 August 1918. P.P., f.150, UAA.
62 Miss G.A. Revell, *op.cit.*; and *Medical Alumni Bulletin*, 8 May 1942.
63 Revell, "The Medical Faculty." *op.cit.* p. 73.
64 FCM, 22 March 1915.
65 Minutes of Senate Meeting, 6 March 1915. UAA.
66 W.H. Alexander, *The University of Alberta. A Retrospect, 1908-1929.* pp. 20-21.
67 FCM, 15 February 1916.
68 Statistics extracted from the presidents' reports to the Senate in the Minutes. The figures include the registration for all three years of the course, including those registered for dentistry and pharmacy, plus those in the arts and medicine programme.
69 Alexander, *The University, op.cit.*, pp. 24-25.
70 S.P. No. 457, 1921. PAA.
71 Letter, Revell to Kerr, 2 August 1918, P.P., f.150. UAA.
72 Walter H. Johns, *A History of the University of Alberta. 1908-1969*, (Edmonton: The University of Alberta Press, 1981), p. 74.
73 Miss Revell, *op.cit.*
74 *The Gateway*, Graduation Number, May 1920.
75 Inspection Report, 5 November 1919, P.P., f.148. UAA.
76 Letter, Tory to Colwell, 7 June 1920, P.P., f. 148. UAA.
77 S.P. No. 355, 1919. PAA.
78 S.P. No. 400, 1920. PAA.
79 Premiers' Papers, file 120. PAA.
80 Miss Revell, *op.cit.*
81 Daniel G. Revell, "The Department of Anatomy, University of Alberta," *Methods and Problems of Medical Education* (New York: The Rockefeller Foundation, 1930), pp. 1-2.
82 J.W. Scott, "Department of Biochemistry, University of Alberta," *ibid.*, p. 3.
83 H.M. Tory, *The Gateway*, 28 November 1922, p. 1.

Chapter 2
The Years of Struggle
The twenties and the thirties

1 Premiers' Papers, f.142. PAA.
2 Letter, Kerr to Tory, 29 July 1921. P.P., UAA.
3 Premiers' Papers. f.142. PAA.
4 See R. Douglas Francis and Howard Palmer, *The Prairie West, Historical Readings* (Edmonton: Pica Pica Press, 1985), pp. 535-6; and Gerald Friesen, *The Canadian Prairies, A History* (Toronto: University of Toronto Press, 1984), pp. 316-29 and 382-88.

5 Letter, Wallace to E.C. Manning, provincial secretary, 13 Feb 1936, f.71.441/4j. PAA.
6 S.P. f.1851. PAA.
7 Letter, Shaner to Rawlinson, 28 February 1938. Shaner Papers. f.64. UAA.
8 Newton, *op.cit.* p. 284.
9 William G. Rothstein, *American Medical Schools and the Practice of Medicine. A History,* (New York, Oxford: Oxford University Press, 1987), pp. 162-66.
10 Annual Report, University of Alberta, 31 December 1921.
11 P.P., f.10.4. UAA.
12 Telegram, Kerr to Tory, 14 December 1923, *ibid.*
13 H.M. Tory, *The Gateway,* 28 November 1922, p. 1.
14 Senate Minutes, 12 May 1920.
15 Correspondence between Kerr and E. Stanley Ryerson, University of Toronto, and J.A. Nicholson, McGill University, February 1919, P.P., f.142. UAA.
16 A more detailed account of medical education and changes in the curriculum over the years will be found in Chapter 6.
17 FCM, 16 November 1937.
18 Letter, Tory to Dr. Chas. B. Heisler, University of State of New York, 17 December 1927. P.P., f.149. UAA.
19 Pope, "Some Reminiscences," *Medical Alumni Bulletin,* 30 December 1944, p. 1.
20 See H.E. Rawlinson, "Frank Hamilton Mewburn," *Canadian Journal of Surgery* (October 1958), pp. 1-5; R.A. Macbeth, "History of the Department of Surgery, University of Alberta," unpublished manuscript, n.d., pp. 5-9; and Miss Revell, *op.cit.*
21 FCM, 16 March 1931.
22 Interviews with Drs.J.S. Gardner and Herbert Begg; and taped interview of Drs. Gardner and James Nixon by Allan Hepburn, *op.cit.*
23 Leone McGregor Hellstedt, "Background and Experiences of a Girl Born in Carnduff, Saskatchewan in January 1900. The Choice and Course of her Career in Medicine," (Stockholm, Sweden, 1970), unpublished manuscript. p. 39.
24 There were fifty-two professors in the Faculty of Medicine in the academic year 1924-25, the first year of the complete medical programme.
25 P.P., f.149. UAA.
26 Interviews, Gardner, Nixon and Hepburn, *op.cit.*; and *Medical Alumni Bulletin*, Vol. 1, No. 1, April 1946.
27 Ower Diaries, several entries in 1929; and P.P., 3/2/5/3-1.UAA.
28 Letter, Shaner to A.W.Myers, Stanford University, 23 May 1922. Shaner Papers, f.3. UAA.
29 Letter, Shaner to E.A.Boyden, University of Alabama, 12 September 1930. *ibid.*

30 One said that Shaner spoke so quietly that he wasn't always able to hear him. (*ibid.* f.1)
31 Interview with Gardner, et al., *op.cit.*
32 *Medical Alumni Bulletin*, 30 December 1944.
33 FCM, September 8th, 1966; and University of Alberta Calendar, 1920/21. p.13.
34 Donald R. Wilson, "James Bertram Collip," *op.cit.*, p. 21; and several interviews.
35 In this era, with the exception of a few demonstrators, all medical faculty members were male.
36 Donald McLeod was one of Edmonton's early pioneers.
37 In 1922, the university made a grant of $500 towards the general upkeep of the General Hospital on condition that the medical school had a primary claim on twelve beds. (Letter, Tory to Mother Superior, General Hospital, 25 October 1922, P.P., f. 146.)
38 A "closed" hospital meant that only physicians who were on staff at the medical school and the hospital could admit patients.
39 Report by M.T. MacEachern, director of hospital activities, ACS, 4 October 1924.
40 Dean of Medicine's Report to the Senate, 13 May 1926.
41 Rothstein, *op.cit.*, pp.177-8.
42 Provincial auditor to provincial treasurer, 11 December 1926. Premiers' Papers. f.139. PAA.
43 Letter, Kerr to Tory, 23 November 1926, P.P., f.10.4. UAA.
44 University of Alberta Hospital Board Minutes, 25 October 1928.
45 Angus C. McGugan. *The First Fifty Years.*, *op.cit.*, p. 9; and J. Ross Vant and Tony Chapman, *More Than a Hospital, University of Alberta Hospitals 1906-1986.* (Edmonton: The University Hospitals Board, 1986), p. 85.
46 Annual Report, University of Alberta Hospital, 1929-30.
47 Pope, *The Gateway*, 15 May 1925, p.1.
48 FCM, various meetings.
49 Robert B. Kerr, *History of The Medical Council of Canada*, (The Medical Council of Canada, 1979), Appendix A, p. 6.
50 Dean's Report to Faculty Council, 15 November 1926.
51 Results of MCC examinations in P.P., f.3/2/4/9-1. UAA.
52 FCM, January 1932.
53 Information concerning this Club is from the Minutes of the Meetings of the Mewburn Reporting Club, f.69-28-14. UAA; and Ower's diaries.
54 Letter, Ower to Shaner, 15 March 1960, Shaner Papers, f.300. UAA.
55 Ower Diaries, 1 May 1933.
56 Jamieson Papers, f.25. UAA.
57 Ower Diaries, 25 January 1935.
58 *Evergreen and Gold*, 1924-25. p. 106.
59 Ower was intimately involved in this club also, not only assisting with the programme but also socially. In 1934, he took all members of the club,

twenty-four of them, to the movies (they saw George Arliss in *The House of Rothschild*, which, Ower said, was very good) and then to his home for coffee, sandwiches and ice cream. (Ower Diaries.)

60 Shaner Report in Mewburn Club Papers.

61 John W.Scott, "Memoirs, 1914-1979," unpublished manuscript (March 1979), p. 12.

62 Ower Diaries, 14 March 1931.

63 Coincidentally they both left in 1928.

64 Letter, Collip to Tory, 19 June 1921, P.P., f.144. UAA.

65 *Gateway*, 14 January 1941.

66 Letter, Tory to Rankin, 2 June 1921, P.P., f.144. UAA.

67 Letter, Collip to Tory, 19 June 1921, *ibid*.

68 Letter, Tory to Collip, 29 August 1921, *ibid*.

69 Letter, Collip to Tory, 19 June 1921, *ibid*.

70 Michael Bliss, "J.B.Collip: A Forgotten Member of the Insulin Team," Wendy Mitchinson and Janice Dickin McGinnis, *Essays in the History of Canadian Medicine*. (Toronto: McClelland and Stewart Limited, 1988), p. 112.

71 See, specifically, Michael Bliss, *The Discovery of Insulin* (Toronto: McClelland and Stewart Limited, 1982).

72 Letter, Collip to Tory, 8 January 1922. P.P., f.144. UAA.

73 Letter, Collip to Tory, 25 January 1922. *ibid*.

74 Michael Bliss, "The Aetiology of the Discovery of Insulin," C.G. Roland, *Health, Disease and Medicine: Essays in Canadian History*, (Toronto: Clarke Irwin Inc., 1984), pp. 341-2.

75 Bliss, "Collip." *op.cit.* p.123

76 Bliss, *The Discovery*, *op.cit.* p. 240.

77 Annual Report, University of Alberta. 3 December 1925, p. 49. According to correspondence in the possession of Dr. John B. Collip, J.Bertram Collip's son, the University of Alberta also received a small cheque in the amount of $1,666.67 from the Insulin Committee in 1949, although a much larger one, $39,683.41, went to the University of Western Ontario, where Collip was then employed. No explanation is given for the cheque to Alberta, except that Collip had requested it. (Letter, C.E. Higginbottom, bursar, University of Toronto to J.B. Collip, 9 June 1949.)

78 Telegram, Collip to Tory, 9 May 1922, P.P., f.144. UAA.

79 Letters, George Johnson to Tory, 21 December 1922, 13 April and 13 August 1923. *ibid*.

80 *The Gateway*, 22 January 1924.

81 Letter, Kerr to Dr. R.T.Washburn, medical superintendent, University of Alberta Hospital, 14 December 1923, P.P., f.144. UAA.

82 Bliss, "Collip," *op.cit.*, p. 123.

83 Copy of resolution in Collip Biography file. UAA, Many years later, a bronze tablet commemorating his achievement was placed in the biochemistry department at the university, 12 June 1959.

84 FCM, 16 October 1923.

85 Interview, Dr. John B. Collip, son of Dr. J.B.(Bert) Collip.

86 Letter, Collip to Tory, 19 June 1921, P.P., f.144. UAA.

87 Letter, Kerr to Tory, 11 June 1927, *ibid.*

88 Letter, Collip to Tory, 30 August 1927, *ibid.*

89 Telegrams, Collip to Tory, 16 and 17 September 1927, *ibid.*

90 Minutes, Board of Governors, 12 January 1928.

91 D.R. Wilson, in FCM, 15 November 1965.

92 Department of Biochemistry Papers. UAA.

93 *ibid.*

94 Ower Diaries, 16 December 1931.

95 Notices in Shaner Papers, f.49. UAA.

96 P.P.143. UAA.

97 Shaner Papers, ff.52 and 55. UAA.

98 *ibid.* f.60

99 S.P. 1309, 1933. PAA.

100 By the early 1930s McGill's quota was one hundred and often more than seven hundred applied. (Letter, Rawlinson to Shaner, 19 September c1930. Shaner Papers, f.30. UAA.)

101 FCM, 20 February 1933.

102 Letter, Munroe to Rankin, 22 November 1935, P.P.3/2/4/9-1. UAA.

103 FCM, 21 January 1935; 14 December 1937; and 17 October 1938; and Letter, M.M.Cantor to Dr. A.B. Gray, Seattle, 11 February 1939, Cantor Papers. UAA.

104 FCM; and Board of Governors' Reports, 1924-1940.

105 Letter, Cantor to Al (?), 11 February 1939, Cantor Papers. UAA.

106 R.A. Macbeth, "Alexander Russell Munroe: 1879-1965," *The Canadian Journal of Surgery*, 10, 3-10 (January 1967), p. 1-5.

107 Later a $5 registration fee was instituted, FCM, 17 April 1933.

108 University Hospital Board Minutes, 21 May 1932.

109 P.P. 3/2/4/9-1. UAA.

110 Minutes of the UAH Board, 11 May 1928 and 25 September 1930.

111 Vant and Cashman, *op.cit.*, pp. 91-94.

112 Annual Report, University of Alberta Hospital. 1929-30. p. 11.

113 FCM, 27 October 1930.

114 Acting Dean Ower's Report to the Board of Governors, 1939-40. pp. 28-29.

115 University of Alberta Hospital Board Minutes, 24 June 1932.

116 Letter, Dean of Medicine to the President, 30 November 1937, P.P. f.3/3/4/10-1. UAA.

117 P.P. f.3/2/4/9-1. UAA.

118 Letter, Dean of Medicine to the President, 6 December 1937, P.P. f.3/3/4/10-1. UAA.

119 Report on University of Alberta, Faculty of Medicine, Visited 3, 4 and 5 October 1938, by Fred C. Zappfe, P.P. f.3.3.4.10-3. UAA.

120 *ibid.*, p. 5.

121 *ibid.*, p. 7.
122 Report of the Dean of the Faculty of Medicine (hereinafter referred to as RDM), 1938-39.
123 Vant and Cashman, *op.cit.*, p. 65.
124 Acting Dean Ower's Report to the BOG, 1939-40.
125 From 1925 to 1937, 272 graduated, and of these 150 were located in Alberta and seventy-five in British Columbia and Saskatchewan. (RDM 1937-38.)

Chapter 3
World War II and the Beginning of Expansion
The forties and fifties

1 Letter, Kerr to Rankin, 10 October 1939, P.P. f.3/3/4/10-1. UAA; and FCM, 16 October 1939.
2 Colonel C.P. Stacey, *Six Years of War*, Vol. 1 of the Official History of the Canadian Army in the Second World War (Ottawa: Queen's Printer, 1955), p. 53.
3 *ibid.* p. 206.
4 Report by Ower, attached to FCM, 6 May 1940.
5 W.B. Parsons, "Medicine In Alberta, the War Years," unpublished, undated manuscript. p. 2.
6 The University of Alberta was represented by Dean (Lieutenant-Colonel) Rankin.
7 Minutes of Meeting of the Deans of the Faculties of Medicine, Canadian Universities, in the office of the Director General of Medical Services, 16 May 1941. P.P., f.3/3/4/10-1. UAA.
8 FCM, 26 May 1941.
9 Letter, Ower to Kerr, 16 June 1941, P.P.,f.3/3/4/10-1. UAA.
10 Shaner Papers, f.66. UAA.
11 Johns. *A History. op.cit.*, pp. 185-6; and FCM, 6 May 1942.
12 FCM, 16 February 1942.
13 Parsons, *op.cit.*, p. 1.
14 RDM, May 1940.
15 *ibid.*
16 FCM, 15 February and 15 March 1943.
17 RDM, 12 May 1944.
18 Dr. R.C.B. Corbet, interview.
19 D.R. Wilson, "History of the Department of Medicine, 1954-1969," unpublished, undated manuscript, p. 3.
20 The committee offered to hold a public hearing in Calgary, but received so little response that it cancelled the arrangements. (S.P.2047. Report of the Survey Committee, p. 124.)
21 Johns. *op.cit.*, pp. 173-80.
22 S.P. 2047, p. 83. PAA.
23 *ibid.*, p. 84.
24 *ibid.*, p. 80.

25 *ibid.*, p. 123.
26 FCM, 20 September 1948.
27 RDM, 3 May 1947.
28 RDM, 1 May 1953.
29 RDM, 1 May 1954 and 1955-56.
30 RDM, 1 May 1948 and 30 April 1949; and University of Alberta Annual
    Report, 1958.
31 FCM, 19 February 1945.
32 FCM, 8 May and 30 September 1946.
33 FCM, 20 January 1947.
34 Faculty of Medicine Papers (hereinafter referred to as FMP), f.81-70-134.
    UAA.
35 Letter, Newton to MacKenzie, UBC, 11 March 1947, FMP, f.134. UBC
    was, at this time, contemplating starting its own medical school, and this
    was probably a compelling reason for doing so.
36 RDM, 1 May 1948.
37 RDM, 1 May 1954.
38 FCM, 19 Mar 1956.
39 All four western Canadian medical schools reported a much lower regis-
    tration than usual in 1958. (RDM, 1958-59.)
40 RDM, 1 May 1954 and FCM, 18 January 1954.
41 *The New York Times*, January 14, 1960, p. 31.
42 *Canadian Medical Association Journal*, (hereinafter referred to as CMAJ)
    3 April 1965, p. 729.
43 *ibid.* 1 April 1958, p. 531 and 1 April 1961, p. 739. This may well have
    been the first time that the profession actively sought out women to enter
    the profession.
44 *ibid.*, 6 April 1963, p. 684.
45 Corbet, *op.cit.*
46 Scott. "Memoirs." *op.cit.*, p. 7.
47 Information concerning Dr. M.R. (Levey) Marshall is drawn from several
    sources including *The Gateway*, 14 March 1924 and 20 March 1925; Angus
    C. McGugan, *The First Fifty Years*, *op.cit.*, pp. 63-4; and interviews with
    Drs. R.C.B. Corbet, R.S. Fraser and T. Shnitka.
48 For most of his life, Walter Mackenzie had spelled his name with a capital
    "K". During a trip to Scotland, he learned that his ancestors had spelled
    it with a small "k" and from then on he did too. The latter spelling is used
    throughout this book.
49 FCM, 30 September 1946.
50 His control over graduate trainees was so complete that even their plans
    for marriage had to be discussed with him. (R.S. Fraser, interview)
51 FCM, 15 December 1947 and 20 December 1948.
52 Letter, President Stewart to D.S. Harvie, Calgary, 6 April 1954, P.P. f.1314.
    UAA.
53 Letter, Marshall to Stewart, 15 March 1954, *ibid.*

[54] FCM, 17 March 1958.

[55] Letter, Newton to Scott, 15 October 1948, P.P. f.16, UAA.

[56] Letter, F. Cyril James to Newton, 23 October 1948, *ibid.*

[57] Letter, Walter Johns, assistant to the president, to Alberta Health Survey, 9 March 1950, P.P. f.1051. UAA.

[58] Letter to "geographic full-time professors" from President Johns, 10 April 1959, P.P. f.1793.2. UAA.

[59] Letter, President Newton to Andrew Stewart, dean of business affairs, 4 May 1950, *ibid.*

[60] By 1950, professors in the medical faculty had to be fellows of the RCPSC or certified by other professional bodies before they could expect to receive a promotion. (Letter, Walter Johns, assistant to the president, to Alberta Health Survey, 9 March 1950, P.P. f.1051.)

[61] Minutes of the Advisory Committee to the President on the naming of a professor of medicine, 12 March 1954, P.P. f.1414. UAA.

[62] Wilson, "History of the Department of Medicine." *op.cit.*, pp. 1-3.

[63] Scott, *The History of The Faculty. op.cit.*, p. 28.

[64] Minutes of meeting of geographic full-time staff, 9 October 1957, P.P. f.1793.2. UAA.

[65] Letter, Scott to Stewart, 13 August 1957, P.P. f.1793.2. UAA.

[66] "The John and Mary Markle Foundation," New York, 13 March 1953, in P.P. f. 1050. Alberta's Faculty of Medicine was very successful in getting Markle scholarships, having a Markle scholar on staff continuously for a period of fifteen years.

[67] *ibid.*

[68] Dean Scott was the Canadian representative on an accreditation team in 1958.

[69] Report of Visitation of Medical Faculty of the University of Alberta, 7-10 May 1956. p. 2-4. P.P. f.1415. UAA.

[70] *ibid.*, pp. 84-85.

[71] *ibid.*, pp. 85-86.

[72] *ibid.*, pp. 27-32.

[73] *ibid.*, p. 18.

[74] *ibid.*, p. 37.

[75] *ibid.*, p. 94.

[76] The accreditation team visited the school from 7-10 May 1956.

[77] Letter, Wilson to Scott, 10 July 1956, P.P. f.1415. UAA.

[78] Report of Curriculum Committee, Basic Sciences, July 1956, *ibid.*

[79] The school had been using the outpatient clinic in the government building on 100th Street since 1939.

[80] Report from the University of Alberta to the Association of American Medical Colleges, May 1957, P.P. f.1415. UAA.

[81] *ibid.*, April 1959.

[82] Report of Visitation to the Medical Faculty of the University of Alberta, September 1959, pp. 16-18, FMP, f. 504.

Chapter 4
From Medical School to Health Sciences Centre
The sixties to the present

1   Duncan D. Campbell, *Those Tumultuous Years*, (Edmonton: University of Alberta, 1977), p. 8.
2   *ibid.*, pp. 1-3.
3   *ibid.*, p. 2.
4   See, J.A. MacFarlane, et al. *Medical Education in Canada.*, Royal Commission on Health Services (Ottawa: Queen's Printer, 1965).
5   Press Release from the ACMC, 22 June 1964; FMP, f.69-123-641. UAA.
6   D.F. Cameron, "The Medical Student and the Royal Commission on Health Services," *MUS Journal* (Summer 1964) pp. 4-11.
7   Letter, Scott to Johns, 13 February 1959, P.P. f.68-1-1793. UAA.
8   Letter, Scarlett to Stewart, 12 November 1958, P.P.f.68-1-1792. UAA
9   R.A. Macbeth, "History of the Department of Surgery," *op.cit.*, p. 19.
10   Report of Visitation to the Medical Faculty, November 1959, p. 2.
11   Information concerning Dean Mackenzie is taken from "A Memorial Tribute to Walter C. Mackenzie," *The Canadian Journal of Surgery*, (July 1979), pp. 303-16; R.A. Macbeth, "Meet the Dean, Walter Campbell MacKenzie," *MUS Bulletin* (March 1964), pp. 5-10; Macbeth, "Walter Campbell Mackenzie, Pioneer International Surgical Statesman," *Annals RCPSC* (March 1989), pp. 109-13 and (May 1989), pp. 209-12; and interviews with Dean Cameron and various others.
12   Quoted in the *Calgary Herald*, March 8, 1966.
13   Gardner, *op.cit.*
14   Letter, Mackenzie to President Stewart, 23 December 1958, P.P.f.68-1-1792. UAA.
15   Later, students and graduate trainees had representation on this committee.
16   FCM, 19 May 1966.
17   Letter, Mackenzie to Stewart, 23 December 1958, P.P. f.68-1-1792. UAA.
18   RDM, 1962-63, pp. 10-13.
19   Donald R. Wilson, "History of the Department of Medicine," *op.cit.*, p. 19.
20   Report from University of Alberta to the AAMC and AMA, April 1959. pp. 5-6.
21   RDM, 1960-61, p. 5.
22   Letter, Mackenzie to President Johns, 22 May 1964, FMP. f.69-123-499.
23   FCM, November 15, 1965.
24   Letter, Wallace to Mackenzie, 27 January, 1965. FMP. f. 69-123-972. UAA.
25   "Planning for a Health Sciences Centre to Provide Comprehensive Medical Care," n.d., no author, c.1966, FMP, 85-108-40. UAA.
26   FCM, 15 June 1971.
27   C.B. Stewart, "Reminiscences on the Founding and Early History of the Medical Research Council of Canada," *Annals RCPSC* (September and November 1986), p. 473.
28   Tait McPhedran, *op.cit.*, p. 13.

[29] "Planning for a Health Sciences Centre," *op. cit.*

[30] Letter, Mackenzie to ACMC, 28 February 1969, FMP, f.80-162-1. UAA.

[31] R.S. Fraser, "A Personal View, 1969-1974," unpublished manuscript, 1986, p. 12.

[32] *ibid.*, pp. 13-14.

[33] *ibid.*, pp. 84-86.

[34] Wilson, "History of the Department," *op. cit.*, p. 19.

[35] FCM, 25 May and 15 October 1964.

[36] McGill was the only school to attract a significant number of students from abroad.

[37] Report of the Faculty Admissions Committee, December 1972.

[38] FCM, October in each year.

[39] Report of the Faculty Admissions Committee, December 1972.

[40] This is in the stanine 9-point grading system.

[41] Admissions Criteria, Faculty of Medicine, n.d., c.1978, FMP, 85-108-90. UAA.

[42] Report of the Faculty Admissions Committee, December 1972.

[43] Admissions Criteria, Faculty of Medicine, n.d., c.1978, FMP, 85-108-90. UAA.

[44] FCM, May 1967.

[45] Report, Division of Postgraduate Medical Education, 18 May 1978.

[46] Tait McPhedran, *op. cit.*, p. 11.

[47] Report, Curriculum Advisory Committee, May 1967.

[48] Report from University of Alberta to AAMC and AMA, April 1959.

[49] Faculty Conference on Medical Education, 20-21 October 1961.

[50] Report, Committee on Examinations, n.d., c.1970, FMP, 85-108-92. UAA.

[51] Report, Student Evaluation Board, 22 May 1973.

[52] Report, Student Evaluation Board, 25 May 1972.

[53] Information concerning this centre was obtained from Donald R. Wilson, "R.S. McLaughlin Examination and Research Centre," unpublished manuscript, n.d.; Wilson, "The Gladys and Merrill Muttart Foundation," unpublished manuscript, n.d. pp. 3-4; and U of A Calendar, 1980-81, p. 121.4.

[54] Report on Faculty Participation in Northern Health Care, 10 December 1974.

[55] FCM, 11 January 1973.

[56] Cameron, *op. cit.*

[57] University of Alberta, Faculty of Medicine, Medical Graduates, 1973-85, Survey Results, January 1989.

[58] *ibid.*

Part II
Chapter 5
The Meds and the Co-Meds

[1] U of A Calendar, 1914-15, pp. 131-39.

[2] *The Gateway*, November 1913. p. 28.

3   *ibid.*, April 1914, p. 60.
4   *ibid.*, April 1915, p. 60.
5   John W. Scott, "Early Medical Education," *op.cit.*, p. 8.
6   FCM, 20 May 1970.
7   *Evergreen and Gold*, 1929, p. 145.
8   Begg, *op.cit.*
9   Letter, Revell to Kerr, 31 August 1918, P.P. f.68-9-150. UAA.
10 Morrish, *op.cit.*, pp. 34-37.
11 McGregor Hellstedt, *op.cit.*, pp. 34-35.
12 Gardner, *op.cit.*
13 *The Gateway*, 22 October 1923.
14 This was later changed to crimson, the traditional colour for medicine.
15 S.P. f. 355. PAA.
16 S.P. f. 400 and f.457. PAA.
17 Gardner, *op.cit.*
18 *Evergreen and Gold*, various issues; and Drs. L.O.Bradley, H.E.Duggan
    and W.S.Johns, interview.
19 *Evergreen and Gold*, 1929. p. 145; and Gardner, *op.cit.*
20 In the records, the first president of the MSC was always referred to as Miss
    Curtin. Women were invariably referred to by their title, and often initials
    or first names were excluded.
21 *The Gateway*, 15 November 1917, p. 1.
22 Large, Revell and Cain. *op.cit.*
23 FCM, 15 November 1920.
24 *The Gateway*, 5 November 1924.
25 *Evergreen and Gold*, 1924-25, p. 106.
26 P.P. f.81-104. UAA.
27 *Evergreen and Gold*, 1938, p. 193.
28 *The Gateway*, 25 October 1920.
29 Letter, J. H. Brunton, Medical Students' Club to Tory, 13 November 1924,
    P.P. f. 68-9-138. UAA.
30 *ibid.* 24 and 31 October 1922.
31 *The Gateway*, 5 November 1924.
32 FCM, 7 May 1931.
33 Three other medical students served as president of the Students' Union
    in later years: Lloyd C. Grisdale, Robert A. Macbeth and John N. Chappel.
34 Ower Diaries, 13 and 14 March 1931.
35 *ibid.*, several entries.
36 *The Gateway*, 17 January 1918; and Graduation Number, April 1918. p. 23.
37 *ibid.*, May 1919.
38 *ibid.*, 11 March 1926, p. 3.
39 *ibid.*, 20 January 1927, p. 5.
40 *ibid.*, p.2.
41 *ibid.*, 2 February 1921, pp. 2 and 5.
42 Large, et al., op. cit.

43 *The Gateway*, 20 January 1927, p. 2.

44 *ibid*. p. 1.

45 Pat Simonds, Pat. "Backward Glances," *MUS Bulletin*, (February 1957), p. 12.

46 RDM, 1939.

47 *The Gateway*, 30 October 1919.

48 Johns, *op.cit.*

49 Ower Diaries, 15 April 1931, and several other entries.

50 Bradley, Duggan and Johns, *op.cit.*

51 Letter, R. McMillan, secretary, AKK Club, to Dr. W.G. Hardy, 25 October 1950, P.P. f. 68-1-990. UAA.

52 Minutes of the Committee on Fraternities, 13 November 1950, *ibid*.

53 Annual Report of the Advisory Committee on Fraternities and Residential Clubs, 3 April 1957.

54 A request to announce the society in the university calendar was refused by GFC, however. (FCM, 22 May 1962.)

55 D.R. Wilson, D.R. "History of the Alpha Omega Alpha Honor Medical Society," unpublished manuscript, 1961; *MUS Bulletin* (January/February 1962); and FCM, 30 December 1961.

56 *Evergreen and Gold*, 1926, p. 41.

57 *Evergreen and Gold*, 1927, p. 74.

58 *The CAMSI Journal*, Alberta's Report, April 1944, p. 47.

59 The BOG rescinded this policy in 1947, expressing doubt that it could legally require students to join faculty societies. (Minutes BOG meeting, 23 January 1947.)

60 *Evergreen and Gold*, 1944, p. 173

61 RDM, 10 May 1946; and FCM, 15 Oct 1948.

62 Letter, Scott to Johns, 6 July 1956, P.P. f.68-1-1415. UAA.

63 P.P. f.68-1-1793.1. UAA.

64 *Evergreen and Gold*, 1943, p. 173.

65 S.P. f.2047. PAA.

66 FCM, 15 November 1954.

67 RDM, April 1949.

68 Letter, Scott to Stewart, 17 May 1954, P.P. f.68-1-1415. UAA.

69 FCM, 19 March 1951.

70 U of A Calendar, 1944-45, p. 1; and Shnitka. *op.cit.*

71 Letter, G.D.Molnar, President, MUS to Scott, 18 August 1950, FMP, f.81-70-352; and FCM, 21 January 1952.

72 FMP, f. 81-70-352. UAA.

73 *MUS Bulletin*, October 1958. p. 13.

74 *Mediscope*, October 1966.

75 MUS Papers, f.81.70-352. UAA.

76 Minutes, MUS Executive Meetings, 20 March 1952.

77 Letter, Provost to John Butt, January 1959, MUS Papers, UAA.

78 Letter, Provost to President, MUS, 25 April 1959. *ibid*.

[79] *MUS Bulletin*, January/February 1963.

[80] *Mediscope*, 7 February 1964.

[81] Marion Doberthein, President, MSA, interview.

[82] J.S. Thompson, "The Medical Student—His Background and His Problems," *CMAJ*, (1 April 1958), pp. 493-97.

[83] J.S. Thompson, "Who Can Go to Medical School," *CMAJ*, 15 November 1956, p. 841.

[84] Thompson cites one interesting case. "The husband returned home from classes and spent the evenings looking after the baby and studying while his wife went out on night nursing duty. She somehow managed to keep awake to look after the baby in the daytime. Their sacrifices have paid off, and this spring the husband received his M.D. Unfortunately the university offers no certificate to the wife in a case like this, although she surely deserves one!" (J.S. Thompson, "The Canadian Student—Western Style," *Journal of Medical Education*, (November 1958), p. 795)

[85] *ibid.*

[86] Thompson, "The Medical Student." *op. cit.*

[87] J.S. Thompson, "Who Can Go," *op. cit.* A later survey conducted in 1974, showed that 75% of the students came from a professional/business class background—and only one student came from a farm, a far cry from the origins of the school and even from the 1950s. (FMP, F.80-162-243.)

[88] S.P. f. 3097. PAA.

[89] *Evergreen and Gold*, 1969, pp. 132-33.

[90] FCM, 19 May 1971.

[91] FCM, 13 October 1971.

[92] Report, Frank J. Moffet, President, MSA to executive, Faculty Council, 21 May 1974.

[93] FCM, 1 October 1974.

[94] Information about more recent activities of the MSA was obtained from Marion Doberthein, the 1988 president; University of Alberta Calendar, 1988-89, p. K12; MSA Report to Faculty Council, 12 March 1987; and Michael Caffaro, "The Medical Students Association," *New Trail*, (Spring 1988), p. 20.

[95] This was typical of hospitals across the continent. In the United States, in 1940, only 105 out of 712 accredited hospitals accepted women interns. (Mary Roth Walsh. *Doctors Wanted: No Women Need Apply, Sexual Barriers in the Medical Profession, 1835-1975*, (New Haven and London: Yale University Press, 1977, p. 224).

[96] FCM 16 October 1933; and Ower's Diaries, 29 January 1934.

[97] FCM, 19 October 1942.

[98] FCM, 29 September 1941.

[99] Minutes, Medical Quota Committee, 26 May 1943, FMP, f.81-70-134. UAA.

[100] GFC Minutes, 27 October and 24 November 1941.

[101] Letter, Downs to the president, 21 November 1941, FMP, f. 81-70-134. UAA.
[102] H.E.Rawlinson, chairman, Admissions Committee, to Dean Scott, 4 June 1949, FMP, f. 80-70-134. UAA.
[103] Dean D.F. Cameron, interview.
[104] Gardner, *op.cit.*
[105] *Evergreen and Gold*, 1928, p. 146.
[106] *Evergreen and Gold*, 1929. p. 145.
[107] Ower's Diaries, 7 March 1931.
[108] Minutes, MUS General Meeting, 3 October 1950.
[109] McGregor Hellstedt, *op.cit.*, p. 35-36.
[110] *ibid.*, p. 43.
[111] *The Gateway*, 15 May 1925, p. 1.
[112] *ibid.* 17 March 1927. p. 3.
[113] Ower's Diaries, 3 December 1932, 7 February 1934.
[114] S.P. f.2713 and 3097. PAA.
[115] J.W. Macleod and H. Howes, "Medical Students in Canadian Universities, 1962-63 and 1963-64," *CMAJ*, (4 April 1964) p. 809.
[116] RDM, 1958-59.
[117] J.W. Macleod, "Medical Student Enrolment in Canadian Universities," *CMAJ*, (6 April 1963), pp. 683-90.
[118] *Speculum*, 1969.
[119] Eva Ryten, "Trends in the Study of Medicine in Canada," *CMAJ*, (15 September 1985), p. 589.
[120] *Medical Alumni Bulletin*, 1947, p. 4.
[121] Alex G. Markle, "An Adventure in Medical Alumni Relations," unpublished manuscript, 8 May 1981, p. 2.
[122] McGregor Hellstedt, *op.cit.*, p. 43.
[123] Being a woman she was not allowed to eat in the M.D. dining room at this hospital. *ibid.*, p. 46.
[124] *ibid.*, pp. 43-54; and *New Trail* (July 1943) p. 26.
[125] Letter, Macklin, University of Western Ontario to Shaner, 30 January 1950, Shaner Papers, f.95. UAA.
[126] RDM, 1960-61; and Shaner Papers, f.76. UAA.

Chapter 6
Medical Education

[1] C.D. O'Malley, editor, *The History of Medical Education*, UCLA Forum in Medical Sciences, Number 12 (London: University of California Press, 1970), p. ix.
[2] Philippe Pinel, *The Clinical Training of Doctors*, edited and translated by Dora B. Weiner (Baltimore and London: The Johns Hopkins University Press, 1980).
[3] John P. McGovern and Charles G. Roland, editors, *Wm Osler. The Continuing Education* (Springfield, Illinois: Charles C. Thomas, 1969), pp. 59-70.

4   J.J.R. Macleod, "The Problem of Broadening the Medical Course," *The University of Toronto Monthly* (February 1920), Reprint.

5   Quoted from Osler's "The Leaven of Science" in Brain, Sir Russell, "Osler and Medicine Today," *CMAJ* (20 August 1960), p. 353.

6   Quoted in Ludmerer, *Learning to Heal, op.cit.*, p. 277.

7   Brain, *op.cit.*, p. 354.

8   According to Abraham Flexner, 457 proprietary schools opened their doors in the United States and Canada during the nineteenth century, many had a short life, and "perhaps 50 [were] still-born." Abraham Flexner, *Medical Education in the United States and Canada*, A Report to the Carnegie Foundation for the Advancement of Teaching, Bulletin Number Four, 1910 (New York: Arno Press & The New York Times, Reprint Edition, 1972), p. 6.

9   Abraham Flexner, *Medical Education: A Comparative Study* (New York: The Macmillan Company, 1925), p. 39.

10 Flexner, *Medical Education in the United States and Canada., op.cit.*, pp.14-15.

11 Carleton B. Chapman, "Preprofessional Requirements: An Anachronism," *The Bulletin of the New York Academy of Medicine*, Vol. 61. No. 5. (June 1985), pp. 407-09.

12 *ibid.*, pp. 410-12.

13 Flexner, *Medical Education, op.cit.*, pp. 19-24.

14 Wilburt C. Davidson, "Osler's Influence," *Journal of the Association of American Medical Colleges* (May 1950), p. 166.

15 J.A. MacFarlane, *op.cit.*, p. 19.

16 Paul Starr, *The Social Transformation of American Medicine, The Rise of a Sovereign Profession and the Making of a Vast Industry*, (New York: Basic Books, Inc., Publishers, 1982), p. 118

17 Ludmerer, *op.cit.*, pp 80-84 and 191-205.

18 Flexner, *Medical Education, op.cit.*, pp. 144-5.

19 They could practise in Alberta with an M.D. from the University of Alberta. To practise elsewhere in Canada, they had to write The Medical Council of Canada licensing examinations.

20 H.R. Clouston, "The Medical Curriculum as Viewed by a Country General Practitioner," *CMAJ* (March 1933), p. 317.

21 Ludmerer, *op.cit.*, p. 159.

22 Flexner, *Medical Education, op.cit.*, p. 270.

23 Gerald M. McDougall, editor, *Teachers of Medicine: The Development of Graduate Clinical Medical Education* (Calgary: University of Calgary Printing Services, 1987), p. 3.

24 S.E.D. Shortt, " 'Before the Age of Miracles': The Rise, Fall and Rebirth of General Practice in Canada, 1890-1940," *Health, Disease and Medicine*, Charles G. Roland (Toronto: published for the Hannah Institute for the History of Medicine by Clarke Irwin Inc., 1984), p. 127

25 Ludmerer, *op.cit.*, pp. 260-1.

26 Scientific study of the organs of the body.

27 U of A Calendar, 1914-15, p. 69.
28 Report from President Tory to the Board of Governors, 1911.
29 FCM, 18 October 1922.
30 U of A Calendar, 1924-25, p. 172.
31 *ibid.*, 1924-25, pp. 92-3.
32 FCM, 16 January 1928 and 19 December 1949.
33 FCM, 15 and 19 September 1914.
34 U of A Calendar, 1937-38, pp. 261-65.
35 The minimum language requirement for licensing in Canada was Latin, and French or German (U of A Calendar 1940-41, p. 192.)
36 FCM, 21 September and 16 November 1942.
37 FCM, 27 May 1928.
38 Henry E. Sigerist, "Medical History in the Medical Schools of Canada," and Genevieve Miller, "The Teaching of Medical History," *Bulletin of the History of Medicine*, Vol. VIII, (1940), p. 307 and Vol. XLIII, (1969), p. 577
39 FCM, 15 November 1926 and 17 January 1927.
40 FCM, several meetings 1938-9.
41 Report of survey by H.H. Hepburn to Ower, 14 March 1942. P.P. f.16. UAA.
42 In 1976, this requirement was increased to a two-year graduate internship.
43 Letter, Scott to Stewart, 26 February 1952, P.P. f.1051. UAA.
44 FCM, 19 March and 1 May 1951.
45 Clouston, *op.cit.*, pp. 317-20.
46 Flexner, *Medical Education*, *op.cit.*, p. 266.
47 Ludmerer, *op.cit.*, p. 262.
48 Melvin Konner, *Becoming a Doctor. A Journey of Initiation in Medical School.* (New York: Elisabeth Sifton Books-Viking, 1987), p. 362.
49 H.E. Rawlinson, "The Humanities and Medicine," *CAMSI Journal* (February 1958), pp. 37-8.
50 MacFarlane, *op.cit.*, pp. 287-89.
51 Quoted in Starr, *op.cit.*, p. 355; and elsewhere.
52 Rothstein, *op.cit.*, p. 297; and Tait McPhedran, *op.cit.*, pp. 9-12.
53 Ralph F. Shaner, "The Teaching of the Basic Sciences," *MUS Bulletin*, Vol. 1, No. 1 (February 1957), p. 9.
54 Tait McPhedran, *op.cit.*, pp. 9-12.
55 Rothstein, *op.cit.*, pp. 256-60.
56 Ludmerer, *op.cit.*, p. 279.
57 Egerton L. Pope, "The Examination of Medical Students," *CMAJ* (October 1933), pp. 427-28.
58 Dean D.R. Wilson, interview.
59 *Physicians for the Twenty-First Century.* The GPEP Report. Report of the Panel on the General Professional Education of the Physician and College Preparation for Medicine (Washington, D.C.: Association of American Medical Colleges, 1984), p. 1.

60 In fact, the report called for a "baccalaureate education that encompasses broad study in the natural and the social sciences and in the humanities" for all students, regardless of which profession they wish to enter (*ibid.*, p. 59).

61 *ibid.*, pp. 5-24.

62 *ibid.*, p. 48.

63 *ibid.*, p.47

64 *The Globe and Mail*, November 12 1988, p. 43.

65 J.S. Thompson, "The Revision of the Medical Curriculum," *MUS Bulletin*, Vol. 1. No. 1 (February 1957), pp. 5-7.

66 Various issues of the U of A Calendar, 1959-68.

67 Report from the University of Alberta to the Association of American Medical Colleges and the American Medical Association, April 1959, P.P. f.1793.2, p. 10.

68 *ibid.*, p. 26.

69 Shaner, "The Teaching of the Basic Sciences," *op.cit.*, p. 8-9.

70 Report from the U. of A. *op.cit.*, p. 28.

71 Dean D.F.Cameron, interview.

72 Curriculum Advisory Committee Report, 25 May 1967.

73 Letter, Gilbert to Mackenzie, 16 February 1966, FCM, 23 February 1966.

74 FCM, 29 March 1967.

75 FCM, 25 May 1967.

76 Letter, Gilbert to Mackenzie, 10 May 1968, FMP, f.40. UAA.

77 FCM, 22 May 1968,

78 Curriculum Advisory Committee Report, September 1971, pp. 1-3.

79 FCM, 27 October 1970.

80 *Speculum*, medical student magazine, 1969,

81 Robert S. Fraser, "A Personal View," *op.cit.*, pp. 37-38.

82 Report of the Class of '73 on Student Internship, May 1972.

83 Curriculum Advisory Committee Report, 22 May 1973, p. 5.

84 *ibid.*, 25 May 1975, p. 3.

85 "Curriculum: Where It's Going," *IATROS*, University of Alberta medical journal, (Fall/Winter 1986), p. 33.

86 Report of the Review Committee for the Student Evaluation Board, 11 January 1973. p. 1.

87 Curriculum Advisory Committee Report, 22 May 1973, p. 4.

88 FCM, 9 October 1973.

89 In 1971, thirty-nine American medical colleges out of a total of ninety-nine had a pass/fail grading system for all four years. Relevant figures for Canadian schools were unavailable.

90 FCM, 9 October 1973.

91 Marion Doberthein, President, Medical Students' Association, 1988, interview.

92 Cameron, *op.cit.*

93 Executive meeting of the Faculty Council, 10 December 1974.

94 U of A Calendar, 1988-9; and Doberthein, *op.cit.*
95 FCM, 17 March 1930.
96 *ibid.*, 19 November 1951
97 RDM, 1 May 1952.
98 FCM, 18 May 1978; and U of A Calendar, 1988-9, p. K13.
99 Report of Committee to Consider a Combined M.D. and Ph.D. Program, 21 March 1966.
100 See Chapter 3.
101 Jamieson, *op.cit.*, pp. 56-57.
102 The Medical Profession Act, Ch. 2 of the Revised Statutes of Alberta, 1922, as amended, 1926.
103 John Ruedy, "Specialty Residency Training in Canada—History and Challenges," *Annals RCPSC*, Vol. 19, No.3 (May 1986), pp. 197-202.
104 Meeting of the teaching staff, 27 January 1949.
105 FCM, 9 October 1973.
106 Robert K. Richards, *Continuing Medical Education. Perspectives, Problems, Prognosis* (New Haven & London: Yale University Press, 1978), pp. 24-27.
107 FCM, 9 May 1952.
108 Letter, W. F. Gillespie, chairman, Programme Committee addressed to Dear Doctor, 1 March 1942, FMP, f.77-183-2. UAA.
109 The American forces who constructed the Alaska Highway during the war, established a military base in Edmonton.
110 FCM, 8 May 1951.
111 Minutes of various Faculty Council meetings through the 1950s.
112 S. Kling, director of continuing medical education, "Continuing Medical Education," *MUS Bulletin* (1964), pp. 11-16; and S. Kling, "The Challenge of Continuing Medical Education," *Alberta Medical Bulletin*, Vol. 29, No. 1 (February 1964), pp. 2-9.
113 *ibid.*
114 Report of Continuing Medical Education, 1976-77.
115 Fifteenth Annual Report, CME, 1977-79, FMP, f.85-108-130. UAA.
116 U of A Calendar, 1988-89. p. K15.
117 Dean Wilson, *op.cit.*
118 Ludmerer, *op.cit.*, p. 280.

Chapter 7
The Growth of Research in the Medical School

1 Letter, Tory to Collip, August 29, 1921. P.P. f.68-9-144. UAA.
2 H.M. Tory. "The University's Function in Medicine," *op.cit.* pp. 1304-5.
3 P.P. f.3/2/6/1-1. UAA.
4 C.B. Stewart. "Reminiscences" *op.cit.* p. 386.
5 *ibid.*
6 FCM, November 16, 1937; and March 21, 1939.
7 Stewart. *op.cit.* pp. 387-8.
8 Letter, J.J.Macleod to Tory, May 22, 1922. P.P. f. 68-9-144. UAA.

9 *Edmonton Journal*, May 25, 1923.
10 *The Gateway*, April 21, 1923. pp. 1 and 6.
11 Bliss, "J.B.Collip: A Forgotten Member." *op.cit.* pp.16-17.
12 R.J. Rossiter, "James Berteam Collip" in the *Royal Society of Canada Journal*, 1965. p.77.
13 Annual Report, University of Alberta, December 31, 1925.
14 Al Askey. "Faculty Profile. Dr. R. F. Shaner" in *MUS Bulletin*, March 1959. pp. 13-14.
15 Shaner Papers, f.42. UAA.
16 Cameron, *op.cit.*
17 RDM, 1961-62.
18 *Ladies Home Journal*, March 1931. pp.8,9,71; and P.P. f.3/2/6/1-5. UAA.
19 E. Silver Dowding. "Dr. Harold Orr and Medical Mycology," in *CMAJ*, Vol. 68. 1953. pp. 386-387.
20 *The Gateway*, March 20, 1925. p.1.
21 Letter, D.F.Cameron to Dean Scott, 15 October, 1955. P.P. f.68-1-1415. UAA.
22 C.B. Stewart. "Reminiscences" *op.cit.* pp. 388-389.
23 Donald R. Wilson, "History of the Faculty of Medicine." unpublished manuscript. November 1981. p.10.
24 Shaner Papers, f. 72.
25 John W. Scott, *History of the Faculty. op.cit.* p.26; and *MUS Bulletin*, March 1959, pp.11-12
26 "Constitution of the Medical Research Club of the University of Alberta". P.P. f.68-1-16. UAA.
27 RDM, May 1, 1948.
28 Report, Pearce to Mackenzie, FCM, May 12, 1964.
29 FCM, January 21 and March 18, 1946; and P.P. f.3/3/3/10-1. UAA.
30 Letters between President Newton and Bursar Whidden, May 1950. P.P. f.68-1-1129. UAA.
31 Minutes of Meeting of Committee on Medical Research. April 26, 1966.
32 Policy and Regulations, Committee for Allocation of Medical Research Grants. April, 1966. P.P. f.68-1-2258. UAA.
33 Status of Research Projects, March 8, 1949. P.P. f.68-1-23. UAA.
34 Research Grants from University Trust Funds, March 31, 1962. FMP. f.85-108-42. UAA.
35 Press Release, June 14, 1946. P.P. f/3/4/6/2/18. UAA.
36 Stewart, *op.cit.* p.472-473.
37 RDM, May 1, 1950.
38 Letters, Mrs. M.D. (Gladys) Muttart to Stewart, November 10, 1954 and December 7, 1955. P.P. f.68-1-1414. UAA.
39 S.P. f.2500. 1949-50. PAA.
40 RDM, May 3, 1947.
41 Press Release, dated March 15, 1953. PP.f.68-1-1050. UAA.
42 Donald R. Wilson. "History of the Department of Medicine." p.2.

43 S.P. f.2403; and RDM, April 30, 1949.

44 Wilson, "History of the Department," *op.cit.* p.11.

45 FCM, May 11, 1948; and S.P. f.2500. PAA.

46 Obituary Column, *CMAJ*, February 1948. p. 217.

47 McEachern Laboratory file. P.P. f. 68-1-898. UAA.

48 Letter, Manning to Stewart, April 23, 1951. P.P. f.68-1-898. UAA.

49 RDM, May 1, 1953.

50 Open letter from Shaner, December 9, 1955. P.P. f. 68-1-898. UAA.

51 Ralph Shaner. "Annual Report of the McEachern Cancer Laboratory, 1954-55." p.2. P.P.f.68-1-1272. UAA.

52 Ralph Shaner. "Report of the McEachern Cancer Laboratory for the Year Ending March 31, 1954." p.5. P.P. f.68-1-1272. UAA.

53 Macbeth. "History of the Department of Surgery." *op.cit.* pp. 20-21; and Dr. Garth Warnock, interview.

54 Warnock, *op.cit.*

55 Dr. K.P. Kowalewski, interview.

56 Letter, Talbot to Johns, 19 October, 1962. FMP. f.69-123-144. UAA.

57 Memo, Johns to Board of Governors, October 5, 1962; and FCM, May 22, 1963.

58 RDM, 1960-61.

59 RDM, May 1, 1953.

60 John W. Scott. "Medical Research at the University" in *Medical Alumni Bulletin*, September 1, 1950. p.1.

61 RDM 1960-61.

62 RDM, 1961-62, p.6; and 1962-63, p.5.

63 FCM, 8 May 1950; 8 May 1953; 19 March 1956; 11 May 1959; and 5 October 1962.

64 Fraser, *op.cit.* p.134.

65 *Bulletin*, Faculty of Medicine, Spring, 1988. p.22.

66 RDM, 1969-70, p.6.

67 Personal Communication, Dr. Peter Allen, 20 November, 1989.

68 *Edmonton Journal*, March 11, 1978.

69 Fraser, R.S. "A Personal View", *op.cit.* p.108.

70 Cameron, *op.cit.*

71 J.E. Bradley. "Alberta Heritage Foundation for Medical Research". unp. ms. December 30, 1980. p.2.

72 *AHFMR Newsletter*, November/December, 1988. p.11.

73 Personal communication, Dean Wilson.

74 *From Laboratory to Marketplace*, *op.cit.* p.12.

[75] Donald R. Wilson "James Bertram Collip" *op.cit.* p.23.

[76] Application, "Muttart Diabetes Research and Training Centre at the University of Alberta", FMP. f.85-108-34. UAA.

[77] Information on the Diabetes Research Team was given by Garth Warnock, one of the members of the team.

[78] *ibid.*; and *From Laboratory to Marketplace*, Biotechnology Initiatives at the University of Alberta, Edmonton, Canada. p.31.

[79] Faculty of Medicine, *Research Inventory*, September, 1987. p.4.

[80] Dean Wilson, *op.cit.*

[81] Much of the information concerning this section was obtained from J. S. Colter.

[82] He is now a "scientific adviser" to the Alberta Heritage Foundation for Medical Research.

[83] Report, J. W. Pearce to Mackenzie, FCM, May 22, 1962.

[84] Cyril Kay. "The MRC Group in Protein Structure and Function", n.d.

[85] *Research Inventory. op.cit.* p.4.

[86] "X-Ray Crystallography" in *AHFMR Newsletter*, July/August, 1988. pp.1-2.

[87] R.S. Fraser. "Cardiology at the University of Alberta, 1922 to 1969". Unpublished manuscript. n.d.

[88] Letter, Scott to Markle Foundation, December 16, 1955. P.P. f.68-1-1414. UAA.

[89] R.S. Fraser. "Report on Cardiovascular Unit, November 1956 to June, 1959." P.P. f.68-1-1791. UAA.

[90] Annual Report of University of Alberta Hospital, 1953-54. p.32.

[91] Vant and Cashman. *op.cit.* p. 209.

[92] Les Willox, quoted in John C. Callaghan, *30 Years of Open Heart Surgery at the University of Alberta Hospitals*. Edmonton: University of Alberta Hospitals, 1986. p.19.

[93] Fraser, "Cardiology" *op.cit.* pp. 93-94,

[94] Callaghan, *op.cit.* p.25.

[95] Annual Report, University of Alberta Hospital, 1955-56. p.16.

[96] *ibid.* pp.25-27.

[97] Adrian Jones and Gerald Higgins. "In the Footsteps of the Pioneers" in *New Trail* (Spring 1988) pp. 10-11

[98] *Laboratory to Marketplace, op.cit.* p.21.

[99] Submission to the Board of Governors, November 3, 1948.

[100] "Faculty of Medicine" in *Alberta Medical Bulletin*, August 1955. pp.59-60.

Conclusion

1 The enrolment figures for first year had reached that level in 1972 and had been held there; while a variety of studies on the number of medical practitioners needed in the future had not contributed any firm results, many predicted a surplus of physicians. (Tait McPhedran, *op.cit.*, p. 16.)

2 In 1988, there were 335 full-time faculty members, 304 part-time, and 510 unpaid volunteers.

3 *Alberta Facts*, 1989, Government of Alberta Treasury Department, Bureau of Statistics, August 1989.

4 Ludmerer, *op.cit.*, pp. 277-80.

5 *Bulletin*, Faculty of Medicine, University of Alberta, No. 8 (Spring 1989), p. 1.

* * * * *

Bibliography

Manuscript Collections

Annual Reports of the Dean of the Faculty of Medicine, 1937 to 1963.

Attorney Generals' Files, Provincial Archives of Alberta.

Biography Files, University of Alberta Archives.

Cantor Papers, University of Alberta Archives.

Chancellors' Papers, University of Alberta Archives.

Department of Biochemistry Papers, University of Alberta Archives.

Faculty of Medicine Papers, University of Alberta Archives.

General Faculty Council Minutes, 1941.

Heber C. Jamieson Papers, University of Alberta Archives.

Minute Book, College of Physicians and Surgeons of Alberta, 1906, 1917.

Minutes, Board of Governors of the University of Alberta.

Minutes of the Medical Faculty Council, 1913 to present.

Minutes of the Meetings of the Mewburn Reporting Club, University of Alberta Archives.

Minutes of the University of Alberta Hospital Board.

Minutes of the University of Alberta Senate, University of Alberta Archives.

Diaries of Dean J.J. Ower, University of Alberta Archives.

Premiers' Papers, Provincial Archives of Alberta.

Presidents' Papers, University of Alberta Archives.

Sessional Papers, Provincial Archives of Alberta.

Ralph Shaner Papers, University of Alberta Archives.

Government Documents

Alberta Facts, 1989, Edmonton: Government of Alberta Treasury Department, Bureau of Statistics, 1989.
Journals of the Legislative Assembly of the Province of Alberta, 1906-1910, Edmonton: Jas.E. Richards, Government Printer, 1911.
The Revised Statutes of Alberta, 1922, Edmonton: J.W. Jeffery, King's Printer, 1942.
Sessional Papers. Alberta. Legislative Assembly.
Statutes of the Province of Alberta, 1907, Edmonton: Jas.E. Richards, Government Printer, 1907.
Statutes of the Province of Alberta, 1910, Edmonton: Jas.E. Richards, Government Printer, 1910.

Interviews

Dr. Walter Anderson.
Dr. L.O. Bradley, '38.
Dr. Herbert Begg, '28.
Dean D.F. Cameron '49.
Dr. John B. Collip, '50.
Dr. J.S. Colter.
Dr. R.C.B. Corbet, '46.
Marion Doberthein.
Dr. H.E. Duggan, '38.
Dr. Robert S. Fraser, '46.
Dr. E.D. (Dunn) Gain, '40.
Dr. J.S. Gardner,'34.
Dr. W.S. Johns, '38.

Dr. K.P. Kowalewski.
Dr. N. Tait McPhedran
Dr. W.M. Mulloy.
Drs. James Nixon and J.S. Gardner interviewed by Dr. Allan Hepburn, 1973.
Mrs. Mary (Jamieson) Petley-Jones
Miss G.A. Revell.
Dr. Maryon Robertson, '62.
Dr. T. Shnitka, '53.
Dr. J. Ross Vant.
Dr. Garth Warnock, '76.
Dr. Donald R. Wilson.
Dean Douglas R. Wilson.

Books

Agnew, G.H. *History of Canadian Hospitals 1920-1970 A Dramatic Half-Century.* Toronto: University of Toronto Press, 1974.
Alexander, William Hardy. *The University of Alberta. A Retrospect, 1908-1929.* Edmonton: University Printing Department, 1929.
Alexander, W.H., E.K. Broadus, F.J. Lewis and J.M. MacEachran. *These Twenty-Five Years. A Symposium.* Toronto: Macmillan Company of Canada Limited, 1933.
Andison, Alexander W. and Jacques G. Robichon. (editors) *The Royal College of Physicians and Surgeons of Canada, 50th Anniversary, 1979.* Province of Quebec: 50th Anniversary Publication Committee, 1979.
Barr, Murray L. *A Century of Medicine at Western.* London: University of Western Ontario, 1977.
Bliss, Michael. *The Discovery of Insulin.* Toronto: McClelland and Stewart Limited, 1982.
Callaghan, John C. *30 Years of Open Heart Surgery at the University of Alberta Hospitals.* Edmonton: University of Alberta Hospitals, 1986.

Campbell, Duncan D. *Those Tumultuous Years. The Goals of the President of the University of Alberta during the Decade of the 1960s.* Edmonton: The Library, University of Alberta, 1977.

Corbett, E.A. *Henry Marshall Tory. Beloved Canadian.* Toronto: The Ryerson Press, 1954.

Cosbie, W.G. *The Toronto General Hospital, 1819-1965: A Chronicle.* Toronto: Macmillan of Canada, 1975.

Flexner, Abraham. *Medical Education in the United States and Canada.* A Report to the Carnegie Foundation for the Advancement of Teaching, 1910. Reprint. New York: Arno Press and *The New York Times*, 1972.

_____. *Medical Education: A Comparative Study.* New York: Macmillan Company, 1925.

_____. *An Autobiography.* New York: Simon and Schuster, 1960.

Francis, R. Douglas and Howard Palmer. *The Prairie West, Historical Readings.* Edmonton: Pica Pica Press, 1985.

Friesen, Gerald. *The Canadian Prairies, A History.* Toronto: University of Toronto Press, 1984.

Gifford, James J. Jr. *The Evolution of a Medical Center. A History of Medicine at Duke University to 1941.* Durham, North Carolina: Duke University Press, 1972.

Gilpin, John F. *Edmonton. Gateway to the North.* Produced in cooperation with the Amisk Waskahegan Chapter, Historical Society of Alberta, and Windsor Publications (Canada) Ltd., 1984.

Godfrey, Charles M. *Medicine for Ontario, A History.* Belleville, Ontario: Mika Publishing Company, 1979.

Hamowy, Ronald. *Canadian Medicine: A Study in Restricted Entry.* Vancouver: Fraser Institute, 1984.

Heagerty, John J. *Four Centuries of Medical History in Canada and a Sketch of the Medical History of Newfoundland.* Toronto: Macmillan Company of Canada Limited, 1928.

_____. *The Romance of Medicine in Canada.* Toronto: Ryerson Press, 1940.

Jack, Donald. *Rogues, Rebels, and Geniuses. The Story of Canadian Medicine.* Toronto: Doubleday Canada Limited, 1981.

Jamieson, Heber C. *Early Medicine in Alberta, the First Seventy-five Years.* Edmonton: Canadian Medical Association, Alberta Division, 1947.

Jarrell, R.A. and N.R. Ball. (editors) *Science, Technology and Canadian History.* The First Conference on the Study of the History of Canadian Science and Technology, at Kingston, Ontario. Waterloo, Ontario: Wilfrid Laurier University Press, 1980.

Johns, Walter H. *A History of the University of Alberta, 1908-1969.* Edmonton: The University of Alberta Press, 1981.

Kaufman, Martin. *The University of Vermont College of Medicine.* Hanover, New Hampshire: University of Vermont College of Medicine, 1979.

Kerr, Robert B. *History of The Medical Council of Canada,* Ottawa: The Medical Council of Canada. 1979.

Konner, Melvin. *Becoming a Doctor. A Journey of Initiation in Medical School.* New York: Elisabeth Sifton Books-Viking, 1987.

Letts, Harry. *The Edmonton Academy of Medicine. A History.* Edmonton: The Edmonton Academy of Medicine, 1986.

Lewis, D. Sclater. *Official History of the Royal College of Physicians and Surgeons.* Montreal: McGill University Press, 1962.

_____. *Royal Victoria Hospital, 1887-1947.* Montreal: McGill University Press, 1969.

Ludmerer, Kenneth M. *Learning to Heal. The Development of American Medical Education.* New York: Basic Books, Inc., Publishers, 1985.

MacDermot, H.E. *One Hundred Years of Medicine in Canada, 1867-1967.* Toronto/Montreal: McClelland and Stewart Limited, 1967.

Macdonald, John. *The History of the University of Alberta, 1908-1958.* Edmonton: The University of Alberta, 1958.

MacFarlane, J.A., R.C. Dickson, Harold Ettinger, Roger Dufresne, John F. McCreary and J. Wendell Macleod. *Medical Education in Canada.* Royal Commission on Health Services. Ottawa: Queen's Printer, 1965.

McDougall, Gerald M. (editor) *Teachers of Medicine: The Development of Graduate Clinical Medical Education.* Calgary: University of Calgary Printing Services, 1987.

McGovern, John P. and Charles G. Roland. (editors) *Wm. Osler. The Continuing Education.* Springfield, Illinois: Charles C. Thomas, Publisher, 1969.

McGugan, Angus C. *The First Fifty Years. The University of Alberta Hospital, 1914-1964.* Edmonton: The University of Alberta Hospital, 1964.

McKeown, Thomas. *The Role of Medicine: Dream, Mirage or Nemesis?* Princeton, N.J.: Princeton University Press, 1979.

Miller, Benjamin F. and Claire Brackman Keane. *Encyclopedia and Dictionary of Medicine and Nursing.* Philadelphia: W.B. Saunders Company, 1978.

Mitchell, Ross. *Medicine in Manitoba. The Story of Its Beginnings.* Winnipeg: Manitoba Medical Association, 1954.

Mitchinson, Wendy and Janice Dickin McGinnis. (editors) *Essays in the History of Canadian Medicine.* Toronto: McClelland and Stewart, 1988.

O'Malley, C.D. (editor) *The History of Medical Education.* An International Symposium held 5-9 February 1968, sponsored by the UCLA Department of Medical History, School of Medicine. Berkeley: University of California Press, 1970.

Physicians for the Twenty-First Century. The GPEP Report. Report of the Panel on the General Professional Education of the Physician and College Preparation for Medicine. Washington, D.C.: Association of American Medical Colleges, 1984.

Pinel, Philippe. *The Clinical Training of Doctors. An Essay of 1793.* Edited and translated, with an introductory essay, by Dora B. Weiner. Baltimore and London: The Johns Hopkins University Press, 1980.

Reverby, Susan and David Rosner. (editors) *Health Care in America. Essays in Social History.* Philadelphia: Temple University Press, 1979.

Richards, Robert K. *Continuing Medical Education. Perspectives, Problems, Prognosis.* New Haven and London: Yale University Press, 1978.

Roland, Charles G. *An Annotated Bibliography of Canadian Medical Periodicals 1826-1975.* Toronto: The Hannah Institute for the History of Medicine, 1979.

_____. *Health, Disease and Medicine: Essays in Canadian History.* Toronto: Published for the Hannah Institute for the History of Medicine by Clarke Irwin Inc., 1984.

_____. *Secondary Sources on the History of Canadian Medicine: A Bibliography.* Waterloo: Wilfred Laurier University Press, 1984.

_____. *William Osler's The Master-Word in Medicine: A Study in Rhetoric.* Springfield, Illinois: Charles C. Thomas, Publisher, 1972.

Rothstein, William G. *American Medical Schools and the Practice of Medicine. A History.* New York, Oxford: Oxford University Press, 1987.

Scarlett, Earle P. *In Sickness and in Health. Reflections on the Medical Profession.* Edited by Charles G. Roland. Toronto: McClelland and Stewart Limited, 1972.

Scott, John W. *The History of the Faculty of Medicine of the University of Alberta, 1913-1963.* Edmonton: The University of Alberta, 1963.

Shortt, S.E.D. (editor) *Medicine in Canadian Society. Historical Perspectives.* Montreal: McGill-Queen's University Press, 1981.

Stacey, C.P. *Six Years of War.* Volume 1 of the Official History of the Canadian Army in the Second World War. Ottawa: Queen's Printer, 1955.

Starr, Paul. *The Social Transformation of American Medicine. The Rise of a Sovereign Profession and the Making of a Vast Industry.* New York: Basic Books, Inc., Publishers, 1982.

Vant, J. Ross and Tony Cashman. *More Than a Hospital. University of Alberta Hospitals, 1906-1986.* Edmonton: The University Hospitals Board, 1986.

Vevier, Charles. (editor) *Flexner: 75 Years Later. A Current Commentary on Medical Education.* Papers from a Conference. New York: University Press of America. 1987.

Walsh, Mary Roth. *Doctors Wanted: No Women Need Apply. Sexual Barriers in the Medical Profession, 1835-1975.* New Haven and London: Yale University Press, 1977.

Articles, Periodicals and Unpublished Manuscripts

AHFMR Newsletter.

Alexander, William Hardy. "In the Beginning." *Alberta Historical Review,* (Spring 1960).

Alberta Medical Bulletin.

Askey, Al. "Faculty Profile. Dr. R.F. Shaner." *MUS Bulletin* (March 1959).

Bliss, Michael. "The Aetiology of the Discovery of Insulin." In *Health, Disease and Medicine: Essays in Canadian History.* C.G. Roland. Proceedings of the First Hannah Conference on the History of Medicine, McMaster University, 3-5 June 1982.

_____. "J.B. Collip: A Forgotten Member of the Insulin Team." In *Essays in the History of Canadian Medicine*. Wendy Mitchinson and Janice Dickin McGinnis, Toronto: McClelland and Stewart Limited, 1988.

Bradley, J.E. "Alberta Heritage Foundation for Medical Research." Unpublished manuscript, December 1980.

Brain, Sir Russell. "Osler and Medicine Today." *Canadian Medical Association Journal* (August 1960).

Bulletin, (Faculty of Medicine, University of Alberta).

Caffaro, Michael. "The Medical Students' Association." *New Trail* (Spring 1988).

Cameron, D.F. "The Medical Student and the Royal Commission on Health Services." *MUS Journal* (Summer 1964).

Chapman, Carleton B. "Preprofessional Requirements: An Anachronism." *The Bulletin of the New York Academy of Medicine*, Vol. 61. No. 5 (June 1985).

Clouston, H.R. "The Medical Curriculum as Viewed by a Country General Practitioner." *Canadian Medical Association Journal* (March 1933).

"Curriculum: Where It's Going." *IATROS*, University of Alberta medical journal (Fall/Winter 1986).

Davidson, Wilburt C. "Osler's Influence." *Journal of the Association of American Medical Colleges* (May 1950).

Dowding, E. Silver. "Dr. Harold Orr and Medical Mycology." *Canadian Medical Association Journal* (1953).

Evergreen and Gold, University of Alberta Yearbook. Various issues.

Fraser, Robert S. "Cardiology at the University of Alberta, 1922 to 1969." Unpublished manuscript, n.d.

_____. *A Personal View 1969-1974*. Edmonton: University of Alberta, Department of Medicine, unpublished report, 1986.

From Laboratory to Marketplace, Biotechnology Initiatives at the University of Alberta, (Edmonton 1989).

Gardner, J.S. "Earle Parkhill Scarlett." *Canadian Bulletin of Medical History*, Volume 1, No. 1 (Summer 1984).

The Gateway. University of Alberta Student Newspaper. Various issues.

Hellstedt, Leone McGregor. "Background and Experiences of a Girl Born in Carnduff, Saskatchewan in January 1900. The Choice and Course of her Career in Medicine." Unpublished manuscript, Stockholm, Sweden, 1970.

IATROS, University of Alberta Medical Journal.

Jamieson, H.C. *A Short Sketch of Medical Progress in Alberta*. Edmonton: Edmonton Academy of Medicine, 1928.

Jones, Adrian and Gerald Higgins. "In the Footsteps of the Pioneers." *New Trail* (Spring 1988).

Kay, Cyril. "The MRC Group in Protein Structure and Function." Unpublished manuscript, n.d.

Kling, S. "The Challenge of Continuing Medical Education." *Alberta Medical Bulletin* (February 1964).

_____. "Continuing Medical Education." *MUS Bulletin* (1964).

Ladies Home Journal (March 1931).

Large, J.M., D.G. Revell and E.F. Cain. "History of Medical Club and Graduates in Medicine, University of Alberta." Unpublished manuscript, 1929.

Macbeth, R.A. "Alexander Russell Munroe: 1879-1965." *The Canadian Journal of Surgery* (January 1967).

_____. "History of the Department of Surgery." University of Alberta. Unpublished manuscript, n.d.

_____. "Meet the Dean, Walter Campbell MacKenzie." *MUS Bulletin* (March 1964).

_____. "Walter Campbell Mackenzie, Pioneer International Surgical Statesman." *Annals RCPSC* (March 1989).

Macleod, J.J.R. "The Problem of Broadening the Medical Course." *The University of Toronto Monthly* (February 1920).

Macleod, J.W. "Medical Student Enrolment in Canadian Universities." *Canadian Medical Association Journal* (April, 1963).

Macleod, J.W., and H. Howes. "Medical Students in Canadian Universities, 1962-63 and 1963-64." *Canadian Medical Association Journal* (April 1964).

Markle, Alex G. "An Adventure in Medical Alumni Relations." Unpublished manuscript, May 1981.

McPhedran, Alexander. "Undergraduate Training and Requirements for License to Practise." *The Western Medical News*, Volume 4, No. 4 (1912).

McPhedran, N. Tait. "The Evolution of Medical Education in Canada." Faculty of Medicine, University of Calgary. Unpublished manuscript, 1988.

Medical Alumni Bulletin.

"A Memorial Tribute to Walter C. Mackenzie." *The Canadian Journal of Surgery* (July 1979).

Miller, Genevieve. "The Teaching of Medical History." *Bulletin of the History of Medicine*, Volume XLIII (1969).

Morrish, Walter. "Memoirs re Medical and Political Experiences." Unpublished manuscript, c.1963.

Neatby, Hilda. "The Medical Profession in the North-West Territories." *Saskatchewan History*, Volume II, Number 2 (May 1949).

New Trail, University of Alberta Alumni Association magazine.

Newton, Robert. "I Passed This Way, 1889-1964." Unpublished memoir of the fourth president of the University of Alberta, n.d.

Ower, J.J. "Citation." *Medical Alumni Bulletin* (April 1946).

Parsons, W.B. "Medicine in Alberta, the War Years." Unpublished manuscript, n.d.

Pope, E.L. "The Examination of Medical Students." *Canadian Medical Association Journal* (October 1933).

_____. "Some Reminiscences." *Medical Alumni Bulletin* (December 1944).

Rawlinson, H.E. "Frank Hamilton Mewburn." *The Canadian Journal of Surgery* (October 1958).

_____. "The Humanities and Medicine." *CAMSI Journal* (February 1958).

Research Inventory, Faculty of Medicine. University of Alberta (1987).

Revell, D.G. "The Department of Anatomy, University of Alberta." *Methods and Problems of Medical Education.* New York: The Rockefeller Foundation, 1930.

_____. "The Medical Faculty — University of Alberta." *Historical Bulletin,* Calgary Associate Clinic, Volume 13 (February 1949).

Rossiter, R.J. "James Bertram Collip." *Royal Society of Canada Journal* (1965).

Ruedy, John. "Specialty Residency Training in Canada - History and Challenges." *Annals RCPSC* (May 1986).

Ryten, Eva. "Trends in the Study of Medicine in Canada." *Canadian Medical Association Journal* (September 1985).

Scarlett, E.P. "A Doctor's Notebook." *Alberta Medical Bulletin,* Volume 28, No. 4 (November 1963).

Scott, John W. "Department of Biochemistry, University of Alberta." *Methods and Problems of Medical Education.* New York: The Rockefeller Foundation, 1930.

_____. "Early Medical Education and Practice in the Province of Alberta." Unpublished manuscript (1975).

_____. "Medical Research at the University." *Medical Alumni Bulletin* (September 1950).

_____. "Memoirs, 1914-1979." Unpublished manuscript (1979).

Shaner, Ralph. "Dr. Daniel Graisberry Revell." Obituary notice, *Proceedings of American Association of Anatomists.* Volume 122, No.4 (1955).

_____. "The Teaching of the Basic Sciences." *MUS Bulletin* (February 1957).

Shortt, S.E.D. "'Before the Age of Miracles': The Rise, Fall and Rebirth of General Practice in Canada, 1890-1940." In *Health Disease and Medicine.* C.G. Roland, Toronto: Published for the Hannah Institute for the History of Medicine by Clarke Irwin Inc., 1984.

Sigerist, Henry E, "Medical History in the Medical Schools of Canada." *Bulletin of the History of Medicine,* Volume VIII (1940).

Simonds, Pat. "Backward Glances." *MUS Bulletin* (February 1957).

Speculum, Faculty of Medicine student magazine, University of Alberta.

Stanley, G.D. "Dr. Daniel Graisberry Revell." *Historical Bulletin,* Calgary Associate Clinic, Volume 14 (1949).

Stewart C.B. "Reminiscences on the Founding and Early History of the Medical Research Council of Canada." *Annals RCPSC* (September and November 1986).

Thompson, J.S. "The Canadian Student — Western Style." *Journal of Medical Education* (November 1958).

_____. "Medical Education in Canada in 1959." *Journal of Medical Education* (August 1959).

_____. "The Medical Student — His Background and His Problems." *Canadian Medical Association Journal* (April 1958).

_____. "The Revision of the Medical Curriculum." *MUS Bulletin* (February 1957).

_____. "Wanted: More and Better Medical Students." *Canadian Medical Association Journal* (April 1961).

_____. ''Who Can Go to Medical School.'' *Canadian Medical Association Journal* (November 1956).

Tory, H.M. ''The University's Function in Medicine.'' *The Canadian Medical Association Journal* (November 1926).

The University of Alberta Calendar. Various issues.

Wilson, Donald R. ''The Gladys and Merrill Muttart Foundation.'' Unpublished manuscript, n.d.

_____. ''History of the Alpha Omega Alpha Honor Medical Society.'' Unpublished manuscript, 1961.

_____. ''History of the Department of Medicine, 1954-1969.'' Unpublished manuscript, n.d.

_____. ''History of the Faculty of Medicine.'' Unpublished manuscript, 1981.

_____. ''James Bertram Collip.'' *Annual Report of the Alberta Medical Association* (1982).

_____. ''R.S. McLaughlin Examination and Research Centre.'' Unpublished manuscript, n.d.

* * * * *

Index

Large Roman numerals refer to the four photographic sections